NEPHROLOGY RESEARCH AND CLINICAL DEVELOPMENTS

NEPHROTIC SYNDROME

ETIOLOGY, PATHOGENESIS AND PATHOLOGY

NEPHROLOGY RESEARCH AND CLINICAL DEVELOPMENTS

Additional books in this series can be found on Nova's website under the Series tab.

Additional e-books in this series can be found on Nova's website under the e-book tab.

NEPHROLOGY RESEARCH AND CLINICAL DEVELOPMENTS

NEPHROTIC SYNDROME

ETIOLOGY, PATHOGENESIS AND PATHOLOGY

MUHAMMED MUBARAK
EDITOR

NOVA BIOMEDICAL

New York

Library of Congress Cataloging-in-Publication Data

ISBN: 978-1-63482-154-4
Library of Congress Control Number: 2015931777

Published by Nova Science Publishers, Inc. † New York

Contents

Preface		**vii**
Chapter 1	Nephrotic Syndrome: An Overview *Muhammed Mubarak*	**1**
Chapter 2	Plasmin, Urokinase Plasminogen Activator Receptor and Amiloride in the Nephrotic Syndrome *Hernán Trimarchi*	**11**
Chapter 3	Pathogenesis of Idiopathic Membranous Glomerulonephritis *Raja Ramachandran and Ashok Kumar Yadav*	**29**
Chapter 4	Complements and Glomerulonephritis *Sabiha Anis*	**41**
Chapter 5	The Genetics of Primary Focal Segmental Glomerulosclerosis *Aiysha Abid*	**57**
Chapter 6	Approach to Renal Biopsy Diagnosis in Nephrotic Syndrome *Muhammed Mubarak*	**81**
Chapter 7	Pathology of Idiopathic Nephrotic Syndrome in Children *Shaheera Shakeel and Muhammed Mubarak*	**101**
Chapter 8	Pathology of Nephrotic Syndrome in Adults *Lavleen Singh, Geetika Singh and Amit Dinda*	**129**
Chapter 9	Successful Running of an Electron Microscopy Unit in a Developing Country: Problems and Challenges *Javed I. Kazi and Muhammed Mubarak*	**161**
Chapter 10	Focal Segmental Glomerulosclerosis *A. V. Vanikar, K. V. Kanodia, R. D. Patel and L. K. Nigam*	**169**
Index		**203**

Preface

Nephrotic syndrome is the most common clinical presenting feature of medical renal diseases throughout the world. Yet, there are very few books in English language exclusively covering this topic and none from the developing countries. A few comprehensive volumes are too voluminous to serve as a ready and handy guide and often beyond the reach of most of the nephrology and nephropathology community in the developing countries. The objective of this book was to partially fill this vacuum. It is for the readers to decide as to what extent we have succeeded in achieving this objective. We do not claim that the topic of nephrotic syndrome has been thoroughly or comprehensively covered in this handbook, but, we are confident that it definitely constitutes an important contribution to the existing scarcity of books on this topic.

This book covers mainly the basic science aspects of the nephrotic syndrome, as is obvious from a superficial look at the contents of the book. The major part relates to the pathological aspects of nephrotic syndrome, as the majority of the contributors are nephropathologists. The clinical and therapeutic aspects of nephrotic syndrome will be presented in another volume on this topic.

The book contents have been conveniently divided into three sections. The first section deals with the overall introduction of the topic of nephrotic syndrome and its pathogenesis. An overview of the nephrotic syndrome is presented by Muhammed Mubarak, with relevant references to the detailed discussion of different aspects in other book chapters. Recent developments regarding the pathogenesis of nephrotic syndrome are covered by Hernán Trimarchi, with particular emphasis on the role of plasmin, uPAR and amiloride in nephrotic syndrome. A discussion of the role of complement system in the pathogenesis of some common glomerulopathies has been summarized by Sabiha Anis. A complete chapter by Aiysha Abid has been devoted to the role of genetic factors in causing or predisposing to focal segmental glomerulosclerosis, which has recently emerged as the leading cause of idiopathic nephrotic syndrome in adults. The pathogenesis of membranous glomerulopathy has undergone revolutionary changes in the past few years and this has been elegantly summarized by Raja Ramchandarn and Ashok Kumar Yadav.

The second section is related to the pathological diagnosis of diseases underlying nephrotic syndrome. It includes a chapter by Muhammed Mubarak describing the approach to renal biopsy diagnosis. The pathology of idiopathic nephrotic syndrome in children is discussed in a separate chapter by Shaheera Shakeel and Muhammed Mubarak. Lavleen Singh and co-workers have described in detail the pathology of nephrotic syndrome in adults.

They have discussed the pathology of both primary and secondary forms of nephrotic syndrome. Javed Kazi and Muhammed Mubarak have highlighted the difficulties and challenges in successfully running a diagnostic electron microscopy service in a developing country like Pakistan.

The third section contains a chapter describing in detail the histopathological lesion of focal segmental glomerulosclerosis by Aruna Vanikar and her co-workers.

Thus, the contributors of the present work come from different parts of the world, giving the book a truly international outlook. All the authors are experienced workers in their respective fields and it was pleasant exercise for me to have interacted with them during the compiling phase of the book. The authors' origin is skewed toward developing countries, which underscores the increasing attention to the nephrology subspecialty in these countries. This multi-author book will serve as a useful guide for both the nephrologists and nephropathologists alike.

I sincerely thank all the devoted and enthusiastic authors of various chapters, who spared precious time from their busy schedules to contribute to this book and to enlighten the readers with the latest updates in their areas of expertise. The staff at Nova Publishers also deserves gratitude for their continuous help and guidance. I earnestly hope that the book will prove a success in its field, particularly for the residents and junior nephrologists and nephropathologists.

Muhammed Mubarak
Histopathology Department,
Sindh Institute of Urology and Transplantation (SIUT),
Karachi, Pakistan
Email: drmubaraksiut@yahoo.com

In: Nephrotic Syndrome: Etiology, Pathogenesis and Pathology ISBN: 978-1-63482-154-4
Editor: Muhammed Mubarak

Chapter 1

Nephrotic Syndrome: An Overview

Muhammed Mubarak*
Professor of Pathology, Histopathology Department,
Sindh Institute of Urology and Transplantation, Karachi, Pakistan

Abstract

Nephrotic syndrome (NS) is one of the best known and main clinical syndromes associated with a variety of medical diseases of kidney in both adults and children. It is not a single disease, but rather a clinicopathological syndrome, caused by a large number of etiologic agents affecting the kidney. It is defined by both the clinical and laboratory or biochemical features. The primary defect in NS consists of excessive leakage of plasma proteins into the urine, termed proteinuria. The other manifestations of NS are mainly secondary to heavy proteinuria and consist of hypoalbuminemia, edema, and hyperlipidemia. However, other factors also play a part in the pathogenesis of these alterations. The NS can present in a variety of ways, including life-threatening complications resulting from the disease. Hence, prompt diagnosis and treatment of the cause, are essential for optimal treatment of the disease and prevention of the complications. This chapter gives an overview of the NS, its causes, its pathophysiology and pathogenesis. The detailed pathological aspects of NS are discussed in other chapters of this book.

Keywords: Hypoalbuminemia, nephrotic syndrome, proteinuria, hyperlipidemia, glomerular filtration barrier

1. Introduction

Nephrotic syndrome (NS) is one of the best known and main clinical syndromes associated with a variety of medical kidney diseases in both adults and children. [1-4] It is not

* Address of Correspondence: Muhammed Mubarak; Histopathology Department, Sindh Institute of Urology and Transplantation (SIUT), Karachi, Pakistan; Email: drmubaraksiut@yahoo.com.

a single disease, but rather a clinicopathological syndrome, caused by a large number of injurious agents affecting the kidney. It is defined by both the clinical and laboratory or biochemical features. The primary defect in NS consists of excessive leakage of plasma proteins into the urine, termed proteinuria. The threshold of proteinuria for defining the clinical syndrome varies according to the age of the patients. In adults, it is more than 3.5 g per day per 1.73 m^2 surface area, while, in children it is often defined as more than $40mg/m^2/h$. [5-7] The pathologic proteinuria is the defining feature and the most readily quantitated sign of NS. The other manifestations of NS are mainly secondary to heavy proteinuria and consist of hypoalbuminemia, edema, and hyperlipidemia. However, other factors also play a part in the pathogenesis of these alterations. [8-14] The cardinal features of NS are shown in Table 1. Protein in the urine (coagulable urine) was first described in 1821, followed 15 years later by the description of "albuminous urine" by Richard Bright. [3]

The NS is prevalent through out the world. However, the incidence and prevalence rates vary across different parts of the world, mostly due to methodological issues. It has an incidence of three news cases per 100,000 adult patients each year. [3] As compared with renal failure and microalbuminuria, which are often the presenting features of systemic kidney diseases, NS is a relatively rare presenting feature.

Table 1. The cardinal features of nephrotic syndrome

Proteinuria more than 3.5 g/24-hour/1.73 m^2 in adults and more than $40mg/m^2/h$ or spot urine protein:creatinine ratio of >3.5 in children.
Serum albumin <2.5 g/dl
Peripheral edema
Hyperlipidaemia (total cholesterol often >10 mmol/l)

2. Causes of NS

The NS is caused by a large number of both primary and secondary glomerulopathies. [15-20] It is imperative to distinguish between the primary and secondary forms of NS and to further specify the cause, as the clinical presentation, response to treatment and prognosis, depend largely on the underlying cause. In addition, determination of the cause may help in the development of disease-specific treatments. [2, 3] The main renal diseases that cause NS are shown in Table 2.

Table 2. The main causes of primary nephrotic syndrome

Focal segmental glomerulosclerosis
Membranous nephropathy
Minimal-change nephropathy
Mesangial proliferative glomerulonephritis
Membranoproliferative glomerulonephritis
Hereditary nephropathies

2.1. Primary NS

Most cases of NS in both adults (60%) and children (95%) are caused by primary glomerulopathies, as shown in Table 2. However, the relative frequencies of different pathological lesions vary depending on many factors, such as age, race, geographic location, biopsy policies, etc. [3] A description of these diseases is provided in chapter on the pathology of NS in children. Significant changes have occurred in the prevalence of the different glomerular diseases in the past several years. [21, 22] Membranous nephropathy (MN) used to be the most common cause of NS in adults; however, many recent biopsy series, mostly from blacks, show that FSGS has superseded MN as the leading cause of primary NS in adult patients. [22] MN still continues to be the leading cause of primary NS in white adults and elderly patients of all races. [23, 24]

Table 3. The main causes of secondary nephrotic syndrome

Systemic diseases
Diabetes mellitus
Systemic lupus erythematosus
Amyloidosis
Myeloma and lymphoma
Cancer
Drugs
Gold
Penicillamine
Captopril
Lithium
Non-steroidal antiinflammatory drugs
Antimicrobial agents
Tamoxifen
Infections
Hepatitis B and C
HIV
Syphilis
Malaria
Schistosomiasis
Filariasis
Toxoplasmosis
Mycoplasma
Hereditary causes
Congenital nephrotic syndrome of the Finnish type
Alport's syndrome
Pierson's syndrome
Nail-patella syndrome
Denys-Drash syndrome

2.2. Secondary NS

A wide variety of systemic diseases involving the kidney present as secondary NS. [3, 16] Many drugs affecting the kidney manifest as secondary NS. Among these, diabetes mellitus (DM), systemic lupus nephritis (SLE), and amyloidosis are the principal causes, as shown in Table 3. Secondary causes of NS account for 40% of cases of NS in adults and only 5% in children. [2, 3]

3. Pathophysiology of NS

The pathophysiology of NS is as varied as the underlying etiology of the condition. However, the cardinal feature of the disease is the increased permeability of the glomerular filtration barrier (GFB) to the macomolecules, mostly albumin but also other plasma proteins, into the urine. [11-14, 25, 26] This phenomenon is observed in all forms of NS irrespective of etiology. Significant proteinuria leads to a fall in serum albumin levels. This is seen even in the face of increased synthesis of albumin by the liver. A marked decrease in serum albumin leads to a drop in plasma oncotic pressure, which in turn leads to edema formation. [2, 3] There are other mechanisms operative in the formation of edema in kidney diseases also. [15] These are discussed in detail elsewhere in this book.

4. Pathogenesis

The pathogenesis of NS is as varied as the underlying diseases causing the disorder. The principal defect lies in the malfunction of the GFB. This barrier is composed of three layers: from within outwards these consist of; fenestrated endothelial cells, the glomerular basement membrane (GBM), and interdigitating layer of foot processes of podocytes. Among these three layers, podocytes have emerged as the main target of damage leading to NS presentation. This damage may be caused of genetic abnormalities, immune aberrations and circulating factors. [8-10, 27-29]

4.1. Role of Genes

Gene defects are being increasingly recognized as the predisposing or underlying causes of NS. The gene defects are particularly prevalent in NS of early onset. The encoded proteins are constituent parts of slit diaphragm (SD), foot process cytoskeleton, foot process-GBM junctions, GBM or cell body of podocytes. The number of implicated genes is increasing day by day. The gene mutations are found in 80 to100% of cases of congenital NS (CNS), 50 to 60% of infantile-onset steroid resistant NS, 65 to 70% of familial steroid resistant NS, and 25% of sporadic steroid resistant NS, particularly with the use of high throughput, next-generation sequencing. The genetic forms of NS can present at any time from intrauterine life to adulthood, but are mostly found in early-onset cases. The practical importance of identifying the genetic causes is that most of these cases are refractory to the use of steroids or immunosuppressive agents. The hereditary forms of NS also do not recur following transplantation; however, exceptions are reported. [30-35]

4.2. Role of Immune System

The role of immune system is more marked in cases of steroid-sensitive NS. It is hypothesized that the altered cell-mediated immunity and T helper type 2 (Th2) cell predominance causes a release of an as yet uncharacterized circulating factor which increases the permeability characteristics of GFB. The evidence in favor of Th2 role in NS consists of association with atopy, increased serum levels of IgE, decreased expression of Th1 asscociated transcription factor, T-bet, and increased expression of Th2 associated transcription factor, *c-maf.*

More recent studies have shown that the disease activity is caused by an imbalance between the actions of Th 17 cells and T regulatory cells. A deficiency or dysfunction of T regulatory cells results in activation of effector T cells to secrete factors that mediate glomerular hyperpermeability or increase oxidant production by polymorphonuclear cells. On the contrary, a hyperfunction of T regulatory cells has been demonstrated to result in remission of NS.

In addition to the role of specific immune responses, innate immunity has also been shown to play a part in the pathogenesis of NS, especially during relapses of disease following infections. [36-38]

4.3. Circulating Factors

Circulating soluble factor hypothesis has remained the most widely accepted paradigm for the pathogenesis of NS till date. This is supported by the immediate recurrence of nephrotic proteinuria in 20% to 40% of patients with FSGS following transplantation in humans. Animal studies have also shown development of proteinuria and foot process effacement in rats when injected with supernatants of T cells from nephrotic patients. A variety of molecules have been suggested as the putative circulating serum factors responsible for the development of increased permeability of GFB; however, the search is still on and the nature of the molecule has defied all the efforts to identify it so far. [39-42]

5. Clinical Presentation

The NS can present in a diversity of ways to the primary or secondary care, either with edema or one of the complications of NS. The main signs and symptoms of NS are shown in Table 4. Although, it is an important presenting feature of kidney diseases, it is not very common and hence, can easily be misdiagnosed or the diagnosis can be delayed. [3]

Table 4. The main signs and symptoms of nephrotic syndrome

Edema
Periorbital edema
Lower limb edema
Edema of the genitals
Ascites
Pleural effusion
Tiredness
Leuconychia
Breathlessness
Fluid overload
Acute renal failure
Breathlessness with chest pain
Thromboemboli
Eruptive xanthomata
Xanthelasmata
Frothy urine

6. Complications

The NS represents a profound alteration of the hemodynamic homeostasis and has systemic consequences, if not treated promptly or appropriately. [43-48] The complications mainly result from abnormal loss of functional plasma proteins into the urine, with resulting alterations in the protein metabolism. The main complications of NS are shown in Table 5.

It is evident from the table that NS is associated with both renal and extrarenal complications. It appears that prolonged nephrotic-range proteinuria leads to renal scarring and eventually renal failure; although the precise mechanism of the proteinuric damage to renal parenchyma is unresolved. In adults, it has been shown that regardless of the underlying histology, patients with proteinuria of ≥3.8 g/day had a 35% risk of end stage renal disease (ESRD) within 2 years, compared to only a 4% risk for those with proteinuria ≤2.0 g/day. In addition, patients with NS have an increased risk of thromboembolism. Data from studies on MN found the prevalence of thrombotic complications to be 29% for renal vein thrombosis, 17-28% for pulmonary embolism, and 11% for deep vein thrombosis. The risk of coronary heart disease (CHD) increased. This is because various risk factors associated with CHD are more prevalent in the nephrotic population, including hypercholesterolemia, hypertension, hypercoagulability, and exposure to certain atherogenic drugs such as steroids. The risk of developing CHD is four times greater in nephrotic patients than in sex-age age-matched controls. Complications in children with NS include a risk of serious infection, in particular cellulites and spontaneous bacterial peritonitis. [43-48]

Table 5. The main complications of nephrotic syndrome

Thromboembolism	
	Renal vein thrombosis
	Deep vein thrombosis
	Pulmonary embolism
	Arterial thrombosis (very rare)
Infection	
	Cellulitis
	Bacterial infections, such as pneumonia and cellulitis
	Bacterial peritonitis (rare)
	Viral infections in immunocompromised patients
Other complications	
	Coronary heart disease
	Hyperlipidemia
	Loss of vitamin D (via binding protein) leading to bone disease
	Acute renal failure
	Chronic renal failure

Conclusion

In conclusion, NS represents one of the most common and well defined clinical syndrome associated with medical diseases of the kidneys in both children and adults. It is imperative to diagnose it early and manage appropriately to prevent progressive damage to the kidney parenchyma. If not treated, it can lead to a variety of complications, some of which may be life-threatening.

References

[1] Carome MA, Moore J Jr. Nephrotic syndrome in adults. A diagnostic and management challenge. *Postgrad. Med.* 1992;92:209-215.

[2] Hull R, Goldsmith D. Identifying and managing nephrotic syndrome in adults. *Practitioner.* 2008;252:32-34.

[3] Hull RP, Goldsmith DJ. Nephrotic syndrome in adults. *BMJ.* 2008;336:1185-1189.

[4] Kodner C. Nephrotic syndrome in adults: diagnosis and management. *Am. Fam. Physician.* 2009;80:1129-1134.

[5] Chesney RW. The idiopathic nephrotic syndrome. Curr Opin Pediatr. 1999;11:158-161.

[6] Yao LP. Nephrotic syndrome. *Pediatr. Rev.* 2000;21:432-433.

[7] Eddy AA, Schnaper HW. The nephrotic syndrome: from the simple to the complex. *Semin. Nephrol.* 1998;18:304-316.

[8] Palmer BF. Nephrotic edema-pathogenesis and treatment. *Am. J. Med. Sci.* 1993;306:53-67.

[9] Wiseman KC. Nephrotic syndrome: pathophysiology and treatment. *ANNA J.* 1991;18:469-478.

[10] Roth KS, Amaker BH, Chan JC. Nephrotic syndrome: pathogenesis and management. *Pediatr. Rev.* 2002;23:237-248.

[11] Doucet A, Favre G, Deschênes G. Molecular mechanism of edema formation in nephrotic syndrome: therapeutic implications. *Pediatr. Nephrol.* 2007;22:1983-1990.

[12] Kleyman TR, Hughey RP. Plasmin and sodium retention in nephrotic syndrome. *J. Am. Soc. Nephrol.* 2009;20:233-234.

[13] Koomans HA. Pathophysiology of oedema in idiopathic nephrotic syndrome. *Nephrol. Dial. Transplant.* 2003;18 (Suppl 6):vi30-32.

[14] Deschênes G, Feraille E, Doucet A. Mechanisms of oedema in nephrotic syndrome: old theories and new ideas. *Nephrol. Dial. Transplant.* 2003;18:454-456.

[15] Glassock RJ, Cohen AH. The primary glomerulopathies. *Dis. Mon.* 1996;42:329-383.

[16] Madaio MP, Harrington JT. The diagnosis of glomerular diseases: acute glomerulonephritis and the nephrotic syndrome. *Arch. Intern. Med.* 2001;161:25-34.

[17] Gupta K, Iskandar SS, Daeihagh P, Ratliff HL, Bleyer AJ. Distribution of pathologic findings in individuals with nephrotic proteinuria according to serum albumin. *Nephrol. Dial. Transplant.* 2008;23:1595-1599.

[18] Engler DB, Grant JA. 'Idiopathic' nephrotic syndrome is not always idiopathic. *Tex. Med.* 1990;86:4-5.

[19] Adu D. The nephrotic syndrome: does renal biopsy affect management? *Nephrol. Dial .Transplant.* 1996;11:12-14.

[20] Maisonneuve P, Agodoa L, Gellert R, Stewart JH, Buccianti G, Lowenfels AB, Wolfe RA, Jones E, Disney AP, Briggs D, McCredie M, Boyle P. Distribution of primary renal diseases leading to end-stage renal failure in the United States, Europe, and Australia/New Zealand: results from an international comparative study. *Am. J. Kidney Dis.* 2000;35:157-165.

[21] Swaminathan S, Leung N, Lager DJ, Melton LJ 3rd, Bergstralh EJ, Rohlinger A, Fervenza FC. Changing incidence of glomerular disease in Olmsted County, Minnesota: a 30-year renal biopsy study. *Clin. J. Am. Soc. Nephrol.* 2006;1:483-487.

[22] Haas M, Meehan SM, Karrison TG, Spargo BH. Changing etiologies of unexplained adult nephrotic syndrome: a comparison of renal biopsy findings from 1976-1979 and 1995-1997. *Am. J. Kidney Dis.* 1997;30:621-631.

[23] Donadio JV Jr, Torres VE, Velosa JA, Wagoner RD, Holley KE, Okamura M, Ilstrup DM, Chu CP. Idiopathic membranous nephropathy: the natural history of untreated patients. *Kidney Int.* 1988;33:708-715.

[24] Schieppati A, Mosconi L, Perna A, Mecca G, Bertani T, Garattini S, Remuzzi G. Prognosis of untreated patients with idiopathic membranous nephropathy. *N. Engl. J. Med.* 1993;329:85-89.

[25] Jayawardene SA, Scoble JE, Goldsmith DJ. Nephrotic syndrome: more than just oedema. *Int. J. Clin. Pract.* 2002;56:129-131.

[26] Appel GB. Improved outcomes in nephrotic syndrome. *Cleve. Clin. J. Med.* 2006;73:161-167.

[27] Bagga A, Srivastava RN. Nephrotic syndrome and proteinuria. *Indian J. Pediatr.* 2002;69:1053-1054.

[28] De Santo NG, Pollastro RM, Saviano C, Pascale C, Di Stasio V, Chiricone D, Cirillo E, Molino D, Stellato D, Frangiosa A, Favazzi P, Capodicasa L, Bellini L, Anastasio P, Perna A, Sepe J, Cirillo M. Nephrotic edema. *Semin. Nephrol.* 2001;21:262-268.

[29] Verma SP, Madaio MP. Diagnosis and treatment of nephrotic syndrome. *Expert Opin. Investig. Drugs.* 1999;8:787-796.

[30] Niaudet P. Genetic forms of nephrotic syndrome. *Pediatr. Nephrol.* 2004;19:1313-1318.

[31] Gbadegesin RA, Winn MP, Smoyer WE. Genetic testing in nephrotic syndrome--challenges and opportunities. *Nat. Rev. Nephrol.* 2013;9:179-184.

[32] Benoit G, Machuca E, Antignac C. Hereditary nephrotic syndrome: a systematic approach for genetic testing and a review of associated podocyte gene mutations. *Pediatr. Nephrol.* 2010;25:1621-1632.

[33] Santín S, Bullich G, Tazón-Vega B, García-Maset R, Giménez I, Silva I, Ruíz P, Ballarín J, Torra R, Ars E. Clinical utility of genetic testing in children and adults with steroid-resistant nephrotic syndrome. *Clin. J. Am. Soc. Nephrol.* 2011;6:1139-1148.

[34] Papez KE, Smoyer WE. Recent advances in congenital nephrotic syndrome. *Curr. Opin. Pediatr.* 2004;16:165-170.

[35] Lipska BS, Iatropoulos P, Maranta R, Caridi G, Ozaltin F, Anarat A, Balat A, Gellermann J, Trautmann A, Erdogan O, Saeed B, Emre S, Bogdanovic R, Azocar M, Balasz-Chmielewska I, Benetti E, Caliskan S, Mir S, Melk A, Ertan P, Baskin E, Jardim H, Davitaia T, Wasilewska A, Drozdz D, Szczepanska M, Jankauskiene A, Higuita LM, Ardissino G, Ozkaya O, Kuzma-Mroczkowska E, Soylemezoglu O, Ranchin B, Medynska A, Tkaczyk M, Peco-Antic A, Akil I, Jarmolinski T, Firszt-Adamczyk A, Dusek J, Simonetti GD, Gok F, Gheissari A, Emma F, Krmar RT, Fischbach M, Printza N, Simkova E, Mele C, Ghiggeri GM, Schaefer F; PodoNet Consortium. Genetic screening in adolescents with steroid-resistant nephrotic syndrome. *Kidney Int.* 2013;84:206-213.

[36] Pereira Wde F, Brito-Melo GE, Guimarães FT, Carvalho TG, Mateo EC, Simões e Silva AC. The role of the immune system in idiopathic nephrotic syndrome: a review of clinical and experimental studies. *Inflamm. Res.* 2014;63:1-12.

[37] Souto MF, Teixeira AL, Russo RC, Penido MG, Silveira KD, Teixeira MM, Simões E Silva AC. Immune mediators in idiopathic nephrotic syndrome: evidence for a relation between interleukin 8 and proteinuria. *Pediatr. Res.* 2008;64:637-642.

[38] van den Berg JG, Weening JJ. Role of the immune system in the pathogenesis of idiopathic nephrotic syndrome. *Clin. Sci* (Lond). 2004;107:125-136.

[39] Maas RJ, Deegens JK, Wetzels JF. Permeability factors in idiopathic nephrotic syndrome: historical perspectives and lessons for the future. *Nephrol. Dial. Transplant.* 2014;29:2207-2216.

[40] Reiser J, Nast CC, Alachkar N. Permeability factors in focal and segmental glomerulosclerosis. *Adv. Chronic Kidney Dis.* 2014;21:417-421.

[41] Trachtman H, Reiser J. suPAR is the circulating factor in some but not all FSGS. *Nat. Rev. Nephrol.* 2014;10:610.

[42] Trimarchi H. Primary focal and segmental glomerulosclerosis and soluble factor urokinase-type plasminogen activator receptor. *World J. Nephrol.* 2013;2:103-110.

[43] Crew RJ, Radhakrishnan J, Appel G. Complications of the nephrotic syndrome and their treatment. *Clin. Nephrol.* 2004;62:245-259.

[44] Harris RC, Ismail N. Extrarenal complications of the nephrotic syndrome. *Am. J. Kidney Dis.* 1994;23:477-497.
[45] Abrass CK. Clinical spectrum and complications of the nephrotic syndrome. *J. Investig. Med.* 1997;45:143-153.
[46] Singhal R, Brimble KS. Thromboembolic complications in the nephrotic syndrome: pathophysiology and clinical management. *Thromb. Res.* 2006;118:397-407.
[47] Ambler B, Irvine S, Selvarajah V, Isles C. Nephrotic syndrome presenting as deep vein thrombosis or pulmonary embolism. *Emerg. Med. J.* 2008;25:241-242.
[48] Cheng YF, Chuang FR, Chen JB, Liao SC, Lam KK, Hsu KT. Spontaneous cellulitis in adults with idiopathic nephrotic syndrome. *Changgeng Yi. Xue. Za. Zhi.* 1998;21:158-164.

In: Nephrotic Syndrome: Etiology, Pathogenesis and Pathology ISBN: 978-1-63482-154-4
Editor: Muhammed Mubarak

Chapter 2

Plasmin, Urokinase Plasminogen Activator Receptor and Amiloride in the Nephrotic Syndrome

Hernán Trimarchi*
Nephrology Service and Kidney Transplant Unit,
Hospital Británico de Buenos Aires, Argentina

Abstract

Proteinuria is a common feature of acute and chronic nephropathies and a key predictor of declining glomerular filtration rate (GFR). It is an independent factor for tubulointerstitial damage induced by direct toxicity of the filtered protein. Systemically, substantial amounts of proteinuria cause symptoms such as interstitial edema, renal salt and water retention, and hypertension. The potential causes for these disorders have been partly elucidated in models of the nephrotic syndrome (NS), in which a primary insult to the podocytes or to the glomerular basement membrane (GBM) is followed by proteinuria and functional tubular derangements. Salt retention in NS has traditionally been attributed to the hypovolemia concept, implying decreased oncotic pressure following proteinuria, loss of fluid into the interstitium, and activation of the renin–angiotensin–aldosterone (RAA) system. Meanwhile, it has been claimed that the vascular volume in NS often remains unchanged along with the absence of blood pressure and RAA system effects. It has become accepted that primary tubular salt retention may per se produce a substantial systemic volume expansion in proteinuric nephrosis. Potential sites of sodium retention along the renal tubule have mostly been attributed to changes in the proximal or distal tubule. Generally, protein overload may impair proximal tubule structure and consequent handling of proteins. Cytoskeletal changes may interfere with trafficking of transporters and channels, and the effects of inflammatory and profibrotic cytokines have also been implicated.

The diuretic amiloride plays a significant role in reducing podocyte cell motility in vitro and proteinuria in mice. Besides its diuretic properties at the distal tubule blocking

* Corresponding author: Hernán Trimarchi, Chief, Nephrology Service and Kidney Transplant Unit, Hospital Británico de Buenos Aires, Argentina, Email: htrimarchi@hotmail.com.

the absorption of sodium and water at the $ENa^{+}C$ channel, amiloride has been recently shown to inhibit the synthesis of the urokinase receptor, called urokinase plasminogen activator receptor (uPAR), a molecule involved in the αvβ3 integrin activation. This integrin (also known as the vitronectin receptor) anchors the podocyte to the GBM; when activated it causes podocyte contraction and eventually contributes to the detachment of the cell from the glomerulus and its appearance in the urine (a phenomenon known as podocyturia), finally causing proteinuria. Amiloride capacity to inhibit uPAR synthesis and suPAR (the soluble circulating version of uPAR but also with glomerular permeability factor properties) secretion by T lymphocytes, macrophages and neutrophils should be taken into consideration as an adjuvant tool in the treatment of NS. Furthermore, amiloride may further decrease proteinuria by acting on the distal nephron on $ENa^{+}C$ channels, as proteinuria stimulates the activity of these channels by promoting the reabsorption of sodium and water. Tubular plasmin, already high in patients with proteinuria, would act as the mediator in sodium and water reabsorption and amiloride may inhibit its action by blocking uPAR. Thus, this would be another additional and relevant nonimmunosuppressive strategy contributing to the fall in proteinuria in NS individuals, if tolerated hemodynamically and no hyperkalemia ensues.

Keywords: Amiloride, edema, glomerulopathies, nephrosis, plasmin, proteinuria

1. Introduction

Proteinuria is a common and relevant component of acute and chronic glomerulopathies and a key predictor of declining glomerular filtration rate (GFR). Basically, proteinuria can be caused by three different pathophysiological events: a podocytopathy, hyperfiltration situations, and/or scarring and sclerosis due to primary or secondary glomerular filtration membrane derangements. Nevertheless, and independent of the cause, proteinuria has also been viewed as an independent factor for tubulointerstitial damage induced by direct toxicity of filtered protein. [1, 2] At both renal and systemic aspects, the substantial amounts of protein passing through the damaged filter to be lost in the urine are capable of causing interstitial edema, renal salt and water retention, hypertension, progressive renal function decline and is a surrogate of morbidity and mortality caused by cardiovascular events. [3-7] The potential causes for these disorders have been partly elucidated in models of the nephrotic syndrome (NS), in which a primary insult to the podocyte or to the glomerular basement membrane (GBM) is followed by proteinuria and functional tubular derangements. Salt retention in the NS has traditionally been accepted to be caused by the hypovolemia theory. This hypothesis implies that decreased oncotic pressure is due to hypoalbuminemia caused by copious proteinuria, loss of fluid into the interstitium, and activation of the renin–angiotensin–aldosterone (RAA) system. Noteworthy, vascular hyperpermeability itself has also been demonstrated as an additional culprit in edema formation and perpetuation. [8] However, it has been claimed that the vascular volume in most cases of the NS remains basically unchanged, coupled with the absence of effects on systemic blood pressure and on the RAA system. [9, 10] In this regard, it has lately become accepted that primary tubular salt retention by itself may produce a primary substantial systemic volume expansion in proteinuria. [11, 12] This hypothesis underscores the cross-talk between the glomerulus and the tubule as the first step, in which a glomerular podocyte damage translates into a proteinuric tubular fluid with interactions at the tubular cell level with subsequent fluid disbalances. Potential sites of sodium retention along the renal tubule have mostly been attributed to changes in the proximal or distal tubule. Generally, protein overload may impair proximal tubule structure and consequent handling of luminal proteins. Cytoskeletal changes may interfere with trafficking of transporters and channels, and the effects of inflammatory and profibrotic cytokines have also been implicated. [1, 2, 13-15] At the distal nephron, epithelial Na^+ channels (ENa^+C) are normally implicated in the absorption of sodium and water. These channels appear to be upregulated in the NS primarily due to both proteinuria itself and to the increased tubular concentration of plasminogen and plasmin, also augmented in the NS due to the upregulation of urokinase plasminogen activator receptor (uPAR). [9, 10, 16-18]

Finally, amiloride- a potassium-sparing diuretic- may play a significant potential role in the treatment of the NS at different levels. Amiloride acts at the proximal tubule inhibiting the Na^+/H^+ and Na^+/Ca^{++} antiporters [19] and at the distal tubule it interferes with water and salt retention at the above-mentioned ENa^+C. Moreover, amiloride has recently been shown to inhibit the synthesis of the urokinase receptor uPAR. [16, 20-22] This molecule converts plasminogen to plasmin at the cell surface of distal tubular cells, which subsequently upregulates ENa^+C activity, resulting in salt and water retention and edema formation. [16, 23] In addition, amiloride appears to reduce podocyte cell motility in vitro and proteinuria in mice by inhibiting a molecule involved in podocyte contraction, the β3 moiety of the αvβ3 integrin. [24] This integrin (also known as part of the vitronectin receptor-complex, together with uPAR) is one of the molecules involved in the anchoring of the podocyte to the GBM. When this integrin is activated, it would cause podocyte contraction and motility. [25] This cellular volume decrease may at final stages contribute to the critical detachment of the cell from the glomerulus and its appearance in the urine (a phenomenon known as podocyturia). The denuded glomerular filtration membrane would render the pathway for chronic proteinuria unhindered. Amiloride would therefore interfere negatively on β3-composed integrins actions and also inhibiting the synthesis of uPAR. [24] These actions position amiloride -at least at the theoretical level- as a relevant drug to be employed in the management and treatment of edema and proteinuria in the NS. Thus, this would be another additional and relevant non-immunosuppressive strategy contributing to the decrease in proteinuria in nephrotic individuals. [25, 26]

2. Edema Formation in the Nephrotic Syndrome

Edema is the characteristic clinical presentation of the NS. The mechanisms of edema formation in the NS have long been a subject of investigation and are continually debated. The 'underfill' hypothesis states that a decrement in oncotic pressure due to hypoalbuminemia leads to excess filtration of fluid from the intravascular space to the interstitial space (reduced intravascular-to-interstitial albumin gradient), causing hypovolemia, renal hypoperfusion, activation of the RAA system, and secondary renal sodium retention. However, at its pure expression, this situation is applied only to some cases of minimal change disease (MCD) and some cases of extreme hypoalbuminemia.

The 'overfill' hypothesis, on the other hand, states that in the NS there is a cause of primary renal sodium retention, leading to edema, suggesting that an abnormal primary tubular alteration in the handling of water and sodium leads to edema. Proteinuria itself can also upregulate the absorption of fluid at the distal nephron. [16] Interestingly, it has been shown in young analbuminemic Nagase rats that there is no difference in transcapillary colloid osmotic pressure, with preservation of the oncotic pressure gradient due to parallel decreases in serum and interstitial oncotic pressures. [27] This phenomenon has also been demonstrated in humans with the NS [28-30]. It has been proposed that two safeguard factors may protect against edema formation in the presence of hypoalbuminemia. [31] An increase in the passage of fluid from the intravascular space into the interstitial space could dilute the interstitial protein concentration and its oncotic pressure. In addition, an increase in fluid delivery to the interstitial space will produce an increase in lymphatic flow that will 'washout' interstitial proteins and finally delivering the protein load back to the systemic circulation. Both safeguard mechanisms could serve to maintain the plasma to interstitial protein ratio close to normal and thus defend against edema formation. Edema would appear when the interstitial protein concentration became virtually inexistent and no gradient forces could be generated due to the lack of oncotic pressure and the secondary intravascular protein decline. Finally, in the analbuminemic Nagase rats, plasma proteins such as transferrin, several globulins and fibrinogen are synthesized to compensate for the lack of plasmatic albumin, in an attempt to maintain oncotic pressure and to serve as transport molecules, replacing some of the main functions of albumin. It is not known to what extent these proteins are excluded from the interstitial space, but lipoproteins and fibrinogen, for example, which are increased in nephrotic subjects, will probably not traverse the capillary endothelium. This factor may also contribute to the preservation of the oncotic pressure and acting against the generation of edema in the NS. [27]

Finally, capillary permeability is severely altered in most nephrotic patients with primary glomerulonephritis. Capillary hyperpermeability plays a role in the pathophysiology of nephrotic edema associated with primary glomerular disease. It has been postulated that this widespread abnormality in capillary permeability could be related to the release of vascular permeability factors and other cytokines by immune cells, as histamine, endotoxins, anaphylatoxins, catecholamines, estrogens, progesterone, insulin and cytokines as vascular endothelial growth factor, Interleukin-1, Interleukin-2, tumor necrosis factor-alpha and vascular permeability factor. [32-35] This capillary permeability appears to be reverted after successful treatment of the NS. [8] In conclusion, most edematous patients with the NS may have a normal to expanded intravascular volume, whereas a minority of patients presents a depleted intravascular volume, as seen in some stages of MCD nephropathy. [36]

3. Plasmin, Urokinase Plasminogen Activator Receptor and the Nephrotic Syndrome

Many primary glomerulopathies can cause NS. MCD, focal and segmental glomerulosclerosis (FSGS), membranous nephropathy (MN), and membranoproliferative glomerulonephritis (MPGN) are among the most frequently encountered in clinical practice. It has been previously mentioned that a tubular derangement is the main culprit for the salt and water retention that occurs in most of the entities that present with NS, leading to edema formation and, eventually or concomitantly, to hypertension and renal insufficiency. In this respect, a key system to take into consideration is the uPA/uPAR binomium. Briefly, the urokinase plasminogen activator (uPA) and tissue plasminogen activator (tPA) are very similar serine proteases with the same physiological action, the activation of plasminogen. One of the receptors that converts plasminogen to plasmin, uPAR, is an extensively N-glycosylated membrane receptor tethered to the cellular plasma membrane. uPAR orchestrates a wide variety of cellular processes, including extracellular proteolysis, cell migration, adhesion, signaling, and proliferation, both under physiologic and pathologic conditions. On the plasma membrane, uPAR acts as the high-affinity binding site for uPA, promoting plasmin generation at the cell surface. The activation of proteolytic cascades after uPA–uPAR interaction is widely believed to be responsible for the biologic activity of uPAR. This interaction is blocked by amiloride, but tPA action is not modified by amiloride. [37] As reviewed by Sarra-Ferraris and Sidenius, additional studies have documented the existence of a variety of biologic activities induced solely by overexpression of uPAR or by the binding catalytically inactive uPA derivatives. These effects, referred to as the "non-proteolytic" functions of uPAR, rely on direct and functional interaction with other proteins on the plasma membrane or in the pericellular environment. The absence of a cytoplasmic tail makes uPAR unable to directly contact signaling molecules in the cytoplasm, and the signaling activity of uPAR has therefore been ascribed to interactions with a growing number of signaling receptors. It has indeed been shown that uPAR regulates signaling downstream of tyrosine kinase receptors, integrins, and G protein-coupled receptors. In addition, non-proteolytic uPAR functions include the direct effect played by uPAR on cell adhesion through its specific interaction with the extracellular matrix protein vitronectin. The importance of the uPAR-vitronectin interaction in the modulation of cell adhesion is becoming more and more compelling because it seems to be intimately connected to most of uPAR's non-proteolytic functions. uPAR modulates pericellular proteolysis by regulating the activity of the plasminogen system. [38] Interestingly, there is enough evidence to hypothesize that the inflammatory response that proteinuria causes in the renal medullary interstitium of nephrotic subjects could be enhanced by uPAR, plasmin and vitronectin. But there are other links where uPAR and the NS encounter. uPAR appears to play a critical role at least in two different ways. The first one is participating in the activation of distal tubular $ENa^{+}C$ via conversion of plasminogen to plasmin. [16, 23] In addition, this phenomenon may also occur in plasma and on the podocyte surface. [16, 23] The second mechanism is probably more controversial but provocative: Urokinase receptors, located on cell surface of certain cells, are bound to the cell by a glycosylphosphatidylinositol (GPI) molecule, which can be split by immunological factors. Once detached from the cell, uPAR is converted into a soluble circulating molecule, suPAR. [25] In a recent publication, Wei et al. provide ample evidence that elevated suPAR levels may play a role as a circulating factor with permeability properties on the glomerular membrane, leading to podocyte contraction and proteinuria. [23] Once described in primary FSGS, suPAR has thereafter been shown to be non-specific to this entity, having been encountered in other glomerulopathies with or without NS, and even in subjects without kidney disease. [39-43] Interestingly, it has been recently shown that both suPAR and interleukin-2 levels are elevated in patients with FSGS and are associated with the response to treatment. According to a previous study by Al-Atrash et al., interleukin-2 upregulated both uPA and uPAR in natural killer cells. An induction of uPAR mRNA and a reciprocal downregulation of uPAR mRNA-binding proteins were observed after interleukin-2 stimulation. [44] Furthermore, Nykjaer et al. demonstrated that interleukin-2 increased uPAR presentation on 20 to 50% of the T-cell population. [45] Recently, Shishido et al. reported that recurrent FSGS after kidney transplantation, which might be considered to be caused by circulating factors such as suPAR, was successfully treated with immunosuppressive treatments with methylprednisolone and cyclosporine, which could suppress IL-2 levels. [46] Therefore, there is a possibility that elevated interleukin-2 might increase suPAR in patients with primary FSGS and the increased levels of suPAR could be reversed by blocking interleukin-2. [47]

Moreover, Zhang et al. showed that the calcineurin–nuclear factor of activated T cells (NFAT) axis stimulates uPAR expression [48], while Ranjan et al. demonstrated that NFAT also binds to interleukin-2 gene promoter and increases interleukin-2 synthesis and secretion. [49] Thus, the mechanism of interleukin-2 and suPAR elevation and their interaction in primary FSGS both need further investigations, but may represent another component of the inflammatory milieu in which the NS expresses its constituents and complications. As a circulating permeability factor, suPAR is regulated by several cytokines and chemokines. [25] In the pathogenesis of FSGS, Huang et al. found that elevated urinary suPAR could activate β3 integrin on cultured human podocytes in vitro, suggesting that suPAR may have a direct role in mediating podocyte injury and disease development. [50] With respect to other glomerulopathies causing NS, the involvement of plasmin and uPAR in the edema generation have also been shown, as will be discussed below. However, the role suPAR may play as a generator of proteinuria is under intense debate. In this regard, elevated plasmin levels frequently occurring in the NS scene can interact with either circulating suPAR and/or cell surface attached uPAR to undertake its actions. [25] Presumably, by systemic circulation interactions, it could affect vascular sodium handling through $ENa^{+}C$ activation. By glomerular filtration, it could induce podocyte contraction and proteinuria. Finally, by tubular luminal interactions, it could induce water and sodium reabsorption and edema generation stimulating $ENa^{+}C$.

4. The Podocyte and Amiloride

Urokinase receptors, expressed on the cell surface of various cells, are committed to the pericellular proteolysis of plasminogen, are essential for the remodeling of the extracellular matrix, and are involved in vasculogenesis and cell migration processes. [51] uPAR is linked to the cell membrane by GPI and has a molecular weight of about 45-55 kDa. [51, 52] uPAR is present in various immunologically active cells, including monocytes, macrophages and activated T cells, and also in endothelial cells, keratinocytes, fibroblasts, smooth muscle cells, megakaryocytes, certain tumor cell lines, podocytes and renal tubular cells. [53-57] uPAR can be activated by various molecules, such as uPA (urokinase-type plasminogen activator, or simply urokinase), plasminogen, chymotrypsin, various metalloproteinases and some elastases. [58-61] uPAR is capable of catalyzing the conversion of plasminogen to plasmin, an important molecule in fibrinolytic processes and in the activation of several matrix metalloproteinases, in the recycling and degradation of the extracellular matrix, in cell activation, migration, contraction, vasculogenesis and in vitronectin interaction and degradation. [51, 62-66] This phenomenon may occur in plasma, on the podocyte surface or in renal distal tubular cells. [16, 23] Patients with NS present elevated serum levels of plasminogen and plasmin. [67] In turn, after being filtered, urinary plasminogen is converted to plasmin by podocyte or distal renal tubular epithelial uPAR; at this distal location, plasmin has been reported to function as a regulator of water and sodium absorption, a key event in the pathogenesis of edema in the NS, and also as a mediator in calcium tubular transport. [16, 68, 69] Cell migration across the endothelium and into tissues is a critical component in inflammation, in immune responses against infections, and in tissue repair and remodeling after injury. The uPA/uPAR system is directly involved in these mechanisms of adhesion, migration and chemotaxis. [57, 65] For example, the adhesion and migration of monocytes involves a functional interaction between cellular uPAR and matrix integrins [70] and in uPAR-dependent changes in integrin-mediated adhesion to fibrinogen, collagen and vitronectin. [23, 71, 72] It is known that uPAR is needed to activate the integrin αvβ3 in podocytes, which promotes cell motility and activation of small GTPases that control cell division. Thus, if the αvβ3 integrin was then activated, the podocyte could contract and proteinuria would be a straight forward result. [24]

A recent study has shown that podocyte uPAR expression can be reduced using amiloride. Amiloride plays a significant role in reducing podocyte cell motility in vitro and proteinuria in mice. [24] Amiloride inhibits the synthesis of uPAR and uPAR mRNA and consequently the αvβ3 integrin activation mediated by uPAR on αvβ3 integrin. Amiloride capacity to inhibit uPAR synthesis by T lymphocytes should be of particular interest in different causes of NS, because blocking their activation would inhibit αvβ3 integrin activation and the development of proteinuria with final renal dysfunction. [23-25]

5. The Tubule and Amiloride

It is well known that although sodium handling occurs along the entire nephron, it is the distal tubule where the fine tuning of sodium adjustment takes part. The ENa^+C located in the distal tubule is one of the main pathways by which sodium and water are absorbed. These channels are positively upregulated by plasmin and by proteinuria, and inhibited by amiloride.[16, 24, 73]

Ichikawa et al. created a unilateral puromicin amoninucleoside nephrosis (PAN) model in the rat such that one kidney was nephrotic and the other functioned normally. They showed that although the nephrotic kidney was proteinuric and sodium avid, the contralateral normal kidney had no proteinuria and handled sodium normally as in control rats. This suggested that an intrarenal defect caused sodium retention. There was a significant increase in sodium reabsorption beyond the distal convoluted tubule in the nephrotic kidney. [74]

An increase in cortical collecting duct Na^+/K^+ ATPase activity and amount has been shown in the PAN model of NS. [75-78] An inverse linear relationship between cortical collecting duct Na^+/K^+ ATPase activity and urinary sodium excretion has been noted. [76] The expression and apical targeting of ENa^+C has been shown to be increased in the cortical collecting duct in the PAN model of the NS and is aldosterone dependent. [10, 78-80] A linear correlation between plasma aldosterone and ENa^+C abundance was found in the PAN model of nephrosis [78], and treatment with amiloride prevented the sodium retention in the rat PAN model of nephrosis whereas treatment with an aldosterone receptor blocker did not. [77, 78] It is noteworthy that in adrenalectomized nephrotic rats, amiloride returned sodium excretion to normal despite the fact that ENa^+C expression was not increased. The observed increase in ENa^+C that occurs in animal models of the NS is due to aldosterone, but the development of nephrotic edema is not dependent on aldosterone. The importance of the ENa^+C channel in the development of nephrotic edema, however, is underscored by the reversal of sodium retention by amiloride in the above animal models. Evidence suggests that the Na^+/K^+-ATPase activity is increased in the NS and appears to be important in the sodium retention seen in the NS. Regulation of ENa^+C occurs through two primary mechanisms: regulation of channel density at the apical membrane and regulation of the open channel probability. [81] The ENa^+C receptor density is regulated by both aldosterone and vasopressin. Open channel probability is regulated by proteolytic processing [65] and by anionic phospholipids present on the inner cell membrane. Noteworthy, it has been reported that both plasminogen and plasmin are present in the urine of proteinuric rats with the metabolic syndrome and heavy proteinuria but not in control rats. [82, 83] As mentioned above, Svenningsen et al. have shown that plasmin present in the urine of nephrotic rats and humans can activate ENa^+C. [16] Additionally, they showed that uPA activator present in the rat and human kidney can convert inactive plasminogen (which is filtered by the nephrotic kidney) to the active-form plasmin. In the rat PAN nephrosis model, they demonstrated that amiloride increases urine sodium excretion due to the ability of amiloride to inhibit ENa^+C and the ability of amiloride to inhibit uPA and thus reduce the amount of active plasmin present. The above mentioned proteolytic processing of ENa^+C is undertaken by nephrotic urinary serine proteases, of which plasmin appears to play a main role. [16]

The above mentioned statements suggest a dominant role of ENa^+C in sodium and water retention in the NS and provide a rationale for specific diuretic blockade of ENa^+C. These important findings provide a mechanism of an intrinsic renal defect whereby abnormally filtered proteins in nephrotic patients can cause sodium retention via ENa^+C activation. It also explains the predictable course of recovery seen in MCD patients treated with steroids. First, there is a decrement in urinary protein excretion, then a reduction in aldosterone (urine and serum), followed by natriuresis, and then diuresis. [36, 84-88]

Another interesting aspect of this topic is the one that relates plasmin to calcium handling in the NS and another potential protective role for amiloride. [68] In the kidney, the fine regulation of calcium balance occurs through the activity of the epithelial calcium channel Transient Receptor Potential ion channel called TRPV5. [89] TRPV5 is mostly expressed in the distal convoluted tubule and connecting tubule of the nephron, where it constitutes the apical entry mechanism for transcellular calcium reabsorption. TRPV5 is a constitutively active ion channel that bears unique electrophysiologic characteristics, including calmodulin and calcium-dependent inactivation and high selectivity for calcium. [90, 91] The activity of TRPV5 is tightly controlled at multiple levels by an array of different factors, including parathyroid hormone and the serine protease tissue kallikrein. Both parathyroid hormone and tissue kallikrein initiate the phosphorylation of TRPV5. [92, 93] Pathologic leakage of glomerular proteins causes multiple tubulointerstitial abnormalities, such as interstitial inflammation and eventually fibrosis, but does not affect tubular structure. [94] However, tubular transport processes could be affected by direct effect of urinary protein on membrane transporters at the luminal side of the distal convoluted tubule, such as ENa^+C. [16] The observation of nephrocalcinosis in patients with nephrotic-range proteinuria, associated with impaired transcellular calcium reabsorption via TRPV5 in a mouse model, suggests that proteinuria might affect tubular calcium handling. [95-97] Patients with NS present elevated serum plasminogen levels. [67] After leakage into the urine, plasminogen is converted into active plasmin by tubular uPA. [16, 98] Tudpor et al. demonstrated that plasmin inhibits TRPV5 activity through the activation of uPAR. [68] Urinary plasmin, by inhibiting TRPV5 activity, could potentially be involved in disturbances in renal calcium handling found in nephrotic patients and may play a role in the tubulo-toxic effects of proteinuric urine. Plasmin inhibition by amiloride could therefore contribute to further tubulointerstitial protection by the inhibition of calcium cortico-medullar deposition, besides the already mentioned podocyte relaxation via uPAR inhibition of β_3 action. [65, 68]

6. The Endothelium and Amiloride

Dietary sodium and potassium contribute in part to the control of the blood pressure. Endothelial cells are targets for aldosterone, which activates the apically located ENa^+C. The activity of these channels is negatively correlated with the release of nitric oxide (NO) and determines endothelial function. [99] A mediating factor between channel activity and NO release is the mechanical stiffness of the cell's plasma membrane, including the submembranous actin network (the cell's 'shell'). Changes in plasma sodium and potassium, within the physiological range, regulate the viscosity of this shell and thus control the shear stress- dependent activity of the endothelial NO synthase located in the shell's 'pockets' (caveolae). High plasma sodium gelates the shell of the endothelial cell, whereas the shell is fluidized by high potassium. Accordingly, this concept envisages that communications between extracellular ions and intracellular enzymes occur at the plasma membrane barrier, whereas 90% of the total cell mass remains uninvolved in these changes. Endothelial cells are highly sensitive to extracellular sodium and potassium. This sensitivity may serve as a physiological feedback mechanism to regulate local blood flow. It may also have pathophysiological relevance when sodium/potassium homeostasis is disturbed. [99]

Endothelial NO synthase (eNOS) is located at the caveolae of the apical cell membrane and its expression and/or activity is regulated by various factors. It appears to be likely that sodium ions control eNOS activity, which is also inhibited by aldosterone, possibly indirectly through ENa^+C-mediated sodium influx. [100] Conversely, inhibition of ENa^+C-mediated sodium influx by amiloride activates eNOS. [101] An increase in the intake of salt induces the production of asymmetrical dimethyl-L-arginine, which is a competitive eNOS inhibitor, and increasing extracellular sodium downregulates eNOS expression and angiogenesis. [102, 103] It is noteworthy that there exists a negative correlation between stiffness and eNOS activity, that extracellular sodium concentration strongly determines stiffness and eNOS function, and also that extracellular potassium concentration influences eNOS activity and stiffness only at low sodium concentrations. Vascular endothelial cells undergo large changes in shape and can best adjust to such alterations if the deformability (physical compliance) of the cells is high. The cortical cytoskeleton of vascular endothelial cells is highly 'dynamic' and the state of polymerization of cortical actin determines the structure and mechanical properties of this layer. [104, 105] Monomeric globular actin (G-actin), which can rapidly polymerize into filamentous actin (F-actin), can cause a rapid increase in local viscosity (gelation). Alternatively, switching from F-actin to G-actin is associated with solation of the cortex, which in other words refers to the submembranous multimeric actin filament meshwork disaggregating into actin monomers. [106] G-actin is known to colocalize with eNOS and to increase eNOS activity. [107] It is possible that in this system potassium is an agonist, while sodium is a functional antagonist. Sodium influx, mediated by aldosterone-activated ENa^+C, stiffens the cytoskeleton by increasing the viscosity of the submembranous layer. It is hypothesized that when sodium is in the high physiological range, filamentous actin dominates over monomeric actin. This would explain the sodium-induced increase in cell stiffness. When potassium is elevated, actin filaments disaggregate into actin monomers and endothelial cells soften. Both F-actin and G-actin are negatively charged molecules and their interaction with positively charged ions as sodium and potassium will finally depend on the local concentrations and specific affinities of the respective ions. These changes are supposed to take place at the cytosolic submembranous zone, the cell shell (caveolae). [108] The solation-gelation hypothesis, based on the different interactions between sodium and potassium with the submembranous actin network, is supported by the observation that sodium has a greater affinity to protein surfaces than potassium. [109] It is assumed that when sodium enters the cell (e.g., through ENa^+C activation) it binds with high affinity to actin displacing potassium from the carboxylate groups within the amino-acid side chains. Thus, increasing the concentration of sodium, which has a higher affinity to actin as compared to potassium, effectively modulates its protein–protein interaction strength. [25] These small changes in sodium or potassium in the submembranous zone should control the state of actin polymerization and thus the cell stiffness and functionality. [99]

As mentioned previously, the genesis of edema in the the NS, can be mainly due to three factors: tubular retention of water and sodium stimulated by plasmin and proteinuria; vascular tone dysregulation and increased permeability secondary to capillary dilation; and hypoalbuminemia and a decreased oncotic pressure, particularly at some stages of acute MCD. In this regard, the first two causes are mainly due to ENa+C activity, which can be managed or ameliorated by amiloride.

Another interesting cellular site in the endothelial cell at which amiloride can be indirectly useful (as any antiproteinuruc agent) is at the endothelial glycocalyx. It has already been mentioned that proteinuria is a marker of cardiovascular morbidity and mortality and NS subjects belong to this clinical situation. It has been beautifully demonstrated by Salmon et al. that in Munich-Wistar-Fromter rats, a primary insult to the endothelial GBM glycocalyx translates with time to a systemic widespread loss of this layer in other organic vascular beds, such as the coronary and mesenteric vessels. This phenomenon was accompanied by local defects in water and sodium permeability. Therefore, this could be another mechanism of edema in the NS. Additionally, considering the relevant role the glycocalyx plays in the endothelium as a primary sensor for the secretion of NO, as a mechanotransductor, as a leukocyte adhesion molecule, as a stimulator for endothelial paracrine functions implicated in vascular medial smooth muscle and myofibroblasts actions, its loss could also link proteinuria to vascular dysfunction. [110-113] Loss of endothelial glycocalyx has been shown to accelerate atherosclerosis. [114] Whether amiloride has direct effects on the endothelial glycocalyx has not been assessed, but its antiproteinuric actions may also prove to be protective for the endothelium and the systemic vascular bed.

7. The Nephrotic Syndrome and Amiloride. Final Considerations

7.1. Tubular Aspects

The asymmetry of volume expansion, which has been traditionally attributed to the decrease in plasma oncotic pressure, is more likely due to an alteration of the capillary hydraulic conductivity, possibly linked to functional changes at the level of intercellular junctions. The low plasma oncotic pressure does not unbalance the transcapillary oncotic gradient and cannot be considered as a determining factor in edema generation or as a resistance factor for edema resorption. Therefore, diuretics preventing renal sodium retention remain the cornerstone of the treatment of nephrotic edema. Accordingly, the association of amiloride and furosemide provides a powerful treatment allowing progressive removal of edema from nephrotic patients. [115, 116] As to the dose to be employed to commit these goals, it varies between 5 and 10 mg/day, depending on the clinical picture, concomitant drugs employed, laboratory results and patient tolerance.

7.2. Glomerulo-tubular Aspects

On the basis of the temporal association among an initial glomerular insult, the appearance of plasmin in urine and primary, renal $ENa^{+}C$-mediated sodium hyper-reabsorption, these findings provide a putative novel mechanistic link between damage to the glomerular filtration barrier, proteinuria, and stimulation of sodium reabsorption in distal tubules and collecting ducts in the NS. This aspect is a target for amiloride. Moreover, the role amiloride plays on podocyte's integrin β_3 is important to reducing cellular contraction and proteinuria. Amiloride offers itself as a low-cost, non-immunosuppressant and complementary tool acting both at the glomerular and tubular level, for the management of complications of the NS as proteinuria, edema and hypertension.

References

[1] Abbate M, Zoja C, Remuzzi G. How does proteinuria cause progressive renal damage? *J. Am. Soc. Nephrol.* 2006;17:2974-2984.

[2] Gekle M. Renal tubule albumin transport. *Annu. Rev. Physiol.* 2005;67:573-594.

[3] Orth SR, Ritz E. Nephrotic syndrome. *Internist* (Berl). 1998;39:1246-1252.

[4] Doucet A, Favre G, Deschenes G. Molecular mechanism of edema formation in nephrotic syndrome therapeutic implications. *Pediatr. Nephrol.* 2007;22:1983-1990.

[5] de Zeeuw D. Albuminuria: a target for treatment of type 2 diabetic nephropathy. *Semin. Nephrol.* 2007;27:172-181.

[6] Matsushita K, van der Velde M, Astor BC, Woodward M, Levey AS, de Jong PE, Coresh J, Gansevoort RT. Chronic Kidney Disease Prognosis Consortium: Association of estimated glomerular filtration rate and albuminuria with all-cause and

cardiovascular mortality in general population cohorts: A collaborative meta-analysis. *Lancet*. 2010;375:2073-2081.

[7] Hillege HL, Fidler V, Diercks GF, van Gilst WH, de Zeeuw D, van Veldhuisen DJ, Gans RO, Janssen WM, Grobbee DE, de Jong PE. Prevention of Renal and Vascular End Stage Disease (PREVEND) Study Group. Urinary albumin excretion predicts cardiovascular and noncardiovascular mortality in general population. *Circulation*. 2002;106:1777-1782.

[8] Rostoker G, Behar A, Lagrue G. Vascular hyperpermeability in nephrotic edema. *Nephron*. 2000;85:194-200.

[9] Lourdel S, Loffing J, Favre G, Paulais M, Nissant A, Fakitsas P, Créminon C, Féraille E, Verrey F, Teulon J, Doucet A, Deschênes G. Hyperaldosteronemia and activation of the epithelial sodium channel are not required for sodium retention in puromycin-induced nephrosis. *J. Am. Soc. Nephrol*. 2005;16:3642-3650.

[10] Audigé A, Yu ZR, Frey BM, Uehlinger DE, Frey FJ, Vogt B. Epithelial sodium channel (ENaC) subunit mRNA and protein expression in rats with puromycin aminonucleoside-induced nephrotic syndrome. *Clin. Sci* (Lond). 2003;104:389-395.

[11] Hricik DE, Chung-Park M, Sedor JR. Glomerulonephritis. *N. Engl. J. Med*. 1998;339: 888-899.

[12] Bengrine A, Li J, Hamm LL, Awayda MS. Indirect activation of the epithelial Na+ channel by trypsin. *J. Biol. Chem*. 2007;282:26884-26896.

[13] Theilig F, Kriz W, Jerichow T, Schrade P, Hähnel B, Willnow T, Le Hir M, Bachmann S. Abrogation of protein uptake through megalin-deficient proximal tubules does not safeguard against tubulointerstitial injury. *J. Am. Soc. Nephrol*. 2007;18:1824-1834.

[14] Lötscher M, Kaissling B, Biber J, Murer H, Levi M. Role of microtubules in the rapid regulation of renal phosphate transport in response to acute alterations in dietary phosphate content. *J. Clin. Invest*. 1997;99:1302-1312.

[15] Tian YC, Fraser D, Attisano L, Phillips AO. TGF-beta1-mediated alterations of renal proximal tubular epithelial cell phenotype. *Am. J. Physiol. Renal Physiol*. 2003;285: F130-142.

[16] Svenningsen P, Bistrup C, Friis UG, Bertog M, Haerteis S, Krueger B, Stubbe J, Nørregaard Jensen O, Thiesson HC, Uhrenholt TR, Jespersen B, Jensen BL, Korbmacher C, Skøtt O. Plasmin in Nephrotic Urine Activates the Epithelial Sodium Channel. *J. Am. Soc. Nephrol*. 2009;20:299-310.

[17] Kim SW, de Seigneux S, Sassen MC, Lee J, Kim J, Knepper MA, Frøkiaer J, Nielsen S. Increased apical targeting of renal ENaC subunits and decreased expression of 11betaHSD2 in HgCl2-induced nephrotic syndrome in rats. *Am. J. Physiol. Renal Physiol*. 2006;290:F674-687.

[18] Deschênes G, Wittner M, Stefano A, Jounier S, Doucet A. Collecting duct is a site of sodium retention in PAN nephrosis: a rationale for amiloride therapy. *J. Am. Soc. Nephrol*. 2001;12:598-601.

[19] Kleyman TR, Cragoe EJ Jr. Amiloride and its analogs as tools in the study of ion transport. *J. Membr. Biol*. 1988;105:1-21.

[20] Edwards S, Lalor PF, Tuncer C, Adams DH. Vitronectin in human hepatic tumours contributes to the recruitment of lymphocytes in an alpha v beta3-independent manner. *Br. J. Cancer*. 2006;95:1545-1554.

[21] Wu S, Murrell GA, Wang Y. Interferon-alpha (Intron A) upregulates urokinase-type plasminogen activator receptor gene expression. *Cancer Immunol. Immunother.* 2002; 51:248-254.

[22] Wang Y, Jones CJ, Dang J, Liang X, Olsen JE, Doe WF. Human urokinase receptor expression is inhibited by amiloride and induced by tumor necrosis factor and phorbol ester in colon cancer cells. *FEBS Lett.* 1994;353:138-142.

[23] Wei C, Möller CC, Altintas MM, Li J, Schwarz K, Zacchigna S, Xie L, Henger A, Schmid H, Rastaldi MP, Cowan P, Kretzler M, Parrilla R, Bendayan M, Gupta V, Nikolic B, Kalluri R, Carmeliet P, Mundel P, Reiser J. Modification of kidney barrier function by the urokinase receptor. *Nat. Med.* 2008;14:55-63.

[24] Zhang B, Xie S, Shi W, Yang Y. Amiloride off-target effect inhibits podocyte urokinase receptor expression and reduces proteinuria. *Nephrol. Dial. Transplant.* 2012; 27:1746-1755.

[25] Trimarchi H. Primary focal and segmental glomerulosclerosis and soluble factor urokinase-type plasminogen activator receptor. *World J. Nephrol.* 2013;2:103-110.

[26] Gadau J, Peters H, Kastner C, Kühn H, Nieminen-Kelha M, Khadzhynov D, Krämer S, Castrop H, Bachmann S, Theilig F. Mechanisms of tubular volume retention in immune-mediated glomerulonephritis. *Kidney Int.* 2009;75:699-710.

[27] Joles JA, Willekes-Koolschijn N, Braam B, Kortlandt W, Koomans HA, Dorhout Mees EJ. Colloid osmotic pressure in young analbuminemic rats. *Am. J. Physiol.* 1989; 257:F23–F28.

[28] Koomans HA, Kortlandt W, Geers AB. Lowered protein content of tissue fluid in patients with the nephrotic syndrome: observations during disease and recovery. *Nephron.* 1985;40:391-395.

[29] Koomans HA, Geers AB, Dorhout Mees EJ, Kortlandt W. Lowered tissue-fluid oncotic pressure protects the blood volume in the nephrotic syndrome. *Nephron.* 1986; 42:317-22.

[30] Fauchald P, Noddeland H, Norseth J. Interstitial fluid volume, plasma volume and colloid osmotic-pressure in patients with nephrotic syndrome. *Scand. J. Clin. Lab. Invest.* 1984;44:661-667.

[31] Aukland K, Nicolaysen G. Interstitial fluid volume: local regulatory mechanisms. *Physiol. Rev.* 1981;61:556-643.

[32] Joles JA, Koomans HA, Kortlandt W, Boer P, Dorhout Mees EJ. Hypoproteinemia and recovery from edema in dogs. *Am. J. Physiol.* 1988;254:F887-894.

[33] Jennette JC, Falk RJ. Adult minimal change glomerulopathy with acute renal failure. *Am. J. Kidney Dis.* 1990;16:432-437.

[34] Furuya R, Kumagai H, Ikegaya N, Kobayashi S, Kimura M, Hishida A, Kaneko E. Reversible acute renal failure in idiopathic nephrotic syndrome. *Intern. Med.* 1993;32: 31-35.

[35] Case records of the Massachusetts General Hospital. Weekly clinicopathological exercise. Case 4-1982. Sudden onset of renal failure and the nephrotic syndrome in a middle-aged woman. *N. Engl. J. Med.* 1982;306:221-231.

[36] Siddall EC, Radhakrishnan J. The pathophysiology of edema formation in the nephrotic syndrome *Kidney Int.* 2012;82:635-642.

[37] Jankun J, Skrzypczak-Jankun E. Molecular basis of specific inhibition of urokinase plasminogen activator by amiloride. *Cancer Biochem. Biophys.* 1999;17:109-123.

[38] Ferraris GM, Sidenius N. Urokinase Plasminogen Activator Receptor: A Functional Integrator of Extracellular Proteolysis, Cell Adhesion, and Signal Transduction. *Semin. Thromb. Hemost.* 2013;39:347-355.

[39] Meijers B, Maas RJH, Sprangers B, Claes K, Poesen R, Bammens B, Naesens M, Deegens JKJ, Dietrich R, Storr M, Wetzels JFM, Evenepoel P, Kuypers D. The soluble urokinase receptor is not a clinical marker for focal segmental glomerulosclerosis. *Kidney Int.* 2014;85:636-640.

[40] Wada T, Nangaku M, Maruyama S, Imai E, Shoji K, Kato S, Endo T, Muso E, Kamata K, Yokoyama H, Fujimoto K6, Obata Y, Nishino T, Kato H, Uchida S, Sasatomi Y, Saito T, Matsuo S. A multicenter cross-sectional study of circulating soluble urokinase receptor in Japanese patients with glomerular disease. *Kidney Int.* 2014;85:641-648.

[41] Sinha A, Bajpai J, Saini S, Bhatia D, Gupta A, Puraswani M, Dinda AK, Agarwal SK, Sopory S, Pandey RM, Hari P, Bagga A. Serum-soluble urokinase receptor levels do not distinguish focal segmental glomerulosclerosis from other causes of nephrotic syndrome in children. *Kidney Int.* 2014;85:649-658.

[42] Sier CF, Sidenius N, Mariani , Aletti G, Agape V, Ferrari A, Casetta G, Stephens RW, Brünner N, Blasi F. Presence of urokinase-type plasminogen activator receptor in urine of cancer patients and its possible clinical relevance. *Lab. Invest.* 1999; 79:717-722.

[43] Stephens RW, Pedersen AN, Nielsen HJ, Hamers MJ, Høyer-Hansen G, Rønne E, Dybkjaer E, Danø K, Brünner N. ELISA determination of soluble urokinase receptor in blood from healthy donors and cancer patients. *Clin. Chem.* 1997;43:1868-1876.

[44] Al-Atrash G, Shetty S, Idell S, Xue Y, Kitson RP, Halady PK, Goldfarb RH. IL-2-mediated upregulation of uPA and uPAR in natural killer cells. *Biochem. Biophys. Res. Commun.* 2002;292:184-189.

[45] Nykjaer A, Müller B, Tod, RF 3rd. Urokinase receptor. An activation antigen in human T lymphocytes. *J. Immunol.* 1994;152:505-516.

[46] Shishido S, Satou H, Muramatsu M. Combination of pulse methylprednisolone infusions with cyclosporine-based immunosuppression is safe and effective to treat recurrent focal segmental glomerulosclerosis after pediatric kidney transplantation. *Clin. Transplant.* 2013;27:E143-E150.

[47] Park SJ, Saleem MA, Shin JI. Elevated soluble urokinase receptors in focal segmental glomerulosclerosis: a role for IL-2? *Kidney Int.* 2014;85:1469-1470.

[48] Zhang B, Shi W, Ma J. The calcineurin-NFAT pathway allows for urokinase receptor-mediated beta3 integrin signaling to cause podocyte injury. *J. Mol. Med* (Berl). 2012;90:1407-1420.

[49] Ranjan D, Chen C, Johnston TD. Curcumin inhibits mitogen stimulated lymphocyte proliferation, NFkB activation, and IL-2 signaling. *J. Surg. Res.* 2004;121:171-177.

[50] Huang J, Liu G, Zhang YM, Cui Z, Wang F, Liu XJ, Chu R, Chen Y, Zhao MH. Plasma soluble urokinase receptor levels are increased but do not distinguish primary from secondary focal segmental glomerulosclerosis. *Kidney Int.* 2013;84:366-372.

[51] Wei Y, Waltz DA, Rao N, Drummond RJ, Rosenberg S, Chapman HA. Identification of the urokinase receptor as an adhesion receptor for vitronectin. *J. Biol. Chem.* 1994;269:32380-32388.

[52] Ploug M, Rønne E, Behrendt N, Jensen AL, Blasi F, Danø K. Cellular receptor for urokinase plasminogen activator. Carboxyl- terminal processing and membrane anchoring by glycosyl- phosphatidylinositol. *J. Biol. Chem.* 1991;266:1926-1933.

[53] de Bock CE, Wang Y. Clinical significance of urokinasetype plasminogen activator receptor (uPAR) expression in cancer. *Med. Res. Rev.* 2004;24:13-39.

[54] Estreicher A, Mühlhauser J, Carpentier JL, Orci L, Vassalli JD. The receptor for urokinase type plasminogen activator polarizes expression of the protease to the leading edge of migrating monocytes and promotes degradation of enzyme inhibitor complexes. *J. Cell Biol.* 1990;111:783-792.

[55] Florquin S, van den Berg JG, Olszyna DP, Claessen N, Opal SM, Weening JJ, van der Poll T. Release of urokinase plasminogen activator receptor during urosepsis and endotoxemia. *Kidney Int.* 2001;59:2054-2061.

[56] Grøndahl-Hansen J, Lund LR, Ralfkiaer E, Ottevanger V, Danø K. Urokinase- and tissue-type plasminogen activators in keratinocytes during wound reepithelialization in vivo. *J. Invest. Dermatol.* 1988;90:790-795.

[57] Thunø M, Macho B, Eugen-Olsen J. suPAR: the molecular crystal ball. *Dis. Markers.* 2009;27:157-172.

[58] Andersen O, Eugen-Olsen J, Kofoed K, Iversen J, Haugaard SB. Soluble urokinase plasminogen activator receptor is a marker of dysmetabolism in HIV-infected patients receiving highly active antiretroviral therapy. *J. Med. Virol.* 2008;80:209-216.

[59] Cunningham O, Andolfo A, Santovito ML, Iuzzolino L, Blasi F, Sidenius N. Dimerization controls the lipid raft partitioning of uPAR/CD87 and regulates its biological functions. *EMBO J.* 2003;22:5994-6003.

[60] Fazioli F, Resnati M, Sidenius N, Higashimoto Y, Appella E, Blasi F. A urokinase-sensitive region of the human urokinase receptor is responsible for its chemotactic activity. *EMBO J.* 1997;16:7279-7286.

[61] Høyer-Hansen G, Ploug M, Behrendt N, Rønne E, Danø K. Cell-surface acceleration of urokinase-catalyzed receptor cleavage. *Eur. J. Biochem.* 1997;243:21-26.

[62] Beaufort N, Leduc D, Rousselle JC, Magdolen V, Luther T, Namane A, Chignard M, Pidard D. Proteolytic regulation of the urokinase receptor/CD87 on monocytic cells by neutrophil elastase and cathepsin G. *J. Immunol.* 2004;172:540-549.

[63] Ossowski L, Aguirre-Ghiso JA. Urokinase receptor and integrin partnership: coordination of signaling for cell adhesion, migration and growth. *Curr. Opin. Cell Biol.* 2000;12:613-620.

[64] Chapman HA. Plasminogen activators, integrins, and the coordinated regulation of cell adhesion and migration. *Curr. Opin. Cell Biol.* 1997;9:714-724.

[65] Blasi F. uPA, uPAR, PAI-1: key intersection of proteolytic, adhesive and chemotactic highways? *Immunol. Today.* 1997;18:415-417.

[66] Waltz DA, Natkin LR, Fujita RM, Wei Y, Chapman HA. Plasmin and plasminogen activator inhibitor type 1 promote cellular motility by regulating the interaction between the urokinase receptor and vitronectin. *J. Clin. Invest.* 1997;100:58-67.

[67] Vaziri ND, Gonzales EC, Shayestehfar B, Barton CH. Plasma levels and urinary excretion of fibrinolytic and protease inhibitory proteins in nephrotic syndrome. *J. Lab. Clin. Med.* 1994;124:118-124.

[68] Tudpor K, Laínez S, Kwakernaak AJ, Kovalevskaya NV, Verkaart S, van Genesen S, van der Kemp A, Navis G, Bindels RJ, Hoenderop JG. Urinary plasmin inhibits TRPV5 in nephrotic-range proteinuria. *J. Am. Soc. Nephrol.* 2012;23:1824-1834.

[69] Andersen RF, Buhl KB, Jensen BL, Svenningsen P, Friis UG, Jespersen B, Rittig S. Remission of nephrotic syndrome diminishes urinary plasmin content and abolishes activation of ENaC. *Pediatr. Nephrol.* 2013;28:1227-1234.

[70] May AE, Kanse SM, Lund LR, Gisler RH, Imhof BA, Preissner KT. Urokinase receptor (CD87) regulates leukocyte recruitment via beta 2 integrins in vivo. *J. Exp. Med.* 1998;188:1029-1037.

[71] Wei Y, Yang X, Liu Q, Wilkins JA, Chapman HA. A role for caveolin and the urokinase receptor in integrin-mediated adhesion and signaling. *J. Cell. Biol.* 1999;144: 1285-1294.

[72] Wei Y, Eble JA, Wang Z, Kreidberg JA, Chapman HA. Urokinase receptors promote beta1 integrin function through interactions with integrin alpha3beta1. *Mol. Biol. Cell.* 2001;12:2975-2986.

[73] Warnock D, Kusche-Virog K, Tarjus A, Sheng Shaohu S, Oberleithner J, Kleyman TR, Jaisser F. Blood pressure and amiloride-sensitive sodium channels in vascular and renal cells. *Nat. Rev. Nephrol.* 2014;10:146-157.

[74] Ichikawa I, Rennke HG, Hoyer JR, Badr KF, Schor N, Troy JL, Lechene CP, Brenner BM. Role for intrarenal mechanisms in the impaired salt excretion of experimental nephrotic syndrome. *J. Clin. Invest.* 1983;71:91-103.

[75] Vogt, B; Favre, H. Na+, K(+)-ATPase activity and hormones in single nephron segments from nephrotic rats. *Clin. Sci* (Lond). 1991;80:599-604.

[76] Deschenes G, Doucet A. Collecting duct (Na+/K+)-ATPase activity is correlated with urinary sodium excretion in rat nephrotic syndromes. *J. Am. Soc. Nephrol.* 2000;11:604-615.

[77] Deschênes G, Gonin S, Zolty E, Cheval L, Rousselot M, Martin PY, Verbavatz JM, Féraille E, Doucet A. Increased synthesis and avp unresponsiveness of Na,K-ATPase in collecting duct from nephrotic rats. *J. Am. Soc. Nephrol.* 2001;12:2241-2252.

[78] Lourdel S, Loffing J, Favre G, Paulais M, Nissant A, Fakitsas P, Créminon C, Féraille E, Verrey F, Teulon J, Doucet A, Deschênes G. Hyperaldosteronemia and activation of the epithelial sodium channel are not required for sodium retention in puromycin-induced nephrosis. *J. Am. Soc. Nephrol.* 2005;16:3642-3650.

[79] de Seigneux S, Kim SW, Hemmingsen SC, Frøkiaer J, Nielsen S. Increased expression but not targeting of ENaC in adrenalectomized rats with PAN-induced nephrotic syndrome. *Am. J. Physiol. Renal Physiol.* 2006;291:F208-217.

[80] Kim SW, Wang W, Nielsen J, Praetorius J, Kwon TH, Knepper MA, Frøkiaer J, Nielsen S. Increased expression and apical targeting of renal ENaC subunits in puromycin aminonucleoside-induced nephrotic syndrome in rats. *Am. J. Physiol. Renal Physiol.* 2004;286:F922-935.

[81] Snyder PM. Minireview: regulation of epithelial Na+ channel trafficking. *Endocrinology*. 2005;146:5079-5085.

[82] Hamm LL, Feng Z, Hering-Smith KS. Regulation of sodium transport by ENaC in the kidney. *Curr. Opin. Nephrol. Hypertens.* 2010;19:98-105.

[83] Ma HP, Eaton DC. Acute regulation of epithelial sodium channel by anionic phospholipids. *J. Am. Soc. Nephrol.* 2005;16:3182-3187.

[84] Oliver WJ. Physiologic responses associated with steroid-induced diuresis in the nephrotic syndrome. *J. Lab. Clin. Med.* 1963;62:449-464.

[85] Koomans HA, Boer WH, Dorhout Mees EJ. Renal function during recovery from minimal lesions nephrotic syndrome. *Nephron*. 1987;47:173-178.
[86] Brown EA, Markandu N, Sagnella GA, Jones BE, MacGregor GA. Sodium retention in nephrotic syndrome is due to an intrarenal defect: evidence from steroid-induced remission. *Nephron*. 1985;39:290-295.
[87] Kumagai H, Onoyama K, Iseki K. Role of renin angiotensin aldosterone on minimal change nephrotic syndrome. *Clin. Nephrol*. 1985;23:229-235.
[88] Oliver WJ, Owings CL. Sodium excretion in the nephrotic syndrome. Relation to serum albumin concentration, glomerular filtration rate, and aldosterone excretion rate. *Am. J. Dis. Child*. 1967;113:352-362.
[89] Hoenderop JG, van der Kemp AW, Hartog A, van de Graaf SF, van Os CH, Willems PH, Bindels RJ. Molecular identification of the apical Ca2+ channel in 1, 25-dihydroxyvitamin D3-responsive epithelia. *J. Biol. Chem*. 1999;274:8375-8378.
[90] Lambers TT, Weidema AF, Nilius B, Hoenderop JG, Bindels RJ. Regulation of the mouse epithelial Ca2(+) channel TRPV6 by the Ca(2 +)-sensor calmodulin. *J. Biol. Chem*. 2004;279:28855-28861.
[91] Nilius B, Vennekens R, Prenen J, Hoenderop JG, Droogmans G, Bindels RJ. The single pore residue Asp542 determines Ca2+ permeation and Mg2+ block of the epithelial Ca2+ channel. *J. Biol. Chem*. 2001;276:1020-1025.
[92] de Groot T, Lee K, Langeslag M, Xi Q, Jalink K, Bindels RJ, Hoenderop JG. Parathyroid hormone activates TRPV5 via PKA-dependent phosphorylation. *J. Am. Soc. Nephrol*. 2009;20:1693-1704.
[93] Gkika D, Topala CN, Chang Q, Picard N, Thébault S, Houillier P, Hoenderop JG, Bindels RJ. Tissue kallikrein stimulates Ca(2+) reabsorption via PKC-dependent plasma membrane accumulation of TRPV5. *EMBO J*. 2006;25:4707-4716.
[94] Kuusniemi AM, Lapatto R, Holmberg C, Karikoski R, Rapola J, Jalanko H. Kidneys with heavy proteinuria show fibrosis, inflammation, and oxidative stress, but no tubular phenotypic change. *Kidney Int*. 2005;68:121-132.
[95] Burke EC, Holley KE, Stickler GB. Familial nephrotic syndrome with nephrocalcinosis and tubular dysfunction. *J. Pediatr*. 1973, 82:202-206.
[96] Mocan H, Yildiran A, Camlibel T, Kuzey GM. Microscopic nephrocalcinosis and hypercalciuria in nephrotic syndrome. *Hum. Pathol*. 2000;31:1363-1367.
[97] Alexander RT, Woudenberg-Vrenken TE, Buurman J, Dijkman H, van der Eerden BC, van Leeuwen JP, Bindels RJ, Hoenderop JG. Klotho prevents renal calcium loss. *J. Am. Soc. Nephrol*. 2009;20:2371-2379.
[98] Passero CJ, Mueller GM, Rondon-Berrios H, Tofovic SP, Hughey RP, Kleyman TR. Plasmin activates epithelial Na+ channels by cleaving the gamma subunit. *J. Biol. Chem*. 2008;283:36586-36591.
[99] Oberleithner H, Kusche-Vihrog K, Schillers H. Endothelial cells as vascular salt sensors. *Kidney Int*. 2010;77:490-494.
[100] Schiffrin EL. Effects of aldosterone on the vasculature. *Hypertension*. 2006;47:312-318.
[101] Perez FR, Venegas F, Gonzalez M. Endothelial epithelial sodium channel inhibition activates endothelial nitric oxide synthase via phosphoinositide 3-kinase/Akt in small-diameter mesenteric arteries. *Hypertension*. 2009;53:1000-1007.

[102] Fujiwara N, Osanai T, Kamada T. Study on the relationship between plasma nitrite and nitrate level and salt sensitivity in human hypertension: modulation of nitric oxide synthesis by salt intake. *Circulation*. 2000;101:856-861.
[103] Li J, White J, Guo L, Zhao X, Wang J, Smart EJ, Li XA. Salt inactivates endothelial nitric oxide synthase in endothelial cells. *J. Nutr*. 2009;139:447-451.
[104] Kasas S, Wang X, Hirling H. Superficial and deep changes of cellular mechanical properties following cytoskeleton disassembly. *Cell Motil. Cytoskeleton*. 2005;62:124-132.
[105] Pesen D, Hoh JH. Micromechanical architecture of the endothelial cell cortex. *Biophys. J*. 2005;88:670-679.
[106] Oberleithner H, Callies C, Kusche-Vihrog K, Schillers H, Shahin V, Riethmüller C, Macgregor GA, de Wardener HE. Potassium softens vascular endothelium and increases nitric oxide release. *Proc. Natl. Acad. Sci. U S A*. 2009;106:2829-2834.
[107] Su Y, Edwards-Bennett S, Bubb MR, Block ER. Regulation of endothelial nitric oxide synthase by the actin cytoskeleton. *Am. J. Physiol. Cell Physiol*. 2003;284:C1542-1549.
[108] Rizzo V, McIntosh DP, Oh P, Schnitzer JE. In situ flow activates endothelial nitric oxide synthase in luminal caveolae of endothelium with rapid caveolin dissociation and calmodulin association. *J. Biol. Chem*. 1998;273:34724-34729.
[109] Vrbka L, Vondrásek J, Jagoda-Cwiklik B, Vácha R, Jungwirth P. Quantification and rationalization of the higher affinity of sodium over potassium to protein surfaces. *Proc. Natl. Acad. Sci. U S A*. 2006;103:15440-15444.
[110] Salmon AHJ, Ferguson JK, Burford JL, Gevorgyan H, Nakano D, Harper SJ, Bates DO, Peti-Peterdi J. Loss of the endothelial glycocalyx links albuminuria and vascular dysfunction. *J. Am. Soc. Nephrol*. 2012;23:1339-1350.
[111] Kumagai R; Lu X, Kassab GS. Role of glycocalyx in flow-induced production of nitric oxide and reactive oxygen species. *Free Radic. Biol. Med*. 2009;47:600-607.
[112] Michel CC, Curry FE. Microvascular permeability. *Physiol. Rev*. 1999;79:703-761.
[113] Weinbaum S, Tarbell JM, Damiano ER. The structure and function of the endothelial glycocalyx layer. *Annu. Rev. Biomed. Eng*. 2007;9:121-167.
[114] Nagy N, Freudenberger T, Melchior-Becker A, Röck K, Ter Braak M, Jastrow H, Kinzig M, Lucke S, Suvorava T, Kojda G, Weber AA, Sörgel F, Levkau B, Ergün S, Fischer JW. Inhibition of hyaluronan synthesis accelerates murine atherosclerosis. Novel insights into the role of hyaluronan synthesis. *Circulation*. 2010;122:2313-2322.
[115] Reubi FC, Weidmann P, Gluck Z. Interrelationships between sodium clearance, plasma aldosterone, plasma renin activity, renal hemodynamics and blood pressure in renal disease. *Klin. Wochenschr*. 1979;57:1273-1285.
[116] Deschenes G, Feraille E, Doucet A. Mechanisms of edema in nephrotic syndrome: old theories and new ideas. *Nephrol. Dial. Transplant*. 2003;18:454-456.

In: Nephrotic Syndrome: Etiology, Pathogenesis and Pathology ISBN: 978-1-63482-154-4
Editor: Muhammed Mubarak

Chapter 3

Pathogenesis of Idiopathic Membranous Glomerulonephritis

Raja Ramachandran* and Ashok Kumar Yadav
Department of Nephrology, Postgraduate Institute of Medical Education and Research, Chandigarh, India

Abstract

Membranous nephropathy is one of the major causes of adult nephrotic syndrome and the leading cause of nephrotic syndrome in Caucasian adults and elderly patients. Etiologically, it is divided into idiopathic and secondary types. The exact etiology and pathogenesis of the idiopathic form is still not completely understood. The preponderance of evidence suggests that idiopathic membranous nephropathy is an auto-immune disease. Pathologically, the disease is characterized by the accumulation of immune deposits on the subepithelial side of the glomerular basement membrane, with resultant diffuse thickening of the peripheral capillary walls and functional derangement of the glomerular filtration barrier with resultant proteinuria. These immune deposits consist of immunoglobulin IgG subclasses and complement components. The identity of the target antigens remained elusive till recent past. However, during the recent past, a series of discoveries related to the target antigens involved in the immune complex formation has led to a better understanding of the molecular pathophysiology of the disease and paved the way for targeted molecular-based therapeutic strategies. In this chapter, we will discuss the recent developments in understanding the molecular pathogenesis of the disease, in context of Heymann nephritis. Detailed discussion of other aspects of the disease is beyond the scope of this chapter.

Keywords: Autoimmune, Heymann nephritis, immune complexes, membranous nephropathy, nephrotic syndrome, pathogenesis

---

* Corresponding author: Dr. Raja Ramachandran, Assistant Professor, Department of Nephrology, Postgraduate institute of Medical Education and Research, Chandigarh-160012, India, Email: drraja_1980@yahoo.co.in.

1. Introduction

Membranous nephropathy (MN) is one of the most common causes of adult nephrotic syndrome (NS), accounting for about one-third of the cases. [1,2] MN is 'idiopathic', if there is no identifiable cause (two-third of the cases), or secondary to systemic diseases, including infections (hepatitis B and hepatitis C), lupus nephritis, drugs and malignancy.

Idiopathic MN (IMN) is characterized by the deposition of immune complexes in the subepithelial space, resulting in thickening of the glomerular basement membrane (GBM) on Hematoxylin and Eosin (H&E) staining (Figure 1A). The immune deposits consist of IgG, complement-3 (C3) and the membrane attack complex (MAC) (C5b-9) (Figure 1B). IgG4 is the most prominent IgG subclass deposited in IMN, followed by IgG1 and IgG3; by contrast, deposition of IgG2 and IgG3 exceeds deposition of IgG4 in MN secondary to malignancy. [3, 4] The above mentioned immune deposits result in functional impairment of the GBM resulting in proteinuria.

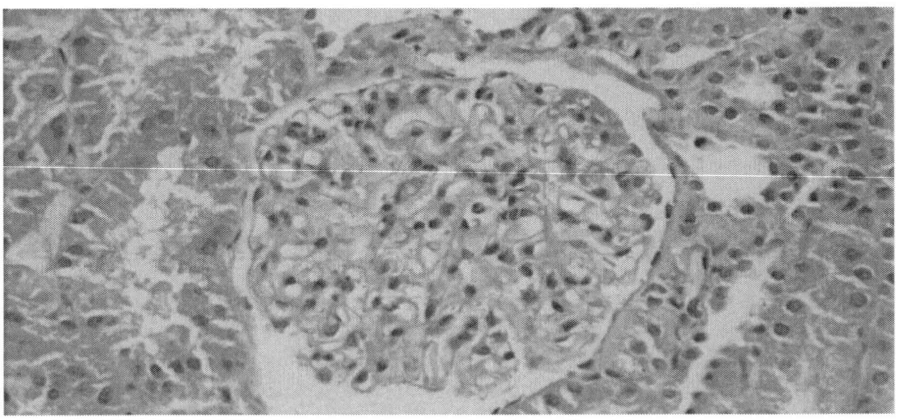

Figure 1A. Glomerulus showing thickened basement membrane in a case of IMN. (H&E, ×20).

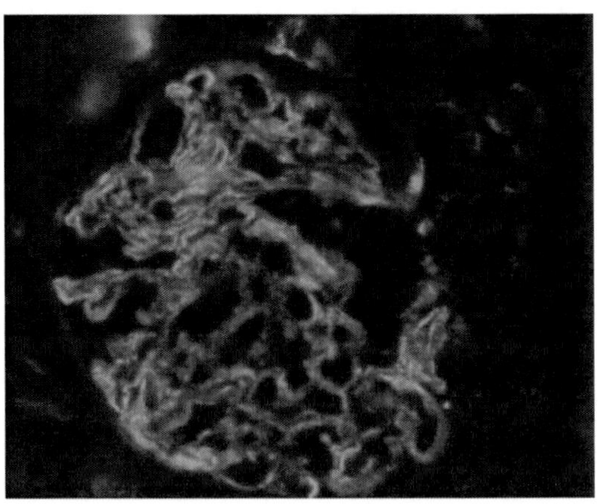

Figure 1B. Moderate granular staining along glomerular basement membrane with IgG in a case of IMN (Immunofluorescence, FITC, ×20).

There are at least 3 probable mechanisms that can explain the formation of immune deposits in experimental and human IMN. The first mechanism is the deposition of circulating immune complexes (CICs) in the GBM (e.g., chronic serum sickness). The second mechanism involves in-situ formation of immune complex of a circulating antibody with a native podocyte antigen and third mechanism is in-situ formation of immune complex of a circulating antibody with a 'planted' exogenous antigen bound to the GBM.

Great progress in the understanding of the pathogenesis of human IMN has been made over the last 5 years. The first convincing experimental model of IMN was the Heymann nephritis [5, 6] followed by cationic bovine serum albumin (BSA). [7] Heymann nephritis model showed that a podocyte antigen could be the target of the circulating antibodies resulting in IMN. In the year 2002, Debiec et al. demonstrated antibodies to neutral endopeptidase (NEP) in a case of neonatal IMN and provided the proof of concept that a podocyte antigen could be responsible for human IMN. [8] Beck et al. identified autoantibodies to podocyte antigen, M-type receptor for phospholipase A2 (PLA2R1) in patients of IMN. [9] A strong association of single nucleotide polymorphism (SNP) in the PLA2R1 gene and IMN further strengthened the above hypothesis. [10] The role of antibodies to other podocyte antigens like aldose reductase (AR), superoxide dismutase-2 (SOD2) and alpha enolase are also being evaluated in IMN. [11] Exogenous antigens like cationic BSA have been implicated in pediatric IMN. All the above-mentioned antibodies have made a paradigm shift in the diagnosis and the management of pediatric and adult IMN.

2. Experimental Studies

2.1. Heymann Nephritis

Heymann et al. [5] described a rat model of IMN, which was referred to as active Heymann nephritis. IMN was induced by immunization of Lewis rats with crude kidney extracts. Fractions of renal brush border membrane were isolated from the subepithelial deposits of the Lewis rats and a hypothesis of glomerular trapping of CICs was made. However, development of IMN in the passive Heymann nephritis model in which, Lewis rats injected with anti-rat brush-border antibodies argued against deposition of the CICs in IMN . [6] Van Damme et al. and Couser et al. [6, 12] demonstrated binding of rabbit anti-rat brush-border antibodies to podocyte antigens, indicating that IMN was caused by the in-situ formation and deposition of immune complexes rather than by CICs.

In 1980s, Heymann nephritis antigen was identified as a rat podocyte transmembrane protein called megalin (LDL receptor-related protein 2, molecular weight 600 KDa). [13, 14] Megalin [15, 16] is present in the podocyte foot processes in clathrin-coated pits and epitope mapping of the megalin showed that full-blown NS was induced by binding of the antibodies to the first ligand-binding domain of megalin. Antibodies to depeptidyl peptidase 4 were reported to cause IMN similar to Heymann nephritis in rats and mice. [17-20] Although, studies of Heymann nephritis have contributed to our understanding of the pathogenesis of IMN, there is no convincing evidence that megalin is involved in human IMN.

2.2. Complement-Mediated Injury

Formation of MAC as a result of the immune complex deposition and complement activation plays a vital role in podocyte injury resulting in proteinuria. [21-23] MAC in sublytic quantities activates various cytokines and protein kinases, which effect the podocyte metabolic pathways and functioning of key cytoskeletal proteins. MAC also up-regulates NADPH oxidoreductase, which results in local production of reactive oxygen species (ROS). The ROSs damage podocyte proteins, lipids and other GBM components. [21-24]

2.3. Serum Sickness

Chronic serum sickness is characterized by deposition of CICs in various tissues/ organs. [25] The location of the immune deposits in the glomeruli depends on the antigen characteristics (size and charge), antibody response and the size of the immune complexes. If the antigens outnumber the antibodies, deposits are usually in the subepithelial space. [26, 27] Other possible mechanisms include dissociation of immune complexes on the subendothelial side and reassociation on the subepithelial aspect of the capillary wall.

3. Autoantibodies in IMN

3.1. PLA2R1 in Pathogenesis of IMN

PLA2R1 is a 180 KDa peptide, expressed on the membrane surface of the podocyte. [9] PLA2R1 is a receptor for phospholipase A2 and consists of a long extracellular domain and a short membrane-spanning intracellular domain. The nephritogenic epitope is located in the methionine-rich extracellular domain. [28-30] The function of the PLA2R1 is not very clear; however, it is hypothesized that it may be involved in cellular senescence. Antibodies to the PLA2R1 are detected in 70% of the cases of IMN by western-blot. [9] A small minority of patients with malignancies and viral infection related MN might have antibodies demonstrable to PLA2R1.

The evidence of the pathogenicity of PLA2R1 antibodies in IMN is very strong: anti-PLA2R1 antibodies co-localize with PLA2R1 antigen in the glomeruli (Figure 1C); anti-PLA2R1 antibodies have been eluted from the kidneys affected by IMN; PLA2R1 antibodies correlate with clinical activity, disappear with remission and reappear during relapse of the disease; recurrence of IMN in the transplant kidneys have been reported in patients with persistent PLA2R1 antibodies just prior to transplant. [9, 31-33] PLA2R1 antibodies decline prior to clinical remission, i.e., there is immunological recovery prior to clinical recovery. There is a very good correlation between serum PLA2R1 antibodies and glomerular deposits of PLA2R1 in IMN cases. [7] However, there have been reports of discrepancies between PLA2R antigen in the glomeruli and circulating PLA2R1 antibodies. Debiec et al. evaluated 42 cases of IMN and reported presence of both PLA2R1 in glomerular deposits and circulating PLA2R1 antibodies in 50% of the cases; 7% had PLA2R1 antibodies in circulation only; 24% had only PLA2R1 in glomerular deposits and 19% were negative for both PLA2R1 in glomeruli and circulating autoantibodies. [7] We have analysed 114 cases of IMN and found that 60% of the cases were positive for both antigen in the glomeruli and autoantibodies in the serum, 16% had only glomerular PLA2R1, 7% had only circulating autoantibodies and 17% were negative for both (Unpublished).

The factors responsible for 'anti- PLA2R negative' IMN include poor sensitivity of the current assays, heterogeneity of the conformational PLA2R epitope, immunological recovery before clinical remission and probably involvement of other antibodies like SOD, AR, NEP and BSA. Presence of PLA2R1 antibodies without detectable glomerular PLA2R may be explained by poorly accessible PLA2R epitopes in the glomeruli at the time of staining and presence of glomerular PLA2R without serum antibodies can be due to rapid clearance of antibodies from the blood and deposition in the glomeruli or due to delayed presentation where the NS might be due to irreversible changes in the kidney.

IMN is characterized by IgG4 subclass dominant circulating autoantibodies (T-Helper-2-Type immune response) and immune deposits in the glomeruli. IMN is regarded as an IgG4 associated disease. [34, 35] IgG4 poorly fixes complement by classical or alternate pathway and complement activation and formation of MAC is a prerequisite for proteinuria in experimental models. Mannose binding lectin (MBL) is also deposited along with IgG in IMN and MBL pathway of complement activation (by activating C4) could play an important role in the complement activation and pathogenesis of human IMN. [36] Other plausible explanation could be activation of alternate pathway of complement activation or activation of the classical pathway by the IgG1 co-deposited along with IgG4. In the neonatal IMN, alloantibodies of the IgG1 subclass to NEP were demonstrated to cause proteinuria rather than the IgG1 subclass. [8] In case of malignancy associated MN, IgG1/2 antibodies are thought to be the dominant subclass in the subepithelial deposits. Hence, the role of IgG4 in the pathogenesis of IMN is not clear and needs more research. The stimuli for autoantibody production in IMN are not known, one probable hypothesis is molecular mimicry to an exogenous antigen in patients genetically susceptible (SNP in HLA-DQA1 and PLA2R gene) to IMN.

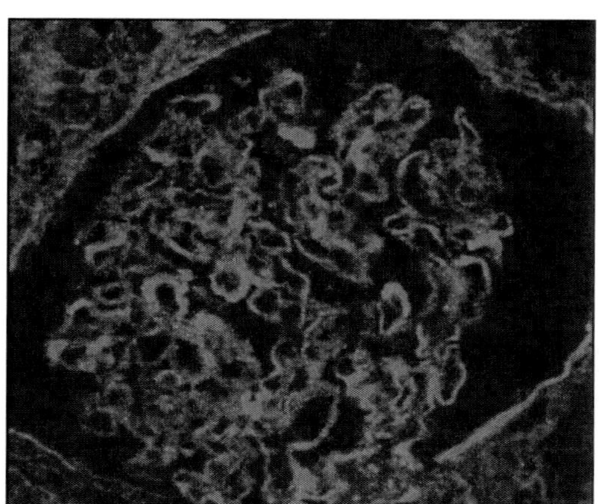

Figure 1C. Granular positivity of PLA2R deposits on the glomerular basement membranes in a case of IMN (Immunofluorescence, TRITC, ×20).

Table 1. Summary of studies of PLA2R in IMN

Author	Country	Number (N)	Serum for PLA2R positive (%)	Tissue PLA2R sensitivity (%)
Beck et al. 2009	USA	37	70%	-
Debiec et al. 2011	France	42	57%	74%
Yun Jung oh et al. 2013	South Korea	100	69%	-
Hoxha et al. 2011	Germany	100	52%	-
Hofstra et al. 2011	Netherlands	18	77%	-
Hoxha et al. 2012	Germany	88	69.3%	68.1%

3.1.1. PLA2R autoantibodies in IMN Diagnosis and monitoring

Beck et al. demonstrated PLA2R1 autoantibodies by western-blot in 70% of the patients with IMN. [9] The PLA2R antibodies are also demonstrable by enzymes like immunosorbent assay (ELISA) and indirect immunofluorescence (IIF). Serum PLA2R1 antibodies are demonstrable in 52-82% of the IMN cases using either of the above mentioned techniques. [37, 38] In addition studies by Hofstra et al. and Hoxha et al. reported a very good correlation of antibody detection by ELISA and IIF. [33, 39] Commercial kits (FDA approved) are available for detection of PLA2R1 antibodies by ELISA and IIF techniques. Hoxha et al. had evaluated 133 cases of PLA2R1 antibody positive IMN and found 81% reduction in PLA2R1 antibody titers with 3 months of immunosuppressive treatment. Patients with remission of proteinuria had significant reduction in the PLA2R1 antibody titers compared to patients with persistent proteinuria. [33] The authors also reported a significant association of PLA2R1 antibodies with proteinuria. To conclude PLA2R1 antibodies play an important role in the diagnosis and the management of IMN. The summary of all the studies of PLA2R antibodies in IMN is mentioned in Table 1.

3.2. Other Autoantibodies in IMN

The other antigens to which autoantibodies in IMN have been demonstrated include SOD2, AR, α-enolase, NEP and BSA. The data regarding the other podocyte antibodies in the pathogenesis of IMN is limited.

3.2.1. SOD2

The SOD2 is a mitochondrial enzyme involved in transformation of superoxide ions into hydrogen peroxide and diatomic oxygen. This enzyme is widely expressed in tubular epithelial cells, where it plays an important role in preserving the kidney during ischemia/reperfusion. The enzyme is not expressed in the human glomeruli, but is neo-expressed in podocytes and in sub-epithelial immune deposits of patients with IMN. [40] The above mentioned phenomenon suggests that hyperexpression and membrane displacement may be implicated in the pathogenesis of IMN. [11] However, only a couple of studies have looked for autoantibodies to SOD2 in IMN and reported prevalence in 41% of cases. [11]

3.2.2. AR

AR is a cytoplasmic enzyme involved in the breakdown of NADPH-dependent reduction of aliphatic and aromatic aldehydes and ketones. It is involved in regulation of tissue tonicity and osmolarity. As in case of SOD2, AR is limited to tubular epithelial cells in normal healthy individuals and is absent in the glomeruli. [41] However, in IMN cases, it is detectable in the subepithelial deposits in the glomeruli. [42] Prunotto et al. had reported a prevalence of AR antibodies in 12.5% of patients with active IMN. [11]

3.2.3. Alpha Enolase

Alpha enolase is one of the most abundant proteins in the cytoplasm and is a key enzyme of glycolysis. Alpha enolase is expressed in tubular epithelial cells of the kidney. [43] Autoantibodies to alpha enolase have been reported in various diseases; however, their exact pathogenic role is not very clear. [44] Similar to AR and SOD2, neo-expression of alpha enolase in the glomeruli of IMN cases and its co-localization with IgG4 in the subepithelial deposits strengthens the hypothesis of autoantibodies to alpha enolase in IMN pathogenesis. Murtas et al. had reported a prevalence of anti-alpha enolase antibodies in 43% of patients with active IMN. [45]

3.2.4. NEP

Ronco et al. reported human counterpart to the Heymann nephritis antigen in a case with neonatal MN. [8] Pregnancy-induced immunization of the mother with transplacental passage of nephritogenic antibodies was hypothesized to result in neonatal IMN. The IMN was replicated by incubating rabbit and rat kidney sections with the patient's serum. NEP was identified as the target antigen to the autoantibodies by western blot and immunoprecipitaion. The anti-NEP antibody from the mother was responsible for inducing intra-glomerular deposits and proteinuria both in the neonate and in the experimental animal (rabbit). Furthermore, the antigen (NEP) was also demonstrated by the confocal microscopy in the immune deposits of both the neonate and the rabbits injected with the maternal serum. In spite of having very high titers of anti-NEP, the mother had no proteinuria or renal manifestations. On further evaluation, it was found that the mother was deficient for NEP and a previous miscarriage had alloimmunized her by NEP expressed on the syncytiotrophoblasts and fetal cells to produce anti-NEP autoantibodies. [8] Following the report by Ronco et al. there are at least two more reports of IMN by similar mechanism. [46]

3.2.5. BSA

Debiec et al. reported high titers of circulating antibodies to BSA in 22% of the cases with IMN. Eighty percent of cases with pediatric (<5 years) IMN had very high titers of antibodies to BSA. [7] Unlike in case of allergy to BSA, where IgE antibodies predominate, BSA was mainly of the IgG1 and IgG4 subclasses in IMN. BSA was detected in the subepithelial deposits of patients with high levels of circulating serum BSA and BSA specific antibodies. To conclude, BSA is found in a minority of cases with PLA2R1 antibody negative IMN and in vast majority of pediatric IMN. [7]

4. Genetics in IMN

Insufficient data exist to define the influence of the genetic factors on the glomerular disease pathogenesis. Recent genome wide association study (GWAS) found that PLA2R1 and HLA-DQ1 genes contributed significantly to the risk of IMN in French, Dutch and British populations. [10] These genetic alterations predispose the patients to produce anti PLA2R autoantibody (Figure 2). [10] Subsequent studies from Korea, China, India (unpublished) and Taiwan reported a similar trend of association in their respective cohorts. [47-49] The results of the last decade suggest that as many as 0.14% of Asians and 0.54% of Europeans are homozygous for risk alleles (PLA2R & HLA-DQ) and are at highest risk for IMN. [10] Identification of new genetic loci and prospective follow-up will help in defining the natural history of disease, progression, remission and response to therapy.

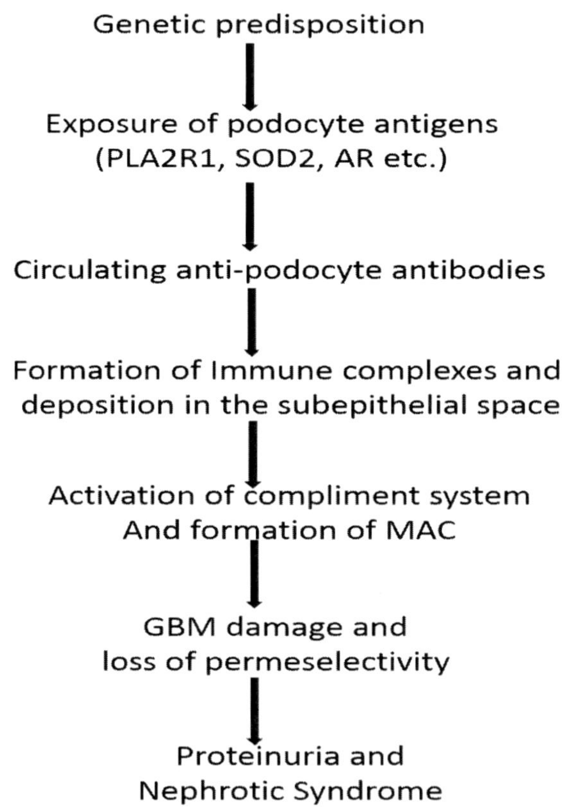

Figure 2. Pathogenesis of idiopathic membranous nephropathy. PLA2R, phospholipase A2 receptor 1; SOD, superoxide dismutase; AR, aldose reductase; MAC, membrane attack complex; GBM, glomerular basement membrane.

Conclusion

Over the years there have been considerable advances in the understanding of the pathogenesis of IMN. The present consensus is that IMN is an antibody-mediated disease, with antigen being identified as PLA2R1 in the majority followed by SOD2, NEP, AR and BSA in a minority. In the future, these antibodies shall have an important role in the diagnosis and therapeutic management of the disease.

References

[1] Glassock RJ. The pathogenesis of idiopathic membranous nephropathy: a 50-year odyssey. *Am. J. Kidney Dis.* 2010 ;56 :157-167.

[2] Rathi M, Bhagat RL, Mukhopadhyay P, Kohli HS, Jha V, Gupta KL, Sakhuja V, Joshi, K. Changing histologic spectrum of adult nephrotic syndrome over five decades in north India: A single center experience. *Indian J. Nephrol.* 2014;24:86-91.

[3] Imai H, Hamai K, Komatsuda A, Ohtani H, Miura AB. IgG subclasses in patients with membranoproliferative glomerulonephritis, membranous nephropathy, and lupus nephritis. *Kidney Int.* 1997;51:270-276.

[4] Kuroki A, Shibata T, Honda H, Totsuka D, Kobayashi K, Sugisaki T. Glomerular and serum IgG subclasses in diffuse proliferative lupus nephritis, membranous lupus nephritis, and idiopathic membranous nephropathy. *Intern. Med.* 2002; 41:936-942.

[5] Heymann W, Hackel Db, Harwood S, Wilson Sg, Hunter Jl. Production of nephrotic syndrome in rats by Freund's adjuvants and rat kidney suspensions. *Proc. Soc. Exp. Biol. Med.* 1959;100:660-664.

[6] Van Damme BJ, Fleuren GJ, Bakker WW, Vernier RL, Hoedemaeker PJ. Experimental glomerulonephritis in the rat induced by antibodies directed against tubular antigens. V. Fixed glomerular antigens in the pathogenesis of heterologous immune complex glomerulonephritis. *Lab. Invest.* 1978; 38:502-510.

[7] Debiec H, Guigonis V, Mougenot B, Decobert F, Haymann JP, Bensman A, Deschênes G, Ronco PM. Antenatal membranous glomerulonephritis due to anti-neutral endopeptidase antibodies. *N. Engl. J. Med.* 2002;346:2053-2060.

[8] Beck LH Jr, Bonegio RG, Lambeau G, Beck DM, Powell DW, Cummins TD, Klein JB, Salant DJ. M-type phospholipase A2 receptor as target antigen in idiopathic membranous nephropathy. *N. Engl. J. Med.* 2009;361:11-21.

[9] Stanescu HC, Arcos-Burgos M, Medlar A, Bockenhauer D, Kottgen A, Dragomirescu L, Voinescu C, Patel N, Pearce K, Hubank M, Stephens HA, Laundy V, Padmanabhan S, Zawadzka A, Hofstra JM, Coenen MJ, den Heijer M, Kiemeney LA, Bacq-Daian D, Stengel B, Powis SH, Brenchley P, Feehally J, Rees AJ, Debiec H, Wetzels JF, Ronco P, Mathieson PW, Kleta R. Risk HLA-DQA1 and PLA(2)R1 alleles in idiopathic membranous nephropathy. *N. Engl. J. Med.* 2011;364: 616-626.

[10] Prunotto M, Carnevali ML, Candiano G, Murtas C, Bruschi M, Corradini E, Trivelli A, Magnasco A, Petretto A, Santucci L, Mattei S, Gatti R, Scolari F, Kador P, Allegri L, Ghiggeri GM. Autoimmunity in membranous nephropathy targets aldose reductase and SOD2. *J. Am. Soc. Nephrol.* 2010;21:507-519.

[11] Couser WG, Steinmuller DR, Stilmant MM, Salant DJ, Lowenstein LM. Experimental glomerulonephritis in the isolated perfused rat kidney. *J. Clin. Invest.* 1978;62:1275-1287.

[12] Saito A, Yamazaki H, Rader K, Nakatani A, Ullrich R, Kerjaschki D, Orlando RA, Farquhar MG. Mapping rat megalin: the second cluster of ligand binding repeats contains a 46-amino acid pathogenic epitope involved in the formation of immune deposits in Heymann nephritis. *Proc. Natl. Acad. Sci. U S A*. 1996;93:8601-8605.

[13] Yamazaki H, Ullrich R, Exner M, Saito A, Orlando RA, Kerjaschki D, Farquhar MG. All four putative ligand-binding domains in megalin contain pathogenic epitopes capable of inducing passive Heymann nephritis. *J. Am. Soc. Nephrol.* 1998;9:1638-1644.

[14] Kerjaschki D, Farquhar MG. Immunocytochemical localization of the Heymann nephritis antigen (GP330) in glomerular epithelial cells of normal Lewis rats. *J. Exp. Med.* 1983;157:667-686.

[15] Assmann, KJ; Tangelder, MM; Lange, WP; Tadema, TM; Koene, RA. Membranous glomerulonephritis in the mouse. *Kidney Int.* 1983;24:303-312.

[16] Ronco P, Allegri L, Melcion C, Pirotsky E, Appay MD, Bariety J, Pontillon F, Verroust P. A monoclonal antibody to brush border and passive Heymann nephritis. *Clin. Exp. Immunol.* 1984;55:319-332.

[17] Assmann KJ, Ronco P, Tangelder MM, Lange WP, Verroust P, Koene RA. Involvement of an antigen distinct from the Heymann antigen in membranous glomerulonephritis in the mouse. *Lab. Invest.* 1989;60:138-146.

[18] Cybulsky AV, Quigg RJ, Salant DJ. Experimental membranous nephropathy redux. *Am. J. Physiol. Renal Physiol.* 2005;289:F660-71.

[19] Assmann KJ, Ronco P, Tangelder MM, Lange WP, Verroust P, Koene RA. Comparison of antigenic targets involved in antibody-mediated membranous glomerulonephritis in the mouse and rat. *Am. J. Pathol.* 1985;121:112-122.

[20] Assmann KJ, Ronco P, Tangelder MM, Lange WP, Verroust P, Koene RA. Involvement of an antigen distinct from the Heymann antigen in membranous glomerulonephritis in the mouse. *Lab. Invest.* 1989;60:138-146.

[21] Cunningham PN, Quigg RJ. Contrasting roles of complement activation and its regulation in membranous nephropathy. *J. Am. Soc. Nephrol.* 2005;16:1214-1222.

[22] Cybulsky AV, Quigg RJ, Salant DJ. Experimental membranous nephropathy redux. *Am. J. Physiol. Renal Physiol.* 2005;289:F660-671.

[23] Nangaku M, Shankland SJ, Couser WG. Cellular response to injury in membranous nephropathy. *J. Am. Soc. Nephrol.* 2005;16:1195-1204.

[24] Kerjaschki D. Pathogenetic concepts of membranous glomerulopathy (MGN). *J. Nephrol.* 2000;13(Suppl 3):S96-100.

[25] Couser WG, Salant DJ. In situ immune complex formation and glomerular injury. *Kidney Int.* 1980;17:1-13.

[26] Dixon FI, Feldman JD, Vazquez JJ. Experimental glomerulonephritis. The pathogenesis of a laboratory model resembling the spectrum of human glomerulonephritis. *J. Exp. Med.* 1961;113:899-920.

[27] Wilson CB, Dixon FJ. Quantitation of acute and chronic serum sickness in the rabbit. *J. Exp. Med.* 1971;134:7-18.

[28] East L, Isacke CM. The mannose receptor family. *Biochim. Biophys. Acta.* 2002; 1572:364-386.

[29] West AP Jr, Herr AB, Bjorkman PJ. The chicken yolk sac IgY receptor, a functional equivalent of the mammalian MHC-related Fc receptor, is a phospholipase A2 receptor homolog. *Immunity*. 2004;20:601-610.

[30] Llorca O. Extended and bent conformations of the mannose receptor family. *Cell. Mol. Life Sci*. 2008;65:1302-1310.

[31] Stahl R, Hoxha E, Fechner K. PLA2R autoantibodies and recurrent membranous nephropathy after transplantation. *N. Engl. J. Med*. 2010;363:496-498.

[32] Debiec H, Martin L, Jouanneau C, Dautin G, Mesnard L, Rondeau E, Mousson C, Ronco P. Autoantibodies specific for the phospholipase A2 receptor in recurrent and De Novo membranous nephropathy. *Am. J. Transplant*. 2011;11:2144-2152.

[33] Hoxha E, Thiele I, Zahner G, Panzer U, Harendza S, Stahl RA. Phospholipase A2 receptor autoantibodies and clinical outcome in patients with primary membranous nephropathy. *J. Am. Soc. Nephrol*. 2014;25:1357-1366.

[34] Kuroki A, Iyoda M, Shibata T, Sugisaki T. Th2 cytokines increase and stimulate B cells to produce IgG4 in idiopathic membranous nephropathy. *Kidney Int*. 2005;68: 302-310.

[35] Tipping PG, Kitching AR. Glomerulonephritis, Th1 and Th2: what's new? *Clin. Exp. Immunol*. 2005;142:207-215.

[36] Lhotta K, Würzner R, König P. Glomerular deposition of mannose-binding lectin in human glomerulonephritis. *Nephrol. Dial. Transplant*. 1999;14:881-886.

[37] Hoxha E, Harendza S, Zahner G, Panzer U, Steinmetz O, Fechner K, Helmchen U, Stahl RA. An immunofluorescence test for phospholipase-A2-receptor antibodies and its clinical usefulness in patients with membranous glomerulonephritis. *Nephrol. Dial. Transplant*. 2011;26:2526-2532.

[38] Qin W, Beck LH Jr, Zeng C, Chen Z, Li S, Zuo K, Salant DJ, Liu Z. Anti-phospholipase A2 receptor antibody in membranous nephropathy. *J. Am. Soc. Nephrol*. 2011;22:1137-1143.

[39] Hofstra JM, Debiec H, Short CD, Pellé T, Kleta R, Mathieson PW, Ronco P, Brenchley PE, Wetzels JF. Antiphospholipase A2 receptor antibody titer and subclass in idiopathic membranous nephropathy. *J. Am. Soc. Nephrol*. 2012;23:1735-1743.

[40] Son D, Kojima I, Inagi R, Matsumoto M, Fujita T, Nangaku M. Chronic hypoxia aggravates renal injury via suppression of Cu/Zn-SOD: a proteomic analysis. *Am. J. Physiol. Renal Physiol*. 2008;294:F62-72.

[41] Williamson JR, Chang K, Frangos M, Hasan KS, Ido Y, Kawamura T, Nyengaard JR, van den Enden M, Kilo C, Tilton RG. Hyperglycemic pseudohypoxia and diabetic complications. *Diabetes*. 1993;42:801-813.

[42] Barski OA, Papusha VZ, Ivanova MM, Rudman DM, Finegold MJ. Developmental expression and function of aldehyde reductase in proximal tubules of the kidney. *Am. J. Physiol. Renal Physiol*. 2005;289:F200-207.

[43] Bruschi M, Carnevali ML, Murtas C, Candiano G, Petretto A, Prunotto M, Gatti R, Argentiero L, Magistroni R, Garibotto G, Scolari F, Ravani P, Gesualdo L, Allegri L, Ghiggeri GM. Direct characterization of target podocyte antigens and auto-antibodies in human membranous glomerulonephritis: Alfa-enolase and borderline antigens. *J. Proteomics*. 2011;74:2008-2017.

[44] Miles LA, Dahlberg CM, Plescia J, Felez J, Kato K, Plow EF. Role of cell-surface lysines in plasminogen binding to cells: identification of alpha-enolase as a candidate plasminogen receptor. *Biochemistry*. 1991;30:1682-1691.

[45] Murtas C, Bruschi M, Candiano G, Moroni G, Magistroni R, Magnano A, Bruno F, Radice A, Furci L, Argentiero L, Carnevali ML, Messa P, Scolari F, Sinico RA, Gesualdo L, Fervenza FC, Allegri L, Ravani P, Ghiggeri GM. Coexistence of different circulating anti-podocyte antibodies in membranous nephropathy. *Clin. J. Am. Soc. Nephrol.*, 2012;7:1394-1400.

[46] Debiec H, Nauta J, Coulet F, van der Burg M, Guigonis V, Schurmans T, de Heer E, Soubrier F, Janssen F, Ronco P. Role of truncating mutations in MME gene in fetomaternal alloimmunisation and antenatal glomerulopathies. *Lancet.* 2004;364: 1252-1259.

[47] Liu YH, Chen CH, Chen SY, Lin YJ, Liao WL, Tsai CH, Wan L, Tsai FJ. Association of phospholipase A2 receptor 1 polymorphisms with idiopathic membranous nephropathy in Chinese patients in Taiwan. *J. Biomed. Sci.* 2010;17:81.

[48] Kim S, Chin HJ, Na KY, Kim S, Oh J, Chung W, Noh JW, Lee YK, Cho JT, Lee EK, Chae DW. Progressive Renal Disease and Medical Informatics and Genomics Research (PREMIER) members. Single nucleotide polymorphisms in the phospholipase A2 receptor gene are associated with genetic susceptibility to idiopathic membranous nephropathy. *Nephron Clin. Pract.* 2011;117:c253-258.

[49] Lv J, Hou W, Zhou X, Liu G, Zhou F, Zhao N, Hou P, Zhao M, Zhang H. Interaction between PLA2R1 and HLA-DQA1 variants associates with anti-PLA2R antibodies and membranous nephropathy. *J. Am. Soc. Nephrol.* 2013;24:1323-1329.

In: Nephrotic Syndrome: Etiology, Pathogenesis and Pathology ISBN: 978-1-63482-154-4
Editor: Muhammed Mubarak

Chapter 4

Complements and Glomerulonephritis

Sabiha Anis*
Department of Immunology,
Sindh Institute of Urology and Transplantation (SIUT),
Karachi, Pakistan

Abstract

In the last few years, research into the role of complement in the immunopathogenesis of renal glomerular diseases has broadened our understanding of the delicate balance between the protective and harmful functions of the complement system. An intricate array of molecular mechanisms also exists for regulating the activity of the complement system. Studies in both animal models and humans with immune mediated glomerulopathies have shed light on both the favorable and unfavorable effects of the complement components and have allowed targeted therapeutic interventions to control the tissue damage.

The identification of mutations of complement regulatory molecules has established a role of complement in the hemolytic uremic syndrome and membranoproliferative glomerulonephritis, and genotyping for mutations of the complement system are already making inroads into clinical practice. The recent clinical studies have resulted in the creation of relevant animal models which may provide important information for the development of highly targeted treatment agents. Research into the role of complement in proteinuria has helped to understand pathways of inflammation which ultimately lead to renal insufficiency irrespective of the underlying renal disease and is the major factor responsible for progression of kidney disease for the majority of renal patients. Research into the complement system is a highly exciting area of translational research and hopefully will result in the development of meaningful therapeutic agents in the near future. This chapter describes the role of complement system in the pathogenesis and progression of renal glomerular diseases.

Keywords: Complement, glomerulopathy, immune complexes, pathogenesis, renal failure

* Address of Correspondence: Sabiha Anis; Assistant Professor, Department of Immunology, Sindh Institute of Urology and Transplantation (SIUT), Karachi, Pakistan. Email: sabiha_anis@hotmail.com.

1. Introduction

Glomerulonephritis (GN) is characterized by intra-glomerular inflammation and cell proliferation. The GN can be acute or chronic and primary or secondary to infections, connective tissue disorders or vasculitis. It can present with hematuria, proteinuria, oliguria, edema, hypertension and other systemic manifestations or renal dysfunction. [1]

The pathogenesis of GN involves both innate and adaptive immune systems and cellular and humoral immune responses. [1, 2] In animal models of GN, the role of toll-like receptors (TLRs), interferon response factor [IRF] transcription factors, interferon alpha, other cytokines and macrophages have been proved to cause renal injury. [3] Similarly, antibodies have a major role in causing GN. These antibodies are either present in the antigen-antibody complexes deposited in the renal microvasculature or glomeruli, or they bind directly with the antigens of the renal structures.

Either way, they mostly cause injury by activating complement cascade. Cell mediated immune response is also implicated in renal injury. [1-3]

2. The Complement System

The complement system comprises a large group of proteins including soluble and cell membrane-associated proteins, complement receptors and array of complement regulatory proteins. They are mainly produced by hepatocytes, macrophages and intestinal epithelial cells.

Their main function is to provide protection against microorganisms and other damaging or injurious agents. The complement system also regulates and augments the cellular and adaptive immune responses. The complement proteins are present as inactive precursor proteins or zymogens, also called proenzymes. Upon activation, they become proteases cleaving downstream pro-proteases.

There are three complement activation pathways, namely alternate, classic and lectin pathways (Figure 1).

The complement activation is tightly regulated by a number of complement regulatory proteins that inhibit complement activation at different steps. Some regulatory proteins inhibit specifically the classical or alternate pathways; while, others regulate all activation pathways. The deficiency of these proteins therefore causes excessive stimulation and inflammation causing tissue damage. This has a major role in the pathogenesis of GN either as a part of adaptive immune response or innate immune system.

In this chapter, the role of complement activation and its dysregulation in glomerular injury has been described (Figure 2).

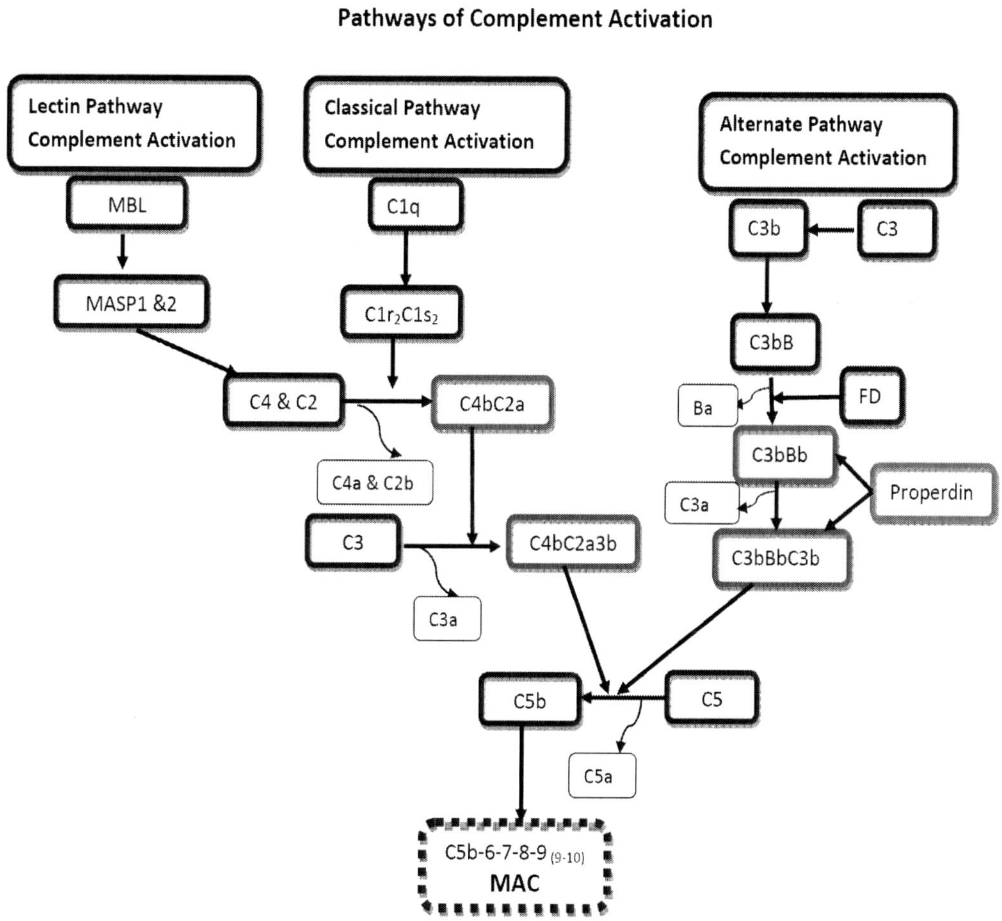

Figure 1. Shows complement activation pathways. Classical pathway is activated upon binding of C1q molecules with Fc portion of at least two molecules of IgG or one molecule of IgM in antigen antibody complexes. This activates two molecules of C1r & C1s which causes further activation of C4 and C2 leading to the formation of classical pathway C3 convertase (C4b2a). C4b2a is also formed by the activation of lectin pathway which is initiated by the binding of mannose binding lectin (MBL) molecules on pathogen surface which in turn activates MBL associated serine proteases (MASP) 1 & 2. The alternate pathway is also activated by microbial surface. C3b is spontaneously and continuously being formed in the circulation by hydrolytic cleavage of C3 proteins. The alternate pathway C3 convertase thus formed is C3bBbC3b. These pathways then converge at C5 convertase (C4b2a3b & C3bBb3b) and progress into membrane attack complex (MAC) formation. Properdin stabilizes alternate pathway C3 and C5 convertases.

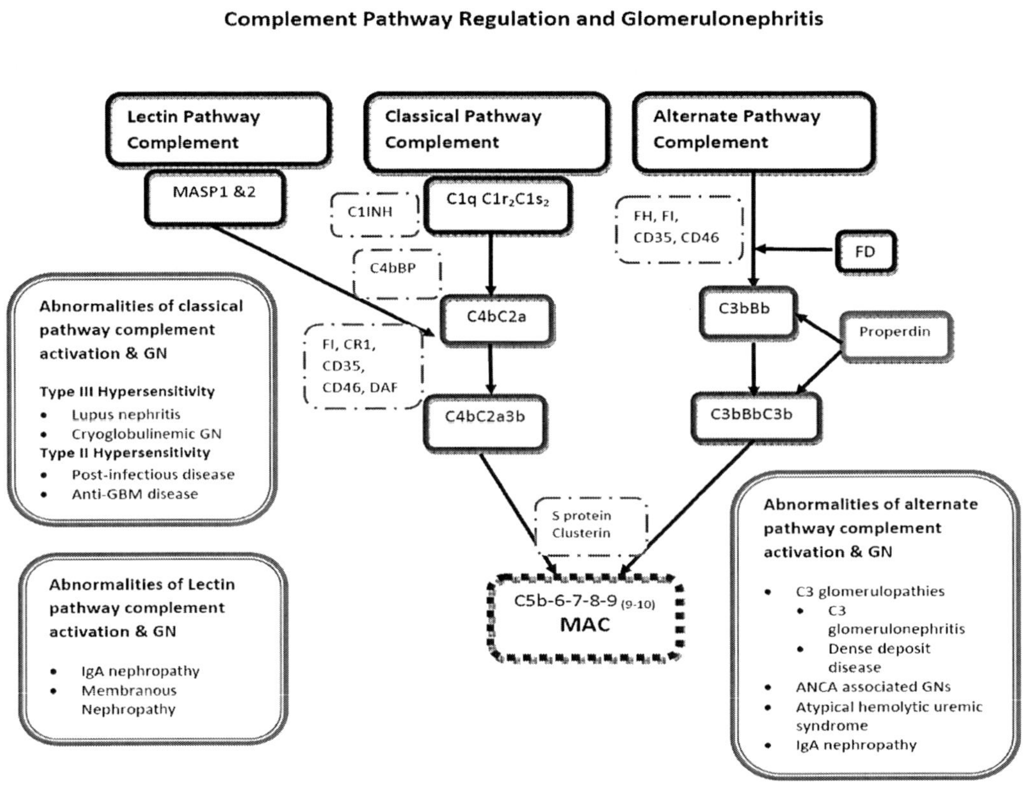

Figure 2. Shows involvement of complement regulatory proteins acting at different stages of activation pathways. Deficiencies of either early complement proteins of classical pathway or of regulatory proteins may be associated with type III hypersensitivity mediated glomerulonephritis (GN). Where as in type II hypersensitivity mediated GN and via lectin pathway, excessive complement activation by some environmental factors is mostly responsible for injury. Abnormalities of alternate pathway usually occur due to mutation or presence of autoantibodies to complement proteins.

2.1. The Classical Complement Pathway Activation

The classical pathway activation proceeds when Fc portion of IgG or IgM antibodies binds to globular head of C1q, a component of early complement protein, C1. The fixing of C1q with antibodies leads to activation of two molecules of other C1 component proteins, C1r and C1s. C1q, C1r and C1s form C1 esterase, which in turn activates downstream proteases by cleaving C4 and C2.

The C1 esterase splits C4 into C4a and C4b and C2 into C2a and C2b. C4a and C2b make C3 convertase, designated as C4b2a. This activated protease splits C3 into C3a and C3b. Thus, the classical pathway C5 convertase is formed designated as C4b2a3b.

The early complement proteins of classical pathway activation are necessary for the clearance of apoptotic cells and immune complexes (ICs). C1q is the main protein that binds specifically to the surface blebs of apoptotic cells. This leads to phagocytosis of the apoptotic cells and ICs and their removal from the circulation. The deficiency of C1q thus may predispose to autoimmunity.

The split products C4a, C2b and C3a are also important in the removal of apoptotic bodies and ICs by opsonization and clearing them from the circulation.

The split products of complement activation, however, are also responsible for causing inflammation. [4, 5]

2.1.1. Classical Pathway Complement Regulation

The regulators of classical pathway complement activation are:

- C1 esterase inhibitor, which dissociates activated C1r and C1s from C1q.
- C3b and C4b, which are the integral components of classical pathway C3 convertase and C5 convertase, are inactivated by a serine protease factor I, which cleaves C3b and C4b into inactive components. Other regulatory proteins including C4b binding proteins (C4BP), CD35 and CD46 act as cofactors for factor I.
- CD35, C4BP and decay-accelerating factor (DAF, CD55) inactivate proteases independently of factor I. [6, 7]

2.2. The Alternate Pathway Complement Activation

The alternate pathway is activated by bacterial cell wall and endotoxins. [4, 5] Low levels of C3b are continuously being formed, due to spontaneous hydrolytic cleavage of C3 in the circulation. If the suitable surface is not available for C3b deposition, it decays and is inactivated rapidly.

Upon binding of C3b on the surface favoring complement activation, it recruits factor B (fB). With the help of factor D (fD), fB is cleaved into Ba and Bb. The alternate pathway C3 convertase is thus formed designated as C3bBb.

Further splitting of C3 results in the formation of alternate pathway C5 convertase, designated as C3bBbC3b. Properdin stabilizes alternate pathway C5 convertase.

2.2.1. The Alternate Pathway Complement Regulation

- Factor H (fH) is the most important fluid phase regulator of alternate pathway complement activation. It accelerates the decay of C3bBb by displacing fB from C3B complex. There are 20 short consensus repeats in fH molecules with at least two binding sites for C3b. High affinity binding of fH to surface bound C3b stops alternate pathway complement activation while low affinity binding leads to the formation of C3 convertase.
- It also acts as a cofactor for fI for the cleavage of C3b. [8, 9]

2.3. The Lectin Pathway

Activation of Lectin pathway takes place when mannose binding lectin (MBL) molecules bind to mannose residues in bacterial cell wall.[10] This leads to activation of MBL associated serine proteases [MASP]-1 and -2. These proteases cleave C4 and C2, leading to the formation of C3 convertase as C4b2a and later C4b2a3b similar to classical pathway C3 convertase and C5 convertase.

2.4. Terminal Pathway Activation

The C5 convertase splits C5 into C5a and C5b. The membrane attack complex (MAC) is formed by the sequential assembly of C6, C7, C8 and then 9 to 10 molecules of C9 with C5b.

2.4.1. Terminal Pathway Regulation

S-protein and clusterin inhibit incorporation of the MAC in the membranes.

3. Abnormalities of Classical Pathway Complement Activation and Renal Diseases

The group of renal diseases is caused by IC formation and activation of classical complement pathway by antibodies mainly IgG. IC -mediated GN can be broadly classified into two types:

Glomerular injury occurring due to type II hypersensitivity reaction, e.g., acute post-streptococcal GN (APSGN) and anti-GBM disease or Goodpasture syndrome

Glomerular injury occurring due to type III hypersensitivity reaction, e.g., systemic lupus erythmatosus (SLE) and cryoglobulinemic GN. [11]

Acute Post Streptococcal Glomerulonephritis (APSGN)

APSGN is usually a childhood disease affecting children between 2 to 10 years of age. However, it can also occur in elderly. [12, 13]

The patients with AAPSGN usually present with hematuria, symptoms of fluid overload and hypertension and sometimes renal insufficiency. Hematuria is typically described as coke colored or smoky urine.

It is characterized by generalized granular or linear IC deposits in the mesangium or in the sub-endothelial or sub-epithelial spaces. The deposits contain ICs of nephritogenic strains of group A beta-hemolytic streptococci and IgG in the walls of capillaries and in glomeruli. Renal biopsy is usually not done due to the usually benign course of the disease. Also evidence of preceding streptococcal infection is usually present.

Immunopathogenesis of APSGN

The most common hypothesis is that there is possible activation of all three pathways of complement cascade in APSGN. The ICs in the glomeruli activate inflammatory process by activating complement cascade with liberation of chemotactic and anaphylatoxic complement split products. Formation of MAC causes injury by cytolysis. The inflammatory cells recruited to the site add to the injury by releasing reactive oxygen species (ROS), cytokines and other inflammatory mediators.

Laboratory Features of APSGN

Serum C3 levels are typically reduced which normalize within 6 to 12 weeks. Serum C4 levels may also be found low but normalize early. In addition, serum C5 and properdin levels may also be found low. Persistence of low C3 levels beyond 12 weeks warrants renal biopsy for proper diagnosis. Serum levels of C1 and C2 are usually normal. At times, both C3 and C4 levels are found normal in the setting of clinical and histopathological features consistent with APSGN. Anti-streptococcal antibodies [ASOT, anti-DNAse B, anti-NAD and ASKase] are found in high titers.

Anti-Glomerular Basement Membrane (GBM) Disease

Anti-glomerular basement membrane (anti-GBM) disease mostly presents as rapidly progressive GN (RPGN) with hematuria and renal dysfunction. It is a rare disease and sometimes accompanied by pulmonary hemorrhage. In most of the cases, IgG anti-GBM antibodies are found in the serum, which are pathogenic. [14-16]

Histopathologically, it is characterized by focal necrotizing GN and crescent formation with linear deposition of IgG and C3 along the glomerular capillary wall and GBM. .

Pathogenesis of Anti-GBM Disease

The auto-antigen for anti-GBM antibodies is called Goodpasture antigen consisting of non-collagenous domain (NC1) of the α-3 chain of type IV collagen. Type II hypersensitivity reaction ensues. The antigen- antibody complexes activate classical pathway complement activation resulting in leukocyte infiltration and crescent formation with proteinuria and renal dysfunction. C5a formed during complement activation promotes severe inflammation. Excessive renal damage is caused by MAC and ROS.

Laboratory Features of Anti-GBM Disease

The complement levels are normal or sometimes raised. Plasma C5b-9 may be used as a potential biomarker for monitoring and predicting the renal injury in clinical practice. Deposition of C5b-9 in renal biopsies and in plasma is associated with more severe manifestation of the disease.

Lupus Nephritis (LN)

Lupus nephritis (LN) occurs in 50% of patients with SLE and 25% of SLE patients present with LN. According to the WHO and revised classification of International Society of Nephrology/Renal Pathology Society (ISN/RPS), LN has six classes that range from mild mesangial involvement (Class I), to diffuse proliferative disease (Class IV), membranous (Class V) and to advanced sclerosis (Class VI). The hallmark is the deposition of IgG, IgM,

IgA, C3 and C4 together with C1q termed as 'full house pattern' of immune deposition. [17, 18]

Pathogenesis of LN

The main pathogenetic mechanism of LN involves impaired handling of ICs with complement deposition. The main mechanism of renal injury is type III hypersensitivity reaction. This results from classical pathway complement activation, and results in excessive inflammation and activation of resident mesangial cells. There are three main mechanisms that lead to IC formation in the glomeruli. [1] Deposition of ICs in the glomeruli formed in the serum. [2] The autoantibodies which are pathognomonic for SLE bind to glomerular antigens in situ such as laminin, annexin II or heparin. [3] Deficiency of early complement components including C1 components, C2 and C4 are associated with lupus due to impaired ICs clearance and breaking of tolerance due to defective clearance of apoptotic bodies leading to breaking of tolerance. This relates to the so called 'waste disposal hypothesis'.

The persistence of apoptotic cells result in the formation of autoantibodies. The most important are anti-dsDNA and anti-C1q antibodies. The co-presence of both in ICs in glomeruli is associated with class III-IV LN.

Laboratory Features of LN

Active SLE and LN are characterized by very low levels of complements (C3 and C4). The C3 and C4 levels in the serum are also used for disease monitoring. Inherited deficiencies of C1q and C4 are strongly associated with the development of SLE in humans.

Autoantibody detection is the most important diagnostic tool in the work-up of SLE and LN.

The hallmark is the anti-nuclear antibodies (ANA) with further detection of anti-dsDNA and anti-extractable nuclear antigen (ENA) antibodies. Besides other autoantibodies such as anti-C1q antibodies, anti-phospholipid antibodies (APL), and rheumatoid factors are also important in the diagnostic work-up. C-reactive protein (CRP) and erythrocyte sedimentation rate (ESR) are also required.

4. Abnormalities of Alternate Pathway Complement Activation and Renal Diseases

Dysregulation of alternate pathway of complement activation is associated with following renal pathologies:

- C3 glomerulopathies
  - C3 glomerulonephritis (C3GN)
  - Dense Deposit disease (DDD)
- Atypical hemolytic uremic syndrome (aHUS)
- IgA nephropathy (IgAN)
- Anti-neutrophil cytoplasmic antibodies (ANCA)-associated glomerulonephritis [17-19]

C3 Glomerulopathies

C3 glomerulopathies by definition, comprise of complement-mediated renal diseases that warrant investigations for the deficiency of complement inhibitors of alternate pathway. Identification of this subgroup of GN has major implications for the treatment strategies because such cases may benefit from anti-complement therapy. [20]

It includes C3 glomerulonephritis (C3GN) and dense deposit disease [DDD] that have a common pathogenetic pathway characterized by the dysregulation of alternate complement pathway activation and low blood C3 levels. The C3 fragments are detected by immune-histochemistry (IHC) or immunofluorescence (IF) irrespective of light or electron microscopic features. The immunoglobulins (Igs) or early complement products of classical pathway such as C1q and C4c or C4d are not found in renal biopsies.

C3 Glomerulonephritis (C3GN)

C3GN occurs at all age groups and in both sexes. It can present with a nephritic–nephrotic picture with most of the patients suffering from hypertension, proteinuria, and hematuria.

It is characterized by mesangial and epimembranous deposits with or without membranoproliferative pattern. Sub-endothelial deposits and crescents can also be found. In all cases, IHC or IF staining shows only C3 deposits without Igs and without dense intra-membranous deposits. It is a less aggressive disease than DDD. The C3 deposits are less discrete and ill- defined, confluent and may blend with extracellular matrix compared to DDD. [20, 21]

Dense Deposit Disease (DDD)

DDD is a C3 glomerulopathy characterized by intramembranous electron-dense deposits with in GBM which stain for C3 only and there is absence of Igs. Earlier it was named as membranoproliferative glomerulonephritis type II (MPGN2), but this terminology is no longer used for DDD. [22, 23]

In DDD, the round C3 deposits are characteristically found within the GBM or in mesangium and in some cases, in Bowman's capsule and tubular basement membranes (TBMs). These deposits may appear as sausage shaped lesions with skip areas of normal GBM. The deposits may thicken and produce hump-shaped sub-epithelial deposits.

Patients with DDD may develop visual impairment secondary to ocular deposits known as drusen in Bruch's membrane.

Pathogenesis of C3 Glomerulopathies

The dysregulation of alternate pathway of complement activation leading to excessive complement activation and inflammation can occur in following ways:

- Autoantibodies against alternate pathway C3 convertase called C3 nephritic factor (C3NeF) or autoantibodies to fH and fB, may result in excessive activation and break down of C3 and fB into their split products. C3NeF binds and stabilizes the fluid phase and the membrane-bound C3 convertases.

- Deficiency of fH due to mutations or increased consumption may lead to C3 glomerulopathy.
- Alteration in other regulatory proteins such as membrane cofactor protein (MCP). [18, 21]

Laboratory Features of C3 Glomerulopathies

Serum complement levels are characterized by very low C3, fB, and fH. C3NeF is found in most patients. ANAs are mostly absent in the serum.

Anti-Neutrophil Cytoplasmic Antibodies (ANCA)-Associated GN

ANCA-associated GN is a manifestation of systemic vasculitis, characterized by the necrotizing inflammation of small vessels in systemic circulation termed as ANCA-associated vasculitis (AAV). These include granulomatosis with polyangiitis, microscopic polyangiitis, and Churg–Strauss syndrome. The target antigens of ANCA in AAV are myeloperoxidase (MPO) which gives a peri-nuclear staining or p-ANCA pattern on neutrophil substrate by indirect IF assay [IFA] and proteinase 3 (PR3) which gives a cytoplasmic staining or c-ANCA pattern by IFA . [24-27]

ANCA-associated GN is characterized by pauci-immune necrotizing, crescentic GN. The IF for Igs and complements in renal biopsy tissue shows negative staining or very little deposition of IgG and/or C3.

Pathogenesis of ANCA-Associated GN

There is ample evidence that in AAV and ANCA-associated GN, the injury is due to alternate pathway complement activation. Deposits of Bb, C3d and C5b-9 complexes can be found in renal capillaries and mesangium and also in urine. IgG-ANCA activates neutrophils, which in turn, liberate mediators that activate alternate pathway complement activation. On the other hand, the absence of C4 split products precludes the involvement of classical and lectin pathways.

Laboratory Features of ANCA-Associated GN

ANCA is a very useful serological marker for pauci-immune crescentic GN. Both c- and p-ANCA patterns by IFA and anti-PR3 and anti-MPO IgG are required to diagnose AAV and ANCA-associated GN. An early diagnosis and prompt treatment is required to save the kidney from the development of end stage renal failure (ESRF).

Other tests are also required to rule out the causes of RPGN including anti-GBM, ANA, ASOT and anti-DNAse B. The infections should also be ruled out before starting the immunosuppressive treatment. Serum complement levels (C3 and C4) are found normal in ANCA-associated GN, despite the activation of alternate pathway of complement system and their involvement in the pathogenesis of the disease.

Atypical Hemolytic Uremic Syndrome [aHUS]

aHUS is a systemic and multifactorial disease characterized by a triad of Coomb's negative hemolytic anemia with fragmented red blood cells (RBCs), thrombocytopenia and renal impairment. Intravascular hemolysis is evident by high serum lactate dehydrogenase

(LDH) and undetectable haptoglobin levels. The lesions are classically described as thrombotic microangiopathy (TMA) that affects the microvasculature of kidneys, heart, brain, lungs and gastrointestinal tract. Prompt diagnosis and treatment is necessary to prevent life threatening complications that occur due to acidosis, hyperkalemia hyponatremia and volume overload. Nearly 50% of the patients with aHUS become dialysis dependent.

Immunopathogenesis of aHUS

The main cause of aHUS is the dysregulation of alternate pathway of complement activation. This may occur due to the abnormality in regulatory complement proteins, namely, fH, fI, MCP (CD46) and thrombomodulin (THBD) or in alternate pathway C3 convertase (C3 and fB) proteins. Mutations in regulatory proteins may lead to defective protection of endothelial cells from the effect of complement activation, thus leading to damage by C5a and MAC formation. The endothelial damage leads to the exposure of sub-endothelial matrix, platelet activation and platelet aggregation and thrombus formation. Mutations in fH can lead to complement activation on the surface of platelets, release of tissue factor causing TMA.

There are two types of fH mutations. Type 1 is associated with reduced fH levels in the serum while type2 is associated with normal but functionally deficient fH levels. Mutations in FH related proteins are also associated with non-functional fH.

Laboratory Features

Serum or plasma C3, C4, fH, fI and fB levels, membrane expression of MCP on blood leucocytes and screening for anti-fH antibodies should be done in patients suspected of aHUS as soon as possible to initiate the treatment promptly. Serum C3 levels are mostly found low. FH is lower in type 1 mutations compared to type 2. Depending upon the type of mutations, MCP may be quantitatively low or may be dysfunctional. Repeated determination of MCP is required.

Mutation Analysis

Mutation of fH is present in 20% to 30% of patients. Certain mutations in fH related proteins (CFHR) are associated with antibody formation against fH and their titers correlated with fH and C3 levels and disease activity. MCP mutation is present in around 15% of children with aHUS and C3 levels are low in these patients. FI mutations can be found in around 10% of patients with aHUS with 30% of patients showing low C3 and fI levels.

FB mutations are very rare, found in only 1% to 4% of aHUS patients. These are gain-of-function mutations with resistance to the action of fH and excessive complement activation. C3 mutations with enhanced capacity to bind fB to C3b are found in 2% to 10% of aHUS patients with low C3 levels in 80% of patients. THBD mutations are found in 3% to 5% of patients with aHUS. Combination of mutations is found in around 12% of aHUS patients.

Screening for mutations and anti-fH antibodies is mandatory before transplantation in these patients.

IgA Nephropathy (IgAN)

IgAN is the most common GN worldwide, characterized by mesangial proliferation on light microscopy and IgA deposition on IF (the hallmark of the disease) with C3, C5-9 and often IgG. It usually follows mucosal viral infections and there are recurrent episodes of nephritic syndrome. C9 and properdin have also been detected in renal biopsies implicating alternate pathway complement activation. The C4d deposits and absence of C1q staining in the mesangium in around 30% of biopsies indicates lectin pathway activation as well. [28-30]

Pathogenesis of IgAN

Polymeric IgA that are produced by mucosal B cells activate alternate pathway of complement cascade and most probably lectin pathway as well. Abnormal glycosylation of IgA1 can activate these complement cascades resulting in inflammation of the glomeruli. The under glycosylation at the hinge region of IgA molecule can occur due to inherited defects or epigenetically.

The abnormal IgA1 tends to self-aggregate and localize in the mesangium. These aggregates then activate complement activation cascades. Activation of lectin pathway is associated with more severe disease in a subset of patients. Binding of abnormally glycosylated IgA1 to CD89 (FcαR), transferrin receptors and TLRs is responsible for recurrent GN. There is increased production of pro-inflammatory cytokines and growth factors that result in mesangial proliferation and matrix expansion. The mesangial cells are activated due to binding of IgA with CD89 [FCαR], transferrin receptors and TLRs. These IgA1 aggregates also bind MBL, ficolin and type 1 collagen resulting in increase in the matrix.

Laboratory Features of IgAN

Despite the evidence of complement activation on renal biopsies, complement levels are normal in the blood. Determination of elevated levels of poorly glycosylated polymeric IgA1 in the serum may be helpful. Detection of anti-under-glycosylated IgA has also been proposed as a useful diagnostic test.

5. Abnormalities of Lectin Pathway Complement Activation and Renal Diseases

In IgAN, besides the renal damage caused by alternative pathway activation, there is also involvement of lectin pathway.

Membranous Nephropathy (MN)

Membranous nephropathy (MN) is the most common cause of nephrotic syndrome in adults. It is characterized by the IC deposition on the outer surface of GBM which thickens. It mainly consists of IgG4, C4d and C5b-9 and consistent with lectin pathway activation. [31]

Pathogenesis of MN

In most of the patients, pathogenesis is mediated by the in situ formation of immune deposits, with the resulting activation of the lectin pathway of complement cascade. In around 70% patients, an autoantibody to M-type phospholipase A2 receptor [anti-PLA2R] is present. It is of IgG4 subclass and claimed to be pathogenic.

Laboratory Features of MN

The serum complement levels are normal. Anti-PLA2R is detected in 70% of patients with idiopathic MN. Stringent work-up is sometimes required to rule out secondary causes of MN such as malignancies.

Conclusion

The complement system activation is an important mechanism of injury in most of the glomerulopathies. This is evident from the fact that in renal biopsies complement products are detected with or without immunoglobulins. The complement activation pathway implicated in renal injury may be of classical pathway activation as occurs in LN or anti-GBM disease. The alternate pathway of complement activation is the important pathogenetic mechanism in many glomerulopathies such as C3 glomerulopathies, ANCA-associated GN, IgAN and aHUS. Lectin pathway activation is involved in IgAN and MN.

Whichever complement activation pathway is involved, the glomerular injury is caused by recruitment and activation of inflammatory cells mediated by complement split products, mainly C5a. The direct lytic injury of glomerular and endothelial cells is caused by MAC (C5b-9) formation implying favorable therapeutic effects of anti-complement products (Eculizumab) in these GN.

References

[1] Hricik DE, Chung-Park M, Sedor JR. Glomerulonephritis. *N. Engl. J. Med.* 1998;339:888-899.

[2] Couser WG, Johnson RJ. The etiology of glomerulonephritis: roles of infection and autoimmunity. *Kidney Int.* 2014;86:905-914.

[3] Pollard KM, Kono DH. Requirements for innate immune pathways in environmentally induced autoimmunity. *BMC Med.* 2013;11:100.

[4] Noris M, Remuzzi G. Overview of complement activation and regulation. *Semin. Nephrol.* 2013;33:479-492.

[5] Blom AM, Volokhina EB, Fransson V, Strömberg P, Berghard L, Viktorelius M, Mollnes TE, López-Trascasa M, van den Heuvel LP, Goodship TH, Marchbank KJ, Okroj M. A novel method for direct measurement of complement convertases activity in human serum. *Clin. Exp. Immunol.* 2014;178:142-153.

[6] Taylor PR, Carugati A, Fadok VA, Cook HT, Andrews M, Carroll MC, Savill JS, Henson PM, Botto M, Walport MJ. A hierarchical role for classical pathway

complement proteins in the clearance of apoptotic cells in vivo. *J. Exp. Med.*. 2000;192:359-366.

[7] Leffler J, Bengtsson AA, Blom AM. The complement system in systemic lupus erythematosus: an update. *Ann. Rheum. Dis*. 2014;73:1601-1606.

[8] Abrera-Abeleda MA, Nishimura C, Frees K, Jones M, Maga T, Katz LM, Zhang Y, Smith RJ. Allelic variants of complement genes associated with dense deposit disease. *J. Am. Soc. Nephrol.* 2011;22:1551-1559.

[9] Loirat C, Fremeaux-Bacchi V. Atypical hemolytic uremic syndrome. *Orphanet J. Rare Dis.* 2011;6:60.

[10] Osthoff M, Trendelenburg M. Impact of mannose-binding lectin deficiency on radiocontrast-induced renal dysfunction. *Biomed. Res. Int.* 2013;2013:962695.

[11] Sturfelt G, Truedsson L. Complement and its breakdown products in SLE. *Rheumatology* (Oxford). 2005;44:1227-1232.

[12] Bastos CA, Santos EP, Oliveira AP, Gomes AP, Cerqueira FR, Santana LA, Ferreira RS, Siqueira-Batista R. Post-streptococcal glomerulonephritis: Immunopathological aspects and perspectives for in silico experiments. *African J. Intern. Med.* 2014;2:98-106.

[13] Nasr SH, Fidler ME, Valeri AM, Cornell LD, Sethi S, Zoller A, Stokes MB, Markowitz GS, D'Agati VD. Postinfectious glomerulonephritis in the elderly. *J. Am. Soc. Nephrol.* 2011;22:187-195.

[14] Chen M, Daha MR, Kallenberg CG. The complement system in systemic autoimmune disease. *J. Autoimmun.* 2010;34:J276-286.

[15] Couser WG. Basic and translational concepts of immune-mediated glomerular diseases. *J. Am. Soc. Nephrol.* 2012;23:381-399.

[16] Ma R, Cui Z, Liao YH, Zhao MH. Complement activation contributes to the injury and outcome of kidney in human anti-glomerular basement membrane disease. *J. Clin. Immunol.* 2013;33:172-178.

[17] Berger SP, Daha MR. Complement in glomerular injury. *Semin. Immunopathol.* 2007;29:375-384.

[18] Nowling TK, Gilkeson GS. Mechanisms of tissue injury in lupus nephritis. *Arthritis Res. Ther.* 2011;13:250.

[19] Berger SP, Roos A, Daha MR. Complement and the kidney: what the nephrologist needs to know in 2006? *Nephrol. Dial. Transplant.* 2005;20:2613-2619.

[20] Barbour TD, Pickering MC, Cook HT. Recent insights into C3 glomerulopathy. *Nephrol. Dial. Transplant.* 2013;28:1685-1693.

[21] Bomback AS, Appel GB. Pathogenesis of the C3 glomerulopathies and reclassification of MPGN. *Nat. Rev. Nephrol.* 2012;8:634-642.

[22] Pickering MC, D'Agati VD, Nester CM, Smith RJ, Haas M, Appel GB, Alpers CE, Bajema IM, Bedrosian C, Braun M, Doyle M, Fakhouri F, Fervenza FC, Fogo AB, Frémeaux-Bacchi V, Gale DP, Goicoechea de Jorge E, Griffin G, Harris CL, Holers VM, Johnson S, Lavin PJ, Medjeral-Thomas N, Paul Morgan B, Nast CC, Noel LH, Peters DK, Rodríguez de Córdoba S, Servais A, Sethi S, Song WC, Tamburini P, Thurman JM, Zavros M, Cook HT. C3 glomerulopathy: consensus report. *Kidney Int.* 2013;84:1079-1089.

[23] Smith RJ, Harris CL, Pickering MC. Dense deposit disease. *Mol. Immunol.* 2011;48:1604-1610.

[24] Charles Jennette J, Xiao H, Hu P. Complement in ANCA-associated vasculitis. *Semin. Nephrol*. 2013;33:557-564.

[25] Ntatsaki E, Carruthers D, Chakravarty K, D'Cruz D, Harper L, Jayne D, Luqmani R, Mills J, Mooney J, Venning M, Watts RA; BSR and BHPR Standards, Guidelines and Audit Working Group. BSR and BHPR guideline for the management of adults with ANCA-associated vasculitis. *Rheumatology* (Oxford). 2014;53:2306-2309.

[26] Gou SJ, Yuan J, Wang C, Zhao MH, Chen M. Alternative complement pathway activation products in urine and kidneys of patients with ANCA-associated GN. *Clin. J. Am. Soc. Nephrol.* 2013;8:1884-1891.

[27] Yuan J, Gou SJ, Huang J, Hao J, Chen M, Zhao MH. C5a and its receptors in human anti-neutrophil cytoplasmic antibody (ANCA)-associated vasculitis. *Arthritis Res. Ther.* 2012;14:R140.

[28] Barratt J, Feehally J. IgA nephropathy. *J. Am. Soc. Nephrol.* 2005;16:2088-2097.

[29] Mubarak M. IgA nephropathy: an update on pathogenesis and classification. *J. Coll. Physicians Surg. Pak.*. 2011;21:230-233.

[30] Glassock RJ. Analyzing antibody activity in IgA nephropathy. *J. Clin. Invest.* 2009;119:1450-1452.

[31] Espinosa-Hernández M, Ortega-Salas R, López-Andreu M, Gómez-Carrasco JM, Pérez-Sáez MJ, Pérez-Seoane C, Aljama-García P. C4d as a diagnostic tool in membranous nephropathy. *Nefrologia.* 2012;32:295-299.

In: Nephrotic Syndrome: Etiology, Pathogenesis and Pathology ISBN: 978-1-63482-154-4
Editor: Muhammed Mubarak

Chapter 5

The Genetics of Primary Focal Segmental Glomerulosclerosis

Aiysha Abid*

Centre for Human Genetics and Molecular Medicine,
Sindh Institute of Urology and Transplantation, Karachi, Pakistan

Abstract

Focal segmental glomerulosclerosis (FSGS) is a heterogeneous disorder resulting from a wide variety of injuries to the glomerular structure. The histopathological lesion of FSGS represents a pattern of glomerular response to injury and not a single disease. The etiologic agents vary from genetic defects in increasing number of glomerular proteins and large number of environmental agents. Often, both the genetic and environmental factors interplay to cause the clinical syndrome of FSGS. The role of genetic factors is increasingly being recognized as an important contributing factor in the causation of FSGS. New insights gained from the molecular genetic studies are also paving the way for specific and targeted therapies of FSGS. This chapter is focussed on the genetic basis of FSGS, the roles played by different genes in causing the disease and the future prospects of genetic research in guiding therapy and prognosis of the disease.

Keywords: FSGS, gene mutations, positional cloning, gene sequencing, nephrotic syndrome, podocyte proteins, slit diaphragm

1. Introduction

Focal segmental glomerulosclerosis (FSGS) is a histopathologic condition of kidney injury characterized by the presence of partial sclerosis (segmental) of some (focal) of the glomeruli. It is one of the leading causes of end stage renal disease (ESRD) worldwide.

* Address of Correspondence: Aiysha Abid, Centre for Human Genetics and Molecular Medicine, Sindh Institute of Urology and Transplantation, Karachi, Pakistan. email: aiyshaabid@gmail.com

Clinically, the destruction of podocytes' architecture and their filtration mechanism results in the presentation of nephrotic syndrome (NS), consisting of proteinuria, hypoalbuminemia, hypercholesterolemia and edema. [1] Other common presentations are hypertension (36% to 63%), microscopic hematuria (29% to 94%) and kidney insufficiency (48% to 59% of adults presenting with a serum creatinine >1.3mg/dL). The effacement of foot processes of the podocytes is another common finding in FSGS. FSGS is the most common underlying cause of NS, particularly in adults. Its incidence is also on the rise in children. At initial presentation, the lesions of glomerulosclerosis are both focal, involving a minority of glomeruli, and segmental, affecting a portion of the glomerular globe. With the progression of disease, widespread and global glomerulosclerosis develops.

Majority of the children with FSGS do not respond to oral glucocorticoid treatment and therefore, are classified as steroid resistant NS (SRNS). Approximately 75% to 90% of the children and 50% to 60% of the adults with biopsy proven FSGS have SRNS while 20% of the children have minimal change nephrotic syndrome (MCNS). Therefore, renal biopsy is recommended in the SRNS children to identify patients with MCNS for whom a positive response to therapy can be achieved and to avoid side effects of long term therapy in the cases of steroid resistance. Most of the early onset SRNS and the familial cases are attributed to the genetic causes (around 95% of the cases have gene mutations) and 40% to 60% of the SRNS children under five years of age have a mutated gene. The incidence of a gene mutation in older children is estimated to be around 20%. [2] Inherited SRNS cases show more rapid progression to ESRD and they respond to immunosuppressive therapy less frequently (8% only) as compared to 40% to 50% of the idiopathic cases. [3] In a recent study, 100% of the familial SRNS cases presenting before two years of age had an identifiable mutation. [4] It was observed that 70% of the patients with familial disease and 15% of sporadic cases had a probably pathogenic variant in 24 genes currently known as SRNS causing genes.

Molecular genetic analyses of the genes mutated in the familial cases revealed that the FSGS is a primary disease of the podocytes. The podocytes constitute the visceral epithelial cell layer of the kidney's glomerular filtration barrier (GFB). The GFB is responsible for the outflow of solutes from the blood capillaries to the urinary space. It consists of three layers: the endothelium, the glomerular basement membrane (GBM) and the podocytes. The endothelial cell layer separates the blood and tissue compartments and is surrounded by the GBM. The GBM is a thick basement membrane and is rich in the negatively charged glycosaminoglycans that are responsible for repelling the proteins from the blood by electrostatic forces during the process of filtration. The podocytes line the outer surface of the GBM. They have highly specialized actin-based cytoplasmic extensions called the foot processes. [5] During the maturation process, they lose their pluripotency and proliferative ability and develop their interdigitating foot processes that are crucial for the formation of early cell-cell contact.

The structural foundation of these foot processes is the actin-based cytoskeleton that forms a firm but highly dynamic structure. The interdigitating foot processes of the adjacent podocytes form pores of about 40 nm in width called the slit diaphragms (SD). An individual SD forms a "zipper-like" cell-cell contact between the podocytes. It is a sophisticated multi-protein complex that maintains the foot process architecture and controls the ultra-filtration of molecules via signalling to the actin cytoskeleton of the podocytes. The podocytes, with their highly dynamic foot processes, and the SD together form the central structure for the barrier function of the glomerulus. They also produce extra-cellular matrix proteins that are responsible for the maintenance of the GBM. They provide mechanical support for the glomerular capillary wall. During the filtration process, the GFB is responsible for the selective permeability of molecules based upon their size and charge. It selectively permits ultra-filtration of water and solutes and is responsible for the production of 130 to 180 L of ultra-filtrate that is free of macromolecules that are >40 KDa such as albumins and clotting factors, etc. Certain structural or functional disorders of the podocytes result in sclerosis of part (segmental) of the glomerular capillaries in a minority (focal) of glomeruli.

FSGS occurs as an acquired (primary acquired FSGS), as a consequence of mutations in the podocyte-specific genes (primary genetic FSGS) and as a secondary disorder [6]. The primary acquired FSGS has been suggested to be caused by certain circulating permeability factors. The presence of these factors as a potential cause of primary acquired FSGS is evident by the rapid recurrence of FSGS after kidney transplantation (30% of cases in adults and 50% in children). It has also been shown that injection of plasma from FSGS patients causes proteinuria in rats. However, the exact mechanism remains to be identified. [7] Among these proposed permeability factors, the soluble urokinase type plasminogen activator receptor (suPAR) and the cardiotrophin like cytokine-1 (CLC-1) have been shown to cause FSGS. [8] Serum levels of suPAR were increased in two-thirds of the patients with FSGS, but not in the patients with other glomerular diseases. A higher serum suPAR concentration before kidney transplantation was associated with an increased risk of recurrence of FSGS after transplantation. [9] The expression of CLC-1 has been shown to decrease nephrin expression by the glomeruli and cultured podocytes. The concentration of the CLC-1 in the circulation of patients with recurrent FSGS may be up to 100 times higher than in the normal subjects. [8]

Primary genetic FSGS (familial FSGS) is a part of inherited glomerulopathies where the exact clinical and histologic presentation may depend on the age of onset, function of the responsible gene and other factors. Clinical presentation and response to treatment may vary depending on the individual's genotype and disease causing gene. Despite the reports of genotype-phenotype correlations, huge genetic and phenotypic heterogeneity exists in the pathogenesis of FSGS.

The secondary FSGS may include a diversified group such as HIV-associated nephropathy (HIVAN), drug-induced FSGS, hypertension and other systemic diseases-associated FSGS and may be caused by a congenital reduction in the renal mass (unilateral agenesis).

Virus induced FSGS usually presents as collapsing variant of FSGS either caused by direct infection of podocytes or by the release of inflammatory cytokines by other virus-infected cells that interact with podocyte receptors.

Several viral proteins such as negative regulatory factor (Nef) and viral protein R (Vpr) are known to cause HIVAN. Similarly, several drugs have been reported to induce FSGS. Interferon γ (IFN- γ) can affect podocytes through the IFN-α and the IFN-β receptors found on podocytes. Pamidronate has been used for the treatment of myeloma and metastatic cancers.

It inhibits the actin-cytoskeleton formation in osteoclasts and may have a similar effect on the podocyte cytoskeleton. Rapamycin has been known to induce FSGS by reducing the expression of nephrin and other SD and cytoskeleton proteins. Several systemic diseases such as hypertension, diabetes and obesity eventually lead to the glomerular hyperfiltration-hypertension which causes mechanical stress to the podocytes.

2. Histopathology of FSGS

The histopathological lesions in FSGS are characterized by mesangial sclerosis, hyalinosis, obliteration of capillaries and adhesion of glomerular tuft and Bowman's capsule. Foot processes effacement on electron microscopy and occasional IgM staining on immunofluorescence are also found. In addition to the classical sclerotic lesions in FSGS, five histological variants have been defined known as the Columbia Classification. This classification is based entirely on light microscopic examination and the variants are; the collapsing variant, the cellular variant, the perihilar variant, the tip variant and FSGS, not otherwise specified (NOS) variant. These variant have different etiologies, pathogenetic mechanisms and diverse clinical behaviour in terms of presentation, progression of disease, therapeutic response and long term outcome and now is widely being used in clinical practice. There are remarkable variations in the prevalence of these variants among different studies. The frequencies of these variants described in the literature are 32% to 72.5% for the NOS variant, 4% to 26% for the perihilar variant, 3% to 25.5% for the cellular variant, 4.8% to 37% for the tip variant and 2% to 24% for the collapsing variant. [10]

3. The Genetics of FSGS

Over the last two decades, the molecular basis of FSGS has been elucidated extensively in the familial as well as in the sporadic cases and mutations in a number of genes encoding podocyte proteins have been described. Most of these genes are mainly expressed in the podocytes and are involved in the organization and function of the SD and the actin cytoskeleton. Mutations in these genes either cause autosomal recessive FSGS (*NPHS1*, *NPHS2*, *PLCE1*, *LAMB2*, *ARGHDIA*, and *MYO1E* genes) or autosomal dominant FSGS (*INF2*, *TRPC6*, *WT1*, *ACTN4*, *CD2AP*, and *ARHGAP24* genes) or mitochondrial disorders (*CoQ6*, $tRNA^{Leu}$, $tRNA^{Tyr}$, $tRNA^{Ile}$). FSGS can also be caused by genes that are widely expressed in other tissues and cell types and cause syndromic FSGS like *WT1*, *PAX2* and *LMX1B*. Among the genes associated with the FSGS, the *NPHS1*, *NPHS2*, *CD2AP*, *TRPC6*, *ACTN4* are cytoskeletal proteins; *LAMB2* is a component of the GBM; *PLCE1* is involved in the podocyte signalling processes; *WT1* and *LMX1B* are transcription factors that control gene regulation and podocyte differentiation and *CoQ6* resides in the mitochondria. Mutations in any of the genes result in the disruption of the complex network of these proteins, foot process effacement and loss of SD. As podocytes have been shown to be involved in the GBM synthesis and fenestration of the endothelial cells, any injury to the podocyte not only affects the structure of the podocyte or SD alone, but also disintegrates the adjacent structures and consequently alters glomerular permeability.

The genetic factors can be divided into the disease-causing genes and common genetic variants associated with the disease phenotype. There has been increased evidence of the notion that common variants may help in understanding the pathogenesis of common diseases like glomerular nephropathies. Most of the cases of familial adult-onset FSGS are inherited as an autosomal dominant disorders and contain gain-of-function mutations; however, penetrance may be incomplete with variable expression of the disease phenotype. Many adult patients with familial FSGS present with non-nephrotic range proteinuria or they may be asymptomatic. Mutations are rare in adults with isolated sporadic FSGS. The most common cause of the autosomal dominant FSGS is the *INF2* gene mutations (16%), followed by mutations in the *TRPC6* (12%) and the *ACTN4* (3.5%) genes. Autosomal recessive mutations are mostly loss–of–function mutations and tend to manifest early in life from first month to early adolescent age and are usually severe in nature and lead to rapid progression to ESRD. Mutations in the *NPHS1*, *NPHS2* and *PLCE1* genes have been found in most of the severe cases of congenital and early onset NS, whereas, mutations in the *LAMB2* and *WT1* genes are found in syndromic NS. In a study with a large European cohort, 66% of the children presenting with NS in their first year of life were found to carry mutations in the *NPHS1*, *NPHS2*, *WT1* and *LAMB2* genes. [11] *WT1* mutations are associated with the Denys-Drash syndrome (DDS) and Frasier syndrome (FS), whereas, mutations in the *LAMB2* gene cause Pierson syndrome. Mitochondrial genes are maternally inherited and they usually follow dominant pattern of inheritance.

Mutations in all the identified genes collectively account for a majority of the cases presenting with the FSGS in their early years of life and also for adult FSGS. Nonetheless, there is a sizeable minority of the cases whose genetic causes are still unknown.

3.1 Autosomal Recessive FSGS

3.1.1. The NPHS1 (Nephrin) Gene

The *NPHS1* gene was first identified in 1998 by positional cloning. It is located on chromosome 19q13.1 and contains 29 exons. It encodes nephrin protein, which is a 185 KDa zipper-like transmembrane protein of the immunoglobin (Ig) superfamily of cell adhesion molecules. It is characterized by the eight C2-type Ig-like domains, a fibronectin type III repeat in the extracellular region, a single transmembrane domain and a cytosolic C-terminal end. It is expressed specifically in the podocytes where its extracellular moiety forms homodimers and bridges the intercellular space between the podocyte foot processes forming the porous structure of the SD. Apart from its role as a structural component of the podocyte and the SD, it also plays an essential role in the intracellular signalling pathways where it interacts with certain other proteins like podocin, CD2 associated protein (CD2AP) and transient receptor potential cation channel subfamily C (TRPC6) proteins. Several other proteins have been reported to be associated with the nephrin- SD complex to form a signalling platform around nephrin. It has been suggested that nephrin is critically involved in the signalling processes that are important for podocyte function, survival and differentiation. [12]

The *NPHS1* gene was first identified as a cause of congenital nephrotic syndrome (CNS) in the Finnish population where two mutations, the Fin_{major} (c.121deCT; p.L41fsX90) and the Fin_{minor} (c.3325C>T; p.R1109X) account for 78% and 16% of the CNS cases respectively in Finland. The CNS of the Finnish type (CNF) is characterized by a severe disease with onset in utero or within the first three months of life. It shows a typical renal histology with immature glomeruli, mesangial cell hypercellularity, pseudocystic dilations of the proximal tubules and foot process effacement. Most of the infants with CNF are born prematurely with low birth weight and an enlarged placenta. Edema is present at birth or appears within the first few days of life. Abnormal glomerular filtration can be detected prenatally as an increase in the maternal α-fetoproteins.

Table 1. Genetic Causes of isolated FSGS/SRNS

Gene	Location	Inheritance	Phenotype	Function/Mechanism
NPHS1	19q13.1	AR	Congenital nephrotic syndrome	Anchoring SD to the cytoplasm
NPHS2	1q25.2	AR	CNS, early onset SRNS; adult onset SRNS in individuals carrying R229Q variant	A key component of the SD
PLCE1	10q23.33	AR	Early onset DMS, familial FSGS	Cell growth and differentiation, gene glomerular development
LAMB2	3p21	AR	Pierson syndrome, isolated FSGS	A key component of the glomerular basement membrane
MYO1E	15q22.2	AR	Familial FSGS/SRNS	A key component of the foot-process cytoskeleton, important for podocyte structure in the glomerulus
ARHGDIA	17q25.3	AR	Childhood onset SRNS	Important for actin cytoskeleton architecture
CUBN	10p13	AR	Childhood onset SRNS	
ADCK4	19q13.2	AR	SRNS with FSGS/collapsing FSGS	C0Q10 biosynthesis pathway
PTPRO	12p12.3	AR	Familial NS	Tumor suppressor
TTC21B	2q24.3	AR	Familial NS	Ciliary protein involved in the regulation of trafficking in the primary cilium, involved in the podocyte cytoskeleton architecture
INF2	14q32.33	AD	Adult onset familial and sporadic FSGS,	Formin proteins accelerate actin filament assembly and regulate actin cytoskeleton
TRPC6	11q22.1	AD	Adult onset familial/sporadic FSGS/SRNS	Ca^{2+} entry during cell proliferation
CD2AP	6p12	AD	Familial FSGS/SRNS	Cytoskeletal remodelling, anchoring SD to the cytoskeleton
ACTN4	19q13	AD	Adult onset familial and sporadic FSGS	Actin filament cross-linking protein
ARHGAP24	4q22.1	AD	Adolescent onset FSGS	
WT1	11p13	AD	Isolated NS; Denys Drash and Frasier syndromes	Transcription factor, acts as a tumor suppressor gene, involved in kidney and gonadal development
PAX2	10q24.31	AD	Papillorenal syndrome, familial FSGS	A transcription factor
ANLN	7p	AD	Familial FSGS	Anillin protein important in cytokinesis and cell growth

SD slit diaphragm; CNS congenital nephrotic syndrome; DMS diffuse mesangial sclerosis; AR autosomal recessive; AD autosomal dominant.

Patients usually develop ESRD within 3 to 8 years. A number of children also die of complications of severe nephrosis (infection, thrombosis, intra-vascular volume depletion).

The Fin_{major} and Fin_{minor} mutations are rarely found in other populations. The *NPHS1* gene screening in non–Finnish populations has revealed that the frequency is lower (~39 to 55%) worldwide compared to the Finnish patients. In total, 236 different mutations have been identified in the *NPHS1* gene in different populations of the world with variable frequencies as described in the Human Genome Mutation Database [HGMD; http://www.hgmd.cf.ac.uk/ac/gene.php?gene=NPHS1]. These mutations include missense, protein-truncating nonsense, frameshift small insertion/deletion mutations and splice-site changes. Genotype-phenotype correlation studies have demonstrated a wide heterogeneity in the clinical course and severity of the disease phenotype associated with different mutations. Besides CNS, the *NPHS1* gene mutations have also been identified in patients with a milder disease of childhood onset with histological findings of FSGS. [13, 14] The clinical course can be explained by in vitro functional assays that have shown that most *NPHS1* missense mutations lead to the retention of protein in the endoplasmic reticulum due to the defective intracellular nephrin trafficking. This results in a complete loss of protein from the cell surface. In some cases, missense mutations with minor modifications that do not alter protein trafficking or dimerization, may produce a milder phenotype with onset of the disease later in life. [13] NS associated with the p.R1160X mutation shows a severe as well as a milder phenotype that appears to be influenced by the gender of the patient as five out of the six patients reported were females. [15] Similarly, two siblings with severe CNS and compound heterozygous mutations in the *NPHS1* gene showed preserved renal function at the ages of 20 and 24 years. [16] It was initially thought that patients with a genetic cause of NS do not respond to drug therapy, however, Patrakka et al., [17] reported their unique observation of significant decrease in proteinuria following the administration of angiotensin converting enzyme inhibitors and indomethacin in a girl with the Fin major mutation. [17] It is now evident that some patients may respond to the therapy and establish a partial or complete remission of proteinuria. [18-23]

3.1.2. NPHS2 Gene Mutations Associated with CNS and Familial SRNS

The *NPHS2* gene was first mapped by the classical linkage analysis in the families with autosomal recessive SRNS to chromosome 1q25-q31. [18] The coding region of the *NPHS2* gene is 1,149 bp in length and contains 8 exons and codes for a 42-KDa podocin protein. It is an integral part of the podocytes and is expressed and localized to the insertion site of the SD. The podocin protein plays an essential role in the regulation of glomerular permeability, and acts as a linker between the plasma membrane and the cytoskeleton. It is an important membrane protein of the stomatin family. It consists of 383 amino acids having a hairpin-like topology consisting of a cytosolic C– and an N– terminal domains and a short transmembrane domain. It also contains a single central hydrophobic domain and the prohibition homology (PHB) domain. This PHB domain allows binding of the podocin protein to cholesterol in the plasma membrane. These complexes directly interact with cholesterol in specialized microdomains of the plasma membrane called lipid rafts. The association of podocin with these lipid raft microdomains is suggested to be a pre-requisite for the recruitment of nephrin into the lipid rafts. [19] It also interacts with the nephrin, CD2AP and TRPC6 proteins and forms an important link between the SD and the podocyte cytoskeleton. The dysfunction of the podocin protein due to mutations in the *NPHS2* gene results in the effacement of the foot processes, disorganization of the GFB and the development of proteinuria.

Initially, the *NPHS2* gene was reported to cause familial early-onset NS with steroid-resistance and rapid progression to ESRD. Later, it was established that mutations in the podocin gene cause SRNS manifesting from birth to adulthood. They are also a frequent cause of CNS manifesting in utero or during the first three months of life (15% to 39%) and infantile NS with onset between 4 months and one year of age (29% to 35%). Renal histology in most of the cases shows FSGS, however, MCNS has also been identified in some cases. Phenotypes associated with the *NPHS2* mutations typically include early childhood onset of the disease, resistance to steroid treatment, progression to ESRD within 5 years of diagnosis, and a low risk of recurrence of the disease after transplantation. [20, 21] Studies with animal models show that *NPHS2* knockout mice present with a phenotype similar to the human disease with foot process effacement, nephrotic range proteinuria and chronic renal insufficiency. [22] To date, more than 170 truncating, missense and splice site mutations have been reported in the *NPHS2* gene in the HGMD (http://www.hgmd.cf.ac.uk/ac/gene.php?gene=NPHS2). The missense mutations represent the largest group distributed throughout the length of the gene and affect different functional domains of the podocin. Most of the commonly found mutations lead to retention of the protein in the endoplasmic reticulum. Some missense mutations although direct the protein correctly to the plasma membrane, affect the signalling properties and/or alter its interaction with other proteins at the SD. The *NPHS2* gene mutations are identified in 10 to 25% of the sporadic NS cases of childhood onset. [22, 23] The incidence in familial SRNS cases has been found to be 30% to 40% in the European and American children, 29% in the Turkish children and 0% in the Japanese, Korean and Pakistani children. [22, 23] Among the most frequent mutations, p.R138Q mutation is typically associated with the early-onset NS. The mutant podocin is shown to be retained in the endoplasmic reticulum and loses its ability to recruit nephrin in the lipid rafts. [19] Some other mutations (e.g., p.V180M and p.R238S) are found in patients with later onset SRNS suggesting that podocin may retain some function in these cases.

A frequently found single nucleotide polymorphism (SNP) in the *NPHS2* gene is p.R229Q. It is shown to be found in varying frequencies in different populations of the world more frequently in the European populations (allele frequency from 2 to 7%) and less frequently in the populations of Asians and African descent from USA and Brazil (0.5 to 2.5% allele frequency). The pathogenic nature of this variant is extensively discussed in the literature. It is found in compound heterozygosity with another pathogenic mutation in the *NPHS2* gene in some cases of the SRNS/FSGS. These patients manifest NS later in life suggesting a reduced pathogenicity of this variant. The mutation was also found in a homozygous state in two children with childhood onset NS. [23] It is therefore considered to be a non-neutral variant that, when found with a second *NPHS2* mutation, tends to increase the chances of susceptibility to FSGS. [24] In vitro studies have demonstrated that the variant podocin shows a decreased binding capacity to the nephrin protein. [24] These observations emphasize the importance of this variant in the proper functioning of the protein. However, there are insufficient data to speculate that gene variants like p.R229Q may also cause FSGS/NS.

A few studies also report a di-genic mode of inheritance where mutations in both the *NPHS1* and *NPHS2* genes are observed simultaneously. [15] These observations provide the evidence of a functional relationship between the nephrin and the podocin proteins and emphasize the critical role of these genes in maintaining the structural and functional integrity of the podocytes and GFB.

3.1.3. PLCE1 Gene Mutations are Implicated in CNS and Recessive FSGS

Homozygosity mapping in the cases of familial NS identified a locus for early onset NS and diffuse mesangial sclerosis (DMS) on chromosome harboring the phospholipase C epsilon 1 (*PLCE1*) gene. The gene spans 334 kb on chromosome 10 and contains 34 exons. It encodes phospholipase C ε 1(PLCε1), a member of phospholipase family of proteins that catalyses the hydrolysis of phosphoinositides and generates second messengers such as inositol-1, 4, 5 triphosphate and diacylglycerol. These second messengers regulate cell growth, differentiation and gene expression etc. The main function of second messenger is the stimulation of calcium release from intracellular storage pools. The PLCE1 protein is involved in the cytoskeletal reorganization and is also shown to modulate the functions of other signal transduction cascade proteins. However, the precise mode of action of PLCE1 in the podocyte remains unclear.

The *PLCE1* gene mutations are the third most common cause of NS in infants after the *NPHS1* and the *NPHS2* genes. [25] Mutations in the *PLCE1* gene have been identified in 10% to 50% of the patients with NS and DMS and in 12% of the recessive familial FSGS cases. [25, 26] All the mutations reported in children with DMS were loss- of-function mutations. Interestingly, the NS patients with the histology of FSGS had missense mutations in the *PLCE1* gene and had a later onset of the disease in contrast to children with the DMS who all had early onset and truncating/loss of function mutations. [25] These findings suggest that *PLCE1* mutations may have a role in the pathogenesis of FSGS either as the cause of the disease or at least as a modifier gene acting in concert with other mutations and environmental factors.

As the genetic forms of NS are thought to be non-responsive to steroid therapy, some patients carrying the *PLCE1* gene mutations show complete remission of proteinuria after treatment with steroids and cyclosporine. [25] Hence, NS caused by the *PLCE1* mutations may be regarded as drug-responsive NS. Another unique observation with *PLCE1* is the identification of homozygous mutations in asymptomatic individuals. A frameshift truncation mutation in exon 3 segregating in a family was also found in an asymptomatic adult. This phenomenon was explained by the presence of an unidentified genetic modifier that may compensate the PLCE1 defect. [27]

3.1.4. LAMB2 Gene Mutations Cause Pierson Syndrome as Well as Isolated NS

The *LAMB2* gene codes for Laminin B2 protein and is crucial for podocyte foot process architecture and stability. It is widely expressed in the GBM, retina, lens capsule, intraocular muscle and the neuromuscular synapses. It is a laminin family member which are heterotrimeric glycoproteins consisting of α, β and γ subunits joined through a coiled coil. [28] They are essential components of all the basement membranes and play crucial roles in maintaining the structures of the basement membranes by forming a monolayer of laminins. They are also shown to mediate matrix-cell interactions that are involved in the cell adhesion, differentiation and migration. The most important β2-containing laminin isoform is laminin-521 which is composed of α5, β2 and γ1 subunits and is specifically expressed in the GBM, intraocular muscles and neuromuscular synapses. Laminin β2 provides cross linking between the basolateral membranes of the podocyte to the GBM in the kidneys. Knock-out mice lacking the β2 chain exhibit proteinuria and die in the perinatal period. [29] Therefore, deficiency in the laminin β2 chain results in the GBM alteration, functional impairment of the GFB and ocular anomalies.

Table 2. Genetic Causes of syndromic SRNS/FSGS

Gene	Location	Disease Association	Protein Function
LAMB2	3p21	Pierson syndrome, isolated FSGS	Key component of the glomerular basement membrane
LMX1B	9q33.3	Nail patella syndrome	Transcription factor
SMARCAL1	2q34-36	Schimke immune-osseous dysplasia	Gene regulation
WT1	11p13	Denys Drash and Frasier syndromes, Isolated NS/FSGS	Transcription factor, acts as a tumor suppressor gene, involved in kidney and gonadal development
COQ2	4q21.23	CoQ10 deficiency with FSGS	CoQ10 biosynthesis pathway, Electron transfer in mitochondrial respiratory chain
ADCK4	19q13.2	SRNS with FSGS/collapsing FSGS	CoQ10 biosynthesis pathway
PAX2	10q24.31	Papillorenal syndrome, familial FSGS	A transcription factor
COQ6	14q24	CoQ10 deficiency with FSGS	CoQ10 biosynthesis pathway

Mutations in the *LAMB2* gene are associated with a rare autosomal recessive syndromic disorder, Pierson syndrome (OMIM #609049). It is characterized by the appearance of early onset NS and variable ocular and neurological defects. The typical ophthalmic signs in Pierson syndrome are microcoria (fixed narrowing of the pupils), abnormal lens shape with cataract and retinal abnormalities. Patients with severe phenotypes exhibit blindness and neuro-developmental defects including hypotonia and delayed motor and cognitive development. [30] Phenotypes of variable severity with less prominent ocular symptoms and isolated NS have also been described. [31, 32] The missense mutations and non-truncating deletion mutations in the *LAMB2* gene exhibit a relatively milder phenotype, while, patients with the protein truncating mutation show a severe phenotype with extra renal manifestations. Further, the patients with the mild phenotype show glomerulopathy with FSGS while, patients with the severe phenotype have DMS.

3.2. Autosomal Dominant FSGS

Adult-onset FSGS is a rare monogenic condition. Mutations in the *ACTN*, *INF2*, *TRPC6* and recently identified *PAX2* gene lead to autosomal dominant kidney disease characterized by proteinuria, progressive chronic kidney disease (CKD) and FSGS. The genes implicated in the adult-onset form of FSGS have yielded significant insight into current understanding of the glomerular filtration.

3.2.1. The INF2 (Inverted Formin 2) Gene

A new locus for autosomal dominant FSGS was recently mapped on chromosome 14q containing the inverted formin 2 (*INF2*) gene by linkage analysis. INF2 is a member of the formin family of actin-regulating proteins that have been shown to accelerate the polymerization and depolymerization of actin in vitro. [33] It has an N-terminal diaphanous-inhibitory domain (DID), the forming homology (FH) domains, FH1 and FH2, and a C-terminal diaphanous-autoregulatory domain (DAD). The disease causing mutations identified in the *INF2* gene are missense mutations that are clustered in the DID and are shown to inhibit actin-depolymerization. [34] *INF2* mutations account for 9% to 16% of the cases of autosomal dominant familial FSGS. It was observed that INF2-related diseases showed variable penetrance with the onset of the disease ranging widely from childhood to adulthood and commonly leading to ESRD in the third and fourth decade of life. Mutations in the *INF2* gene are also shown to be associated with the Charcot-Marie-Tooth disease (CMT). It is a group of inherited disorders affecting peripheral neurons and renal disease with FSGS. [35]

3.2.2. The TRPC6 Gene

The *TRPC6* gene is located on chromosome 11q21-q22. It encodes for the TRPC protein and is expressed in the podocytes, renal tubules and glomeruli. The TRPC6 protein consists of three or four amino-terminal ankyrin repeats, six putative transmembrane domains, a short sequence termed the "TRP box" (of unknown function), and a potential coiled-coil structure in the amino and carboxy sequences. The protein is thought to mediate the intracellular calcium homeostasis of the podocytes. The mutant TRPC6 protein is implicated in impaired calcium signalling and shown to disrupt the glomerular cell function. It was first identified to cause autosomal dominant FSGS through increased channel activity. [36] Mutations in the *TRPC6* gene account for 3% to 7% of the cases of familial adult-onset FSGS with mild to moderate nephrotic range proteinuria, progressing to ESRD. Most of the mutations that have been reported so far are gain-of-function mutations leading to increased activity of ion channels by increasing the calcium current amplitudes or by delaying the channel inactivation. Recently, *TRPC6* mutations have also been detected in patients with early to late onset SRNS with a unique association of collapsing glomerulosclerosis in renal histology in a 6 months old child. [37]

3.2.3. The PAX2 Gene Causes Syndromic As Well As Familial FSGS

The protein product of the *PAX2* gene is a member of paired box (PAX) transcription factor gene family that plays a critical role in the kidney development. [38] Mutations in this gene have been associated with congenital abnormalities of the kidney and urinary tract (CAKUT) as part of a syndrome known as papillorenal syndrome in which ocular manifestations also occur. The inheritance pattern in the families with FSGS was consistent with autosomal dominant inheritance with incomplete penetrance. Heterozygous mutations have been identified in 7 families with FSGS. [39] The ages of onset were from 8 to 68 years in these families but most of the patients had disease onset in the second to fourth decade of their lives. Renal biopsy of one of the patients showed FSGS and diffuse podocytopathy with degenerative changes and focal foot process effacement on electron microscopy. The findings indicated that *PAX2* mutations can cause disease through haploinsufficiency or a dominant-negative effect.

The PAX2 protein is a transcription factor containing an N-terminal DNA-binding paired domain and a transactivation domain at the C terminus. In a recent study, *PAX2* gene mutations were responsible for 4% of the familial FSGS and 8% of CAKUT. [39]

3.2.4. The ACTN4 Gene

The *ACTN4* gene was mapped to chromosome 19q3 by positional cloning in large multiplex families with FSGS. It is an actin-bundling protein of the cytoskeleton and is highly expressed in the podocytes. [40] Initially, mutations in the *ACTN4* gene were identified in familial cases of autosomal dominant FSGS. [41] The affected family members presented with adolescent onset proteinuria progressing to ESRD during adulthood. Renal histology revealed irregular granular staining patterns in the capillary walls of preserved glomeruli. Incomplete penetrance is also observed in some members of these families without the development of renal phenotype suggesting the involvement of other genetic or non-genetic factors in the pathogenesis of *ACTN4* associated FSGS. To date approximately 150 gene mutations have been identified in the *ACTN4* gene (The 1000 genome browser, http://browser.1000genomes.org/Homo_sapiens/Gene/Variation_Gene/) that are thought to interfere with the regulation of the actin cytoskeleton of podocytes. These mutations include missense and splice-site mutations frequently affecting the binding domain of actinin 4. However, mutations in the *ACTN4* gene account for only 4% of the familial cases of FSGS.

FSGS associated mutations in the *ACTN4* gene are mainly localized to the N-terminal actin binding domain of the protein. These mutations cause an increase in the actin-binding affinity of the protein that changes the actin dynamics within the cell. In vitro functional studies have demonstrated an increased binding of the mutant protein to the filamentous actin and the formation of large aggregates and impaired migration patterns. [42, 43] Recently, it has been shown that ACTN4 interacts with retinoic acid receptor (RARα) and enhances its transcriptional activation. In addition, mutant ACTN4 protein not only mislocalized to the cytoplasm, but it also lost its ability to be associated with nuclear receptors. Consequently, the mutant protein fails to potentiate transcriptional activation by the nuclear hormone receptors in podocytes. [44]

3.2.5. WT1 Gene Causes Wilms' Tumor and Syndromic Forms of NS

The *WT1* gene is located on chromosome 11p13 and codes for a zinc-finger transcription factor important for the regulation of several genes involved in kidney and gonadal development. [45, 46] Mutations in the *WT1* gene have been known to cause DDS, FS and isolated NS with DMS. [47] The DDS is characterized by the presence of early onset SRNS, XY pseudohermaphroditism, gonadal dysgenesis and Wilms' tumor (in more than 90% of the cases). The age of onset of SRNS is usually congenital. Patients rapidly progress to ESRD with a renal histology typical of DMS. Electron microscopy shows foot process effacement.

To prevent the development of Wilms' tumor, bilateral nephrectomy is usually recommended before the transplantation. No recurrence of disease has been observed after renal transplantation in the cases of *WT1* gene mutations. Most of the mutations that are associated with the DDS phenotype are missense mutations, predominantly affecting exons 8 and 9 of the *WT1* gene. Among these mutations, p.R394W is the most common mutation that affects the zinc finger domain and therefore reduces the DNA binding capacity of the WT1 protein. Knock-in mice with the heterozygous p.R394W mutation have been shown to have DMS and male genital anomaly phenotypes that are characteristics of human DDS. Isolated DMS has also been described to be associated with recessive *WT1* gene mutations.

The FS is also characterized by the XY pseudohermaphroditism and progressive nephropathy with SRNS. [48] Patients with FS often show late onset proteinuria and a better renal outcome as compared to the patients with DDS. The patients present FSGS on renal biopsy and show good renal function until the second to third decade of life. They present with female external genitalia, streak gonads and XY karyotype. The risk of developing Wilms' tumor is comparatively low in patients with FS. However, the development of gonadoblastoma from gonadal dysgenesis is common. A heterozygous donor splice-site mutation in intron 9 has been associated with the FS phenotype. This mutation affects the KTS (lysine-threonine-serine amino acid residue) region of the WT1 protein and produces the KTS (–) isoform. The KTS (+) isoform of the WT1 protein has an important role in the genitourinary tract and kidney development.

WT1 mutations can also rarely cause isolated NS in an autosomal dominant manner. The truncating mutations in the *WT1* gene have been detected in patients with isolated Wilms' tumor. [49] The Wilms' tumor is among the most common solid tumors in children and accounts for 8% of all the childhood cancers. The *WT1* gene mutations were first identified in the Wilms' tumor, aniridia, genitourinary malformations and mental retardation (WAGR) syndrome which is characterized by the Wilms' tumor, aniridia, genitourinary malformations and mental retardation. Patients with the WAGR syndrome contain a deletion on the short arm of chromosome 11, associated with the complete loss of *WT1* function. [50] Familial type Wilms' tumor is also inherited in an autosomal dominant manner with germline mutations in the *WT1* gene. Patients carrying mutations show remarkable phenotypic heterogeneity. Splice site mutations that are found more frequently in the FS cases, are also identified in some cases of the DDS or in isolated DMS. Similarly, patients with mutations that are typical for DDS may exhibit isolated FSGS or Wilms' tumor. Incomplete penetrance is also evident in some cases of the *WT1* gene mutations. Two monozygotic twins with a heterozygous p.R366P mutation died because of complications of CNS at 23 weeks and 13 months of age, respectively. Surprisingly, their father who was a carrier was asymptomatic and had normal renal function at the age of 41 years. The possible explanation for this observation is described as the presence of somatic mosaicism or genomic imprinting or the lack of heritability. [50, 51]

3.2.6. The CD2AP Gene

The *CD2AP* gene codes for an actin-related protein and in homozygous knock-out mice, mutations in this gene are shown to cause mesangial cell proliferation and glomerulosclerosis and electron microscopy showed extensive foot process effacement. [52] CD2AP$^{+/-}$ mice showed no proteinuria but glomerular lesions were similar to human FSGS. Subsequently, autosomal dominant mutations in the *CD2AP* gene were identified to cause FSGS. [53]

Besides the disease-causing heterozygous mutations, a homozygous *CD2AP* mutation has also been described. Both parents who were heterozygous showed no kidney pathology. CD2AP is a multifunctional adaptor molecule localized to cytoplasm and edges of cells and involved in the cytoskeletal remodelling, cell survival and endocytosis. It interacts with the nephrin and podocin proteins and serves as a linker anchoring SD proteins to the actin cytoskeleton of the podocytes.

4. Mitochondrial Disorders

FSGS associated with mutations in the mitochondrial genes represents a heterogeneous group of multisystem disorders. Mutations in the $tRNA^{Leu(UUR)}$ are usually associated with the MELAS (mitochondrial myopathy, encephalopathy, lactic acidosis and stroke like episodes) syndrome. The most common mutations, p.A3243G is also found in the FSGS patients sometimes associated with maternally inherited diabetes and/or sensorineural hearing loss. In most of the cases, patients showed subnephrotic-range proteinuria and slowly progressing FSGS. Mutations in another mitochondrial gene $tRNA^{Tyr}$ have been associated with FSGS. A patient with p.A5843G mutation presented with mitochondrial cytopathy preceded by steroid resistant FSGS. A A4269G mutation in the $tRNA^{Ile}$ gene has been found in a patient with mitochondrial encephalomyopathy, deafness, epilepsy and FSGS.

Coenzyme Q_{10} (CoQ_{10}) is a cofactor of several enzymes that are involved in several pathways such as mitochondrial respiratory chain and the modulation of apoptosis. There are 13 genes known to be involved in CoQ_{10} biosynthesis pathway. Mutations in at least 8 genes have been associated to cause primary CoQ_{10} deficiency. Symptoms include respiratory chain disorders with or without SRNS. Mutations in the *CoQ2*, *CoQ6*, *ADCK4* and *PDSS2* genes are typically associated with SRNS and a wide variety of clinical manifestations. [54] Homozygous mutations in the *ADCK4* gene have been found to cause SRNS with FSGS or collapsing FSGS. [55]

It was demonstrated that the ADCK4 protein localizes to the mitochondria and foot processes in podocytes, as well as to the proximal tubules and collecting ducts in the kidney. Disease-causing homozygous or compound heterozygous mutations were identified in 11 out of 15 patients from 8 unrelated families. Disease onset in these families was typically between ages 10 and 20 years, although several had earlier onset, including 1 patient with onset in the first year of life.

Histology showed FSGS or collapsing FSGS, and electron microscopy showed effacement of the foot processes of the podocytes. One patient was treated with a high-dose of CoQ10 supplementation which resulted in some clinical improvement in renal function. Patient-derived cells showed CoQ10 deficiency and reduced mitochondrial respiratory enzyme activity.

The *COQ6* gene located on chromosome 14q24, first identified to cause autosomal recessive coenzyme Q10 deficiency, manifests as NS. [56] The patients presented with proteinuria at a median age of 1.2 years and progressed to end-stage renal failure at a median age of 1.7 years. Renal biopsies showed FSGS in 7 patients and DMS in 1 patient. However, subsequent analysis of the *CoQ6* gene in 530 families with NS identified 2 heterozygous truncating mutations in 2 unrelated patients. Homozygosity mapping in patients with FSGS, mild psychomotor delay and optic atrophy revealed disease causing mutation in the *CoQ2* gene. [57] The gene encodes para-hydroxybenzoate-polyprenyl-transferase enzyme which is involved in the CoQ10 biosynthesis pathway.

5. Other Rare Genes Causing Autosomal Recessive/Dominant/Syndromic NS/FSGS

Several other genes have been identified to cause NS or associated glomerulopathies with and without extrarenal manifestations and whose roles in the regulation of the GFB are less clear. Mutations have been identified in the *PTPRO* gene in a study of SRNS families of Turkish and non-Turkish origins. [58] Notably, children with the homozygous *PTPRO* gene mutations are responsive to intensified immunosuppressive treatment. PTPRO is a tyrosine phosphatase and is expressed at the apical membrane of the podocyte foot processes. Tyrosine phosphorylation of tight junction proteins are shown to play a major role in controlling the paracellular permeability, cell signaling, and actin cytoskeleton remodelling. Mutations in the *MYO1E* gene localized on the chromosome 15q21 have been identified to be associated with childhood-onset, glucocorticoid-resistant FSGS. [59] Mutation screening in a panel of 52 patients with FSGS or mesangial sclerosis identified a homozygous truncating mutation (Y695X) in a Turkish girl with FSGS. The MYO1E protein localizes to the plasma membrane of the podocyte and plays a role in normal glomerular filtration. Cellular studies showed that the A159P-mutant protein mislocalized to the cytoplasm, did not co-localize with F-action, and was unable to promote podocyte migration, indicating a defect in normal MYO1E function. Electron microscopy of children with the *MYO1E* mutations showed thickening and disorganization of the GBM. The *ARHGAP24* gene was identified by mutational analysis of candidate genes based on its role in glomerular biology. [60] Analysis in the familial FSGS revealed disease causing mutation in one family. [61] Mutations in the *LMX1B* gene are reported to cause nail-patella syndrome, a rare disorder characterized by dysplasia of the nails, absent or malformed patellae, dysplasia of the elbows, glaucoma and progressive nephropathy. Another syndromic FSGS associated disorder, Schimke immune-osseous dysplasia is known to be caused by mutations in the *SMARCAL1* gene. This autosomal recessive disorder is characterized by spondyloepiphyseal dysplasia causing growth retardation, defective cellular immunity, hyperpigmented macules, dysmorphic facial features and NS due to FSGS. [62]

Recently, in a study of whole exome sequencing and homozygosity mapping of consanguineous families with FSGS revealed a disease-causing p.P209L mutation in the *TTC21B* gene localized to chromosome 2. The patients had late-onset albuminuria with high blood pressure and FSGS and reached ESRD at 15-32 years of age with no recurrence after transplantation. [63] The *TTC21B* gene has previously been reported to be associated with autosomal recessive nephronophthisis belonging to the group of ciliopathies. The p.P209L mutation has been identified in seven of 46 families with a primary diagnosis of late-onset FSGS. It was also observed that patients bearing this mutation are of North African or Portuguese descent and share a common haplotype, indicating a founder effect.

Another study recently identified heterozygous R431C mutation in the *ANLN* gene in a large 4-generation family with autosomal dominant FSGS. [64] The mutation was found by a combination of linkage analysis and whole-exome sequencing focusing on genes known to be enriched in the podocyte. Mutational screening of the *ANLN* gene in 250 families with FSGS identified 1 missense mutation (G618C) that segregated with the disorder in a single family. Overexpression of the R431C mutant in HEK293 cells resulted in reduced and defective binding to CD2AP. The *ANLN* gene codes for the F-actin binding protein anillin, important in cytokinesis and interacts with key proteins such as CD2AP and mDia2 (mouse formin 2) during cell division. It also regulates cell growth by its interaction with the promigratory and prosurvival phosphoinositides 3 kinase/AKT (protein kinase B) pathway.

6. Variants on Chromosome 22 Associated with FSGS

Genome-wide association studies using admixture mapping methods have identified a genetic susceptibility locus for FSGS located on chromosome 22 in African-Americans. This region harbours two potential disease-causing genes, *APOL1* and *MYH9*. [65] Subsequent studies identified two coding variants in the *APOL1* gene, named as G1 and G2 that confer increased risk of developing FSGS, hypertension associated kidney disease, or HIVAN. The ApoL1 protein confers resistance to the African trypanosomiasis (sleeping sickness) by lysing the disease-causing trypanosomes. ApoL1 trypanolytic activity is determined by three C-terminal domains; a pore-forming domain, a pH-sensitive membrane-addressing domain and the serum resistance-associated protein (SRA) - interacting domain. The kidney risk variants of the *APOL1* gene are located in the SRA binding domain. The G1 represents a pair of missense variants $G1^G$ (p.S342G, rs73885319) and $G1^M$ (p.I384M, rs60910145) in the coding region of the *APOL1* gene and are in nearly absolute linkage disequilibrium. The G2 variant denotes a 6 base pair (bp) deletion leading to an in-frame deletion of two amino acids (p.N388/Y389, rs71785313) near the C-terminus of the protein. The two variants arose independently on separate chromosomes and because of the close physical proximity of the two variants (12 bp), they have not undergone physical recombination.

The G1/G2 variants are observed frequently throughout sub-Saharan Africa in variable frequencies and in African Americans. [66] The two alleles are very common in African-Americans with a combined allele frequency of approximately 35%. Individuals having homozygous or compound heterozygous alleles of these variants have a 7- to 10-fold increased risk of developing FSGS or hypertension-associated ESRD. The inheritance of these two alleles show a strong recessive model, where in heterozygous state, the variants protect against trypanosomes, but in the homozygous or compound heterozygous state (recessive), variants confer susceptibility to kidney injury. Several studies have shown that *APOL1* G1 and G2 are strongly associated with non-diabetic ESRD and hypertension associated ESRD (odds ratio ~ 7) but no positive association was found with diabetic ESRD. [67- 69]

In the past few years, genome wide association studies have identified thousands of common genetic variants associated with complex diseases. However, these variants have low frequencies and contributed a little to the overall genetic variance of the disease. Most of the identified common association SNPs have only weak genetic effect (e.g., odds ratio <1.5) with low penetrance, whereas, rare variants have moderate-to-high penetrance. It has now been suggested that rare and low frequency coding variants might have a large effect on complex disease phenotypes. The proposed association of *APOL1* gene variants with the kidney injury reveals its uniqueness as opposed to most other complex disease genes; *APOL1* variants are frequent and have larger effect size (high penetrance). Several case control studies have identified the strong effect size [70] and high frequency (~ 72%) of the cases that carry two APOL1 risk alleles for HIVAN, FSGS, lupus collapsing glomerulopathy, hypertension-attributed nephropathy. [67, 68, 71]

7. MicroRNAs As Biomarkers for FSGS

MicroRNAs (miRNAs) are small noncoding RNA molecules that have been suggested as gene regulators at the posttranscriptional level. It is thought that miRNAs regulate nearly 30% of protein-coding genes and are involved in the developmental, pathogenic and tumorigenesis processes. Recently, the diagnostic value of circulating miRNAs has been demonstrated in various diseases. It has been revealed that miRNAs released by the cells and tissues into the circulation can serve as non-invasive biomarkers for various diseases and tissue injuries. Altered levels of circulating miRNAs have been observed in patients with kidney diseases including acute kidney injury, CKD and lupus nephritis. The elevation of the urinary levels of miR-10a and miR-30d was confirmed in urine samples from patients with FSGS. [72] It has also been shown that miR-186 may be considered as a biomarker for FSGS with nephrotic range proteinuria. [73]

8. Treatment Options and Future Prospects

FSGS is known to be a condition of great genetic heterogeneity, with the number of causative genes increasing constantly. The identification of disease-causing genes in NS/FSGS has greatly helped in understanding the molecular aetiology of the disease. However, there is still a dearth of exact understanding of the pathogenesis of idiopathic FSGS with no curative treatment. The next challenges for the researchers and clinicians are to accurately confer the disease-causing roles of the gene mutations in the correct diagnosis/prognosis of the disease and to develop therapies to slow down the disease progression. For example, for the patients with mutation in the *WT1* gene, careful regular medical examinations are required as they are at a higher risk of developing Wilms' tumor. Similarly, steroid treatment in patients with mutations in the *NPHS2* gene may be discontinued since majority of the patients with the *NPHS2* gene mutations are steroid resistant. Recurrence rates in these patients after kidney transplantation are also very low. Recurrence of proteinuria has been reported in children with *NPHS1* mutations who developed anti-nephrin antibodies. Remission may be achieved in these patients by immunosuppression or plasmapheresis. The outcome of kidney transplantation has been reported to be 5-year patient survival of 90% and 5-year graft survival of over 80%. Partial remission has been shown with calcineurin inhibitors in patients with mutations in the *TRPC6* gene through the suppression of TRPC6-mediated calcineurin overactivation. Similarly, calcineurin inhibitors have been shown to reduce proteinuria in patients with mutations in the

NPHS2 and *WT1* genes. A decrease in proteinuria through the use of angiotensin-converting enzyme inhibitors (ACEIs) and angiotensin-receptor blockers (ARBs) has also been achieved in some cases of CNS patients with *NPHS1* or *NPHS2* gene mutations. It has been widely accepted that the identification of accurate pathogenic variants in the disease causing genes will eventually modify therapeutic approach to avoid unnecessary immunosuppression and also manage treatment of rare conditions such as treatment of CoQ10 enzyme deficiency disorders with enzyme therapy. Mitochondrial disorders cause multi-systemic conditions that also require constant follow up for neurological and renal manifestations.

In future, studies of the podocyte genes in humans as well as in animals will identify new players in the pathogenesis of NS/FSGS. The insights into the podocyte structure and function provided by the studies of the genetic disorders will greatly help explain the effect of treatment regimens used in these disorders.

Conclusion

In conclusion, significant progress has been made in understanding and unravelling the molecular and genetic basis of NS, especially childhood NS. The discovery of new genes and gene variants is still in progress. A complete understanding of the molecular genetic pathogenesis of the disorders will open the avenues for specific and targeted therapy of the disorder in near future.

References

[1] D'Agati, VD, Kaskel FJ, Falk RJ. Focal segmental glomerulosclerosis. *N. Eng. J. Med.* 2011;365:2398-2411.

[2] Rood IM, Deegens JK, Wetzels JF. Genetic causes of focal segmental glomerulosclerosis: implications for clinical practice. *Nephrol. Dial. Transplant.* 2012;27:882-890.

[3] Buscher AK, Kranz B, Buscher R, Hildebrandt F, Dworniczak B, Pennekamp P, Kuwertz-Broking E, Wingen AM, John U, Kemper M, Monnens L, Hoyer PF, Weber S, Konrad M. Immunosuppression and renal outcome in congenital and pediatric steroid resistant nephrotic syndrome. *Clin. J. Am. Soc. Nephrol.* 2010;5:2075-2084.

[4] McCarthy HJ, Bierzynska A, Wherlock M, Ognjanovic M, Kerecuk L, Hegde S, Feather S, Gilbert RD, Krischock L, Jones C, Sinha MD, Webb NJ, Christian M, Williams MM, Marks S, Koziell A, Welsh GI, Saleem MA; RADAR the UK SRNS Study Group. Simultaneous sequencing of 24 genes associated with steroid-resistant nephrotic syndrome. *Clin. J. Am. Soc. Nephrol.* 2013;8:637-648.

[5] Jarad G and Miner JH. Update on the glomerular filtration barrier. *Curr. Opin. Nephrol Hypertens.* 2009;18:226-232.

[6] Barisoni L, Schnaper HW, Kopp JB. Advances in the biology and genetics of the podocytopathies: implications for diagnosis and therapy. *Arch. Pathol. Lab. Med.* 2009;133:201-216.

[7] Savin VJ, McCarthy ET, Sharma M. Permeability factors in focal segmental glomerulosclerosis. *Semin. Nephrol.* 2003;23:147-160.

[8] McCarthy ET, Sharma M, Savin VJ. Circulating permeability factors in idiopathic nephrotic syndrome and focal segmental glomerulosclerosis. *Clin. J. Am. Soc. Nephrol.* 2010;5:2115-2121.

[9] Wei C, El Hindi S, Li J, Fornoni A, Goes N, Sageshima J, Maiguel D, Karumanchi SA, Yap HK, Saleem M, Zhang Q, Nikolic B, Chaudhri A, Daftarian P, Salido E, Torres A, Salifu M, Sarwal MM, Schaefer F, Morath C, Schwenger V, Zeier M, Gupta V, Roth D, Rastaldi MP, Burke G, Ruiz P, Reiser J. Circulating urokinase receptor as a cause of focal segmental glomerulosclerosis. *Nat. Med.* 2010;17:952-960.

[10] Shakeel S, Mubarak M, Kazi JI, Jafry N and Ahmed E. Frequency and clinicopathological characteristics of variants of primary focal segmental glomerulosclerosis in adults presenting with nephrotic syndrome. *J. Nephropathol.* 2013;2:28-35.

[11] Hinkes BG, Mucha B, Vlangos CN, Gbadegesin R, Liu J, Hesselbacher K, Hangan D, Ozaltin F, Zenker M, Hildebrandt F. Nephrotic syndrome in the first year of life: two thirds of cases are caused by mutations in 4 genes (NPHS1, NPHS2, WT1 and LAMB2). *Pediatrics.* 2007;119:e907-e919.

[12] Patrakka J, Tryggvason K. Nephrin- a unique structural and signaling protein of the kidney filter. *Trends Mol. Med.* 2007;13:396-403.

[13] Philippe A, Nevo F, Esquivel EL, Reklaityte D, Gribouval O, Tete MJ, Loirat C, Dantal J, Fischbach M, Pouteil-Noble C, Decramer S, Hoehne M, Benzing T, Charbit M, Niaudet P, Antignac C. Nephrin mutations can cause childhood onset steroid-resistant nephrotic syndrome. *J. Am. Soc. Nephrol.* 2008;19:1871-1878.

[14] Santin S, Garcia-Maset R, Ruiz P, Gimenez I, Zamora I, Pena A, Madrid A, Camacho JA, Fraga G, Sanchez-Moreno A, Cobo MA, Bernis C, Ortiz A, de Pablos AL, Pintos G, Justa ML, Hidalgo-Barquero E, Fernandez-Llama P, Ballarin J, Ars E, Torra R; FSGS Spanish Study Group. Nephrin mutations cause childhood and adult-onset focal segmental glomerulosclerosis. *Kidney Int.* 2009;76:1268-1276.

[15] Koziell A, Grech V, Hussain S, Lee G, Lenkkeri U. Tryggvason K and Scambler P. Genotype/phenotype correlations of NPHS1 and NPHS2 mutations in nephrotic syndrome advocate a functional inter-relationship in glomerular filtration. *Hum. Mol. Genet.* 2002;11:379-388.

[16] Schulteisss M, Ruf RG, Mucha BE, Wiggins R, Fuchshuber A, Lichtenberger A, Hildebrandt F. No evidence for genotype/phenotype correlation in NPHS1 and NPHS2 mutations. *Padiatr. Nephrol.* 2004;19:1340-1348.

[17] Patrakka J, Kestila M, Wartiovaara J, Ruotsalainen V, Tissari P, Lenkkeri U, Mannikko M, Visapaa I, Holmberg C, Rapola J, Tryggvason K, Jalanko H. Congenital nephrotic syndrome (NPHS1); features resulting from different mutations in Finnish patients. *Kidney Int.* 2000;58:972-980.

[18] Fuchshuber A, Jean G, Gribouval O, Gubler MC, Broyer M, Beckmann JS, Niaudet P, Antignac C. Mapping of a gene (SRN1) to chromosome 1q25-q31 in idiopathic nephrotic syndrome confirms a distinct entity of autosomal recessive nephrosis. *Hum. Mol. Genet.* 1995;4:2155-2158.

[19] Huber TB, Simons M, hartleben B, Semetz L, Schmidts M, Gundlach E, Saleem MA, Walz G and Benzing T. Molecular basis of the functional podocin-nephrin complex:

mutations in the NPHS2 gene disrupt nephrin targeting to lipid raft microdomains. *Hum. Mol. Genet.* 2003;12:3397-3405.

[20] Ruf RG, Lichtenberger A, Karle SM, Haas JP, Anacleto FE, Schultheiss M, Zalewski I, Imm A, Ruf EM, Mucha B, Bagga A, Neuhaus T, Fuchshuber A, Bakkaloglu A, Hildebrandt F; Arbeitsgemeinschaft Für Pädiatrische Nephrologie Study Group. Patients with mutations in NPHS2 (podocin) do not respond to standard steroid treatment of nephrotic syndrome. *J. Am. Soc. Nephrol.* 2004;15:722-732.

[21] Weber S Gribouval O, Esquivel EL, Morinière V, Tête MJ, Legendre C, Niaudet P, Antignac C. NPHS2 mutation analysis shows genetic heterogeneity of steroid resistant nephrotic syndrome and low post-transplant recurrence. *Kidney Int.* 2004;66:571-579.

[22] Lowik MM, Groenen PJ, Levtchenko EN, Monnens LA and van den Heuvel LP. Molecular genetic analysis of podocyte genes in focal segmental glomerulosclerosis. *Eur. J. Pediatr.* 2009;168:1291-1304.

[23] Abid A, Khaliq S, Shahid S, Lanewala A, Mubarak M, Hashmi S, Kazi J, Masood T, Hafeez F, Naqvi SAA, Rizvi SA, Mehdi SQ. A spectrum of novel NPHS1 and NPHS2 gene mutations in pediatric nephrotic syndrome patients from Pakistan. *Gene.* 2012;502:133-137.

[24] Tsukaguchi H, Sudhakar A, Le TC, Nguyen T, Yao J, Schwimmer JA, Schachter AD, Poch E, Abreu PF, Appel GB, Pereira AB, Kelluri R, Pollak MR. NPHS2 mutations in late-onset focal segmental glomerulosclerosis: R229Q is a common disease associated allele. *J. Clin. Invest.* 2002;110:1659-1666.

[25] Hinkes B, Wiggins RC, Gbadegesin R, Vlangos CN, Seelow D, Nurnberg G, Garg P, Verma R, Chaib H, Hoskins BE, Ashraf S, Becker C, Hennies HC, Goyal M, Wharram BL, Schachter AD, Mudumana S, Drummond I, Kerjaschki D, Waldherr R, Dietrich A, Ozaltin F, Bakkaloglu A, Cleper R, Basel-Vanagaite L, pohl M, Griebel M, Tsygin AN, Soylu A, Muller D, Sorli CS, Bunney TD, Katan M, Liu J, Attanasio M, O'Toole JF, Hasselbacher K, Mucha B, Otto EA, Airik R, Kispert A, Kelley GG, Smrcka AV, Gudermann T, Holzman LB, Nurnberg P, Hildebrandt F. Positional cloning uncovers mutations in PLCE1 responsible for a nephrotic syndrome variant that may be reversible. *Nat. Genet.* 2006;38:1397-1405.

[26] Boyer O, Benoit G, Gribouval O, Nevo F, Pawtowski A, Bilge I, Bircan Z, Deschenes G, Guay-Woodford LM, Hall M, Macher MA, Soulami K, Stefanidis CJ, Weiss R, Loirat C, Gubler MC, Antignac C. Mutational analysis of the PLCE1 gene in steroid resistant nephrotic syndrome. *J. Med. Genet.* 2012;47:445-452.

[27] Gilbert RD, Turner CL., Gibson J, Bass PS, Haq MR, Cross E, Bunyan DJ, Collins AR, Tapper WJ, Needell JC, Dell B, Morton NE, Temple IK, Robinson DO. Mutations in phospholipase C epsilon 1 are not sufficient to cause diffuse mesangial sclerosis. *Kidney Int.* 2009;75:415-419.

[28] Tunggal P, Smyth N, Paulsson M, Ott MC. Laminins: structure and genetic regulation. *Microsc. Res. Tech.* 2000;51:214-227.

[29] Noakes PG, Miner JH, Gautam M, Cunningham JM, Sanes JR, Merlie JP. The renal glomerulus of mice lacking s-laminin/Laminin β2: nephrosis despite molecular compensation by lamini β1. *Nat. Genet.* 1995;10:400-406.

[30] Wuhl E, Kogan J, Zurowska A, Matejas V, Vandevoorde RG, Aigner T, Wendler O, Lesniewska I, Bouvier R, Reis A, Weis J, Cochat P, Zenker M. Neurodevelopmental

deficits in Pierson (microcoria-congenital nephrosis) syndrome. *Am. J. Med. Genet. A.* 2007;143:311-319.

[31] Choi HJ, Lee BH, Kang JH, Jeong HJ, Moon KC, Ha IS, Yu YS, Matejas V, Zenker M, Choi Y, Cheong HI. Variable phenotype of Pierson syndrome. *Pediatr. Nephrol.* 2008;23:995-1000.

[32] Matejas V, Hinkes B, Alkandari F, Al-Gazali L, Annexstad E, Aytac MB, Barrow m, Blahova K, Bockenhauer D, Cheong HI, Maruniak-Chudek, Cochat P, Dotsch J, Gajjar P, Hennekam RC, Janssen F, Kagan M, Kariminejad A, Kemper MJ, Koenig J, Kogan J, Kroes HY, Kuwertz-Broking E, Lewanda AF, Medeira A, Muscheites J, Niaudet P, Pierson M, Saggar A, Seaver L, Suri M, Tsygin A, Wuhl E, Zurowska A, Uebe S, Hildebrandt F, Antignac C, Zenker M. Mutations in the human Laminin B2 (LAMB2) gene and the associated phenotypic spectrum. *Hum. Mut.* 2010;31:992-1002.

[33] Higgs HN. Formin proteins: a domain-based approach. *Trends Biochem. Sci.* 2005;30: 342-353.

[34] Chhabra ES, Ramabhadran V, Gerber SA, Higgs HN. INF2 is an endoplasmic reticulum-soociated formin protein. *J. Cell. Sci.* 2009;122:1430-1440.

[35] Boyer O, Nevo F, Plaisier E, Funalot B, Gribouval O, Benoit G, Cong EH, Arrondel C, Tête MJ, Montjean R, Richard L, Karras A, Pouteil-Noble C, Balafrej L, Bonnardeaux A, Canaud G, Charasse C, Dantal J, Deschenes G, Deteix P, Dubourg O, Petiot P, Pouthier D, Leguern E, Guiochon-Mantel A, Broutin I, Gubler MC, Saunier S, Ronco P, Vallat JM, Alonso MA, Antignac C, Mollet G. INF2 mutations in Charcot-Marie-Tooth disease with glomerulopathy. *N. Eng. J. Med.* 2011;365:2377-2388.

[36] Winn MP, Conlon PJ, Lynn KL, Farrington MK, Creazzo T, Hawkins AF, daskalakis N, Kwan SY, Ebersviller S, Burchette JL, Pericak-Vance MA, Howell DN, Vance JM, Rosenberg PB. Amutation in the TRPC6 cation channel causes familial focal segmental glomerulosclerosis. *Science.* 2005;308:1801-1804.

[37] Gigante M, Caridi G, Montemurno E, Soccio M, D'Apolito m, Cerullo G, Aucella F, Schirinzi A, Emma F, Massella L, Messina G, de Palo T, ranieri E, Ghiggeri GM, Gesulado L. TRPC6 mutations in children with steroid resistant nephrotic syndrome and atypical phenotype. *Clin. J. Am. Soc. Nephrol.* 2011;6:1626-1634.

[38] Harshman LA, Brophy PD. PAX2 in human kidney malformations and disease. *Pediatr. Nephrol.* 2012;27:1265-1275.

[39] Barua M, Stellacci E, Stella L, Weins A, Genovese G, Muto V, Caputo V, Toka HR, Charoonratana VT, Tartaglia M, Pollak MR. Mutations in PAX2 associate with adultonset FSGS. *J. Am. Soc .Nephrol.* 2014;25:1942-1953.

[40] Mathis BJ, Kim SH, Calabrese K, Haas M, Seidman JG, Seidman CE, pollak MR. A locus for inherited focal segmental glomerulosclerosis maps to chromosome 19q13. *Kidney Int.* 1998;53:282-286.

[41] Kaplan JM, Kim SH, North KN, Rennke H, Correia LA, Tong HQ, Mathis BJ, Rodriguez-Perez JC, Allen PG, Beggs AH, Pollak MR. Mutations in ACTN4, encoding alpha-actinin-4, cause familial focal segmental glomerulosclerosis. *Nat. Genet.* 2000;24:251-256.

[42] Yao J, Le TC, Kos CH, Henderson JM, Allen PG, Denker BM, Pollak MR. Alpha-actinin-4-mediated FSGS: an inherited kidney disease caused by an aggregated and rapidly degraded cytoskeletal protein. *PLoS Biol.* 2004;2:e167.

[43] Michaud JL, Chaisson KM, Parks RJ, Kennedy CR. FSGS-associated alpha-actinin-4 (K256E) impairs cytoskeletal dynamics in podocytes. *Kidney Int.* 2006;70:1054-1061.

[44] Khurana S, Chakraborty S, Lam M, Liu Y, Su YT, Zhao X, Saleem MA, Mathieson PW, Bruggeman LA, Kao HY. Familial focal segmental glomerulosclerosis (FSGS)-linked α-actinin 4 (ACTN4) protein mutants lose ability to activate transcription by nuclear hormone receptors. *J. Biol. Chem.* 2012;287:12027-12035.

[45] Call KM, Glaser T, Ito CY, Buckler AL, Pelletier J, Haber DA, Rose EZ, Kari A, Yeger H, lewis WH, Jones C, Housman DE. Isolation and characterization of zinc finger polypeptide gene at the human chromosome 11 Wilms' tumor locus. *Cell.* 1990;60: 509-520.

[46] Rose EA, Glaser T, Jones C, Smith CL, Lewis WH, Call KM, Minden M, Champagne E, Bonetta L, Yeger H, Housman DE. Complete physical map of the WAGR region of 11p13 localizes a candidate Wilms' tumor gene. *Cell.* 1990;60:495-508.

[47] Jeanpierre C, Denamur E, Henry I, Cabanis MO, Luce S, Cecille A, Elion J, Peuchmaur M, Loirat C, Niaudet P, Gubler MC, Junien C. Identification of constitutional WT1 mutations, in patients with isolated diffuse mesangial sclerosis, and analysis of genotype/phenotype correlations by use of a computerized mutation database. *Am. J. Hum Genet.* 1998;62:824-833.

[48] Moorthy AV, Chesney RW, Lubinsky M. Chronic renal failure and XY gonadal dysgenesis: "Frasier" syndrome – a commentary on reported cases. *Am. J. Med. Genet.* 1987;3:297-302.

[49] Haber DA, Buckler AJ, Glaser T, Call KM, Pelletier J, Sohn RL, Douglass EC, Housmann DE. An internal deletion within an 11p13 zinc finger gene contributes to the development of Wilm's tumor. *Cell.* 1990;61:1257-1269.

[50] Gessler M, Burns GA. Molecular mapping and cloning of the breakpoints of a chromosome 11p14.1-p13 deletion associated with the AGR syndrome. *Genomics.* 1988;3:117-122.

[51] Fencl F, malina M, stara V, Zieg J, Mixova D, Seeman T, Blahova K. Discordant expression of a new WT1 gene mutation in a family with monozygotic twins presenting with congenital nephrotic syndrome. *Eur. J. Pediatr.* 2012;171:121-124.

[52] Shih NY, Li J, Karpitskii V, Nguyen A, Dustin ML, Kanagawa O, Miner JH, Shaw AS. Congenital nephrotic syndrome in mice lacking CD2-associated protein. *Science.* 1999;286:312-315.

[53] Gigante M, Pontrelli P, Montemurno E, Roca L, Aucella F, Penza R, Caridi G, Ranieri E, Ghiggeri GM, Gesualdo L. CD2AP mutations are associated with sporadic nephrotic syndrome and focal segmental glomerulosclerosis (FSGS). *Nephrol. Dial. Transplant.* 2009;24:1858-1864.

[54] Doimo M, Desbats MA, Cerqua C, Cassina M, Trevisson E, Salviati L. Genetics of coenzyme q10 deficiency. *Mol. Syndromol.* 2014;5:156-162.

[55] Ashraf S, Gee HY, Woerner S, Xie LX, Vega-Warner V, Lovric S, Fang H, Song X, Cattran DC, Avila-Casado C, Paterson AD, Nitschke P, Bole-Feysot C, Cochat P, Esteve-Rudd J, Haberberger B, Allen SJ, Zhou W, Airik R, Otto EA, Barua M, Al-Hamed MH, Kari JA, Evans J, Bierzynska A, Saleem MA, Bockenhauer D, Kleta R, El desoky S, hacihamdioglu DO, Gok F, Washburn J, Wiggins RC, Choi M, Lifton RP, Levy S, Han Z, Salviati L, Prokisch H, Williams DS, Pollak M, Clarke CF, Pei Y,

Antignac C, Hildebrandt F. ADCK4 mutations promote steroid-resistant nephrotic syndrome through CoQ10 biosynthesis disruption. *J. Clin. Invest.* 2013;123:5179-5189.

[56] Heeringa SF, Chernin G, Chaki M, Zhou W, Sloan AJ, Ji Z, Xie LX, Salviati L, Hurd TW, Vega-Warner V, Killen PD, Raphael Y, Ashraf S, Ovunc B, Schoeb DS, McLaughlin HM, Airik R, Vlangos CN, Gbadesin R, Hinkes B, Saisawat P, Trevisson E, Doimo M, Casarin A, Pertegato V, Giorgi G, Prokisch H, Rotig A, Nurnberg G, Becker C, Wang S, Ozaltin F, Topaloglu R, Bakkaloglu A, Bakkaloglu SA, Muller D, Beissert A, Mir S, Varpizen S, Zenker M, Matejas V, Santos-Ocana C, Navas P, Kusakabe T, Kispert A, Akman S, Soliman NA, Krick S, Mundel P, Reiser J, Nurnberg P, Clarke CF, Wiggins RC, Faul C, Hildebrandt F. COQ6 mutations in human patients produce nephrotic syndrome with sensorineural deafness. *J. Clin. Invest.* 2011;121: 2013-2024.

[57] Quinzii C, Naini A, Salviati L, Trevisson E, Navas P, Dimauro S, Hirano M. A mutation in para-hydroxybenzoate-polyprenyl transferase (COQ2) causes primary coenzyme Q10 deficiency. *Am. J. Hum. Genet.* 2006;78:345-349.

[58] Ozaltin F, Ibsirlioglu T, Taskiran EZ, Baydar DE, Kaymaz F, Buyukcelik M, Kilic BD, Balat A, Iatropoulos P, Asan E, Akarsu NA, Schaefer F, Yilmaz E, Bakkaloglu A; PodoNet Consortium. Disruption of PTPRO causes childhood onset nephrotic syndrome. *Am. J. Hum. Genet.* 2011;89:139-147.

[59] Mele C, Mele C, Iatropoulos P, Donadelli R, Calabria A, Maranta R, Cassis P, Buelli S, Tomasoni S, Piras R, Krendel M, Bettoni S, Morigi M, Delledonne M, Pecoraro C, Abbate I, Capobianchi MR, Hildebrandt F, Otto E, Schaefer F, Macciardi F, Ozaltin F, Emre S, Ibsirlioglu T, Benigni A, Remuzzi G, Noris M; PodoNet Consortium. MYO1E Mutations and Childhood Familial Focal Segmental Glomerulosclerosis. *N. Eng. J. Med.* 2011;365:295-306.

[60] Akilesh S, Suleiman H, Yu H, Stander MC, Lavin P, Gbadegesin R, Antignac C, Pollak M, Kopp JB, Winn MP, Shaw AS. Arhgap24 inactivates Rac1 in mouse podocytes, and a mutant form is associated with familial focal segmental glomerulosclerosis. *J. Clin. Invest.* 2011;121:4127-4137.

[61] Boyer O, Woerner S, Yang F, Oakeley EJ, Linghu B, Gribouval O, Tete MJ, Duca JS, Klicketein L, Damask AJ, Szustakowski JD, Heibel F, Matignon M, Baudouin V, Chantrel F, Champigneulle J, Martin L, Nitschke P, Gubler MC, Johnson KJ, Chibout SD, Antignac C. LMX1B mutations cause hereditary FSGS without extrarenal involvement. *J. Am. Soc. Nephrol.* 2013;24:1216-1222.

[62] Sarin S, Javidan A, Boivin F, Alexopoulou I, Lukic D, Svajger B, Chu S, Baradaran-Heravi A, Boerkoel CF, Rosenblum ND, Bridgewater D. Insight into the renal pathogenesis in Schimke Immuno-Osseous Dysplasia: A renal histological characterization and expression analysis. *J. Histochem. Cytochem.* 2014. Pii: 0022155414558335.

[63] Cong EH, Bizet AA, Boyer O, Woerner S, Gribouval O, Filhol E, Arrondel C, Thomas S, Silbermann F, Canaud G, Hachicha J, Ben Dhia N, Peraldi MN, Harzallah K, Iftene D, Daniel L, Willems M, Noel LH, Bole-Feysot C, Nitschke P, Gubler MC, Mollet G, Saunier S, Antignac C. A homozygous missense mutation in the ciliary gene TTC21B causes familial FSGS. *J. Am. Soc. Nephrol.* 2014;25:2435-2443.

[64] Gbadegesin RA, Hall G, Adeyemo A, Hanke N, Tossidou I, Burchette J, Wu G, homstad A, Sparks MA, Gomez J, Jiang R, Alonso A, Lavin P, Conlon P, Korstanje R,

Stander MC, Shamsan G, Barua M, Spurney R, Singhal PC, Kopp JB, Haller H, Howell D, Pollak MR, Shaw AS, Schiffer M, Winn MP. Mutations in the gene that encodes the F-actin binding protein anillin cause FSGS. *J. Am. Soc. Nephrol.* 2014;25:1991-2002.

[65] Genovese G, Tonna SJ, Knob AU, Appel GB, Katz A, Bernhardy AJ, Needham AW, Lazarus R, Pollak MR. A risk allele for focal segmental glomerulosclerosis in African Americans is located within a region containing APOL1 and MYH9. *Kidney Int.* 2010;78:698-704.

[66] Limou S, Nelson GW, Kopp JB, Winkler CA. APOL1 kidney risk alleles: Population genetics and disease associations. *Adv. Chronic Kidney Dis.* 2014;21:426-433.

[67] Lipkowitz MS, Freedman BI, Langefeld CD, et al. Apolipoprotein L1 gene variants associate with hypertension-attributed nephropathy and the rate of kidney function decline in African Americans. *Kidney Int.* 2013;83:114-120.

[68] Freedman BI, Kopp JB, Langefeld CD, Genovese G, Friedman DJ, Nelson GW, Winkler CA, Bowden DW, Pollak MR. The apolipoprotein L1 (APOL1) gene and non-diabetic nephropathy in African Americans. *J. Am. Soc. Nephrol.* 2010;21:1422-1426.

[69] Bostrom MA, Kao WH, Li M, Abboud HE, Adler SG, Iyengar SK, Kimmel PL, Hanson RL, Nicholas SB, Rasooly RS, Sedor JR, Coresh J, Kohn OF, Leehey DJ, Thornley-Brown D, Bottinger EP, Lipkowitz MS, Meoni LA, Klag MJ, Lu L, Hicks PJ, Langefeld CD, Parekh RS, Bowden DW, Freedman BI. Genetic association and gene-gene interaction analyses in African American dialysis patients with nondiabetic nephropathy. *Am. J. Kidney Dis.* 2012;59:210-221.

[70] [70] Freedman BI, Langefeld CD, Andringa KK, Croker JA, Williams AH, Garner NE, Birmingham DJ, Hebert LA, Hicks PJ, Segal MS, Edberg JC, Brown EE, Alarcón GS, Costenbader KH, Comeau ME, Criswell LA, Harley JB, James JA, Kamen DL, Lim SS, Merrill JT, Sivils KL, Niewold TB, Patel NM, Petri M, Ramsey-Goldman R, Reveille JD, Salmon JE, Tsao BP, Gibson KL, Byers JR, Vinnikova AK, Lea JP, Julian BA, Kimberly RP; Lupus Nephritis–End Stage Renal Disease Consortium. End-stage renal disease in African Americans with lupus nephritis is associated with APOL1. *Arthritis Rheumatol.* 2014;66:390-396.

[71] Kopp JB, Nelson GW, Sampath K, Johnson RC, Genovese G, An P, Friedman D, Briggs W, Dart R, Korbet S, Mokrzycki MH, Kimmel PL, Limou S, Ahuja TS, Berns JS, Fryc J, Simon EE, Smith MC, Trachtman H, Michel DM, Schelling JR, Vlahov D, Pollak M, Winkler CA. APOL1 genetic variants in focal segmental glomerulosclerosisband HIV-associated nephropathy. *J. Am. Soc. Nephrol.* 2011;22: 2129-2137.

[72] Wang N, Zhou Y, Jiang L, Li D, Yang J, Zhang CY, Zen K. Urinary microRNA-10a and microRNA-30d serve as novel, sensitive and specific biomarkers for kidney injury. *PLoS One*. 2012;7:e51140.

[73] Zhang C, Zhang W, Chen HM, Liu C, Wu J, Shi S, Liu ZH. Plasma microRNA-186 and proteinuria in focal segmental glomerulosclerosis. *Am. J. Kidney Dis.* 2014. pii: S0272-6386(14)01083-X.

In: Nephrotic Syndrome: Etiology, Pathogenesis and Pathology ISBN: 978-1-63482-154-4
Editor: Muhammed Mubarak

Chapter 6

Approach to Renal Biopsy Diagnosis in Nephrotic Syndrome

*Muhammed Mubarak**
Pathology, Histopathology Department,
Sindh Institute of Urology and Transplantation, Karachi, Pakistan

Abstract

Renal biopsy has become an essential diagnostic tool for the investigation of medical renal diseases throughout the world. In general, the approach to renal biopsy diagnosis in the nephrotic syndrome (NS) corresponds to that adopted for the pathological investigation of all medical renal diseases. However, there are some mild differences in the approach depending on the biopsy indications and the prevalent renal diseases and other factors. In fact, NS is the most common indication for performing renal biopsies in nephrology practice worldwide, except for some countries, where asymptomatic urinary abnormalities (AUA), constitute the most common indication. It is well known that the biopsy indications vary from center to center and from country to country and even from one nephrologist to another nephrologist.

In this chapter, we will discuss the approach to be adopted in the interpretation of renal biopsies in patients with NS, both in adults and children. The focus will be on making a complete pathological diagnosis. The final etiological diagnosis of the diseases is beyond the scope of this chapter. The diagnosis of medical disorders of the kidney is a multidisciplinary task; nephrologists and nephropathologists play a crucial role in this task. This chapter is primarily related to the pathological aspects of investigation of the renal biopsy in patients with NS. The extent of pathological evaluation of renal biopsies also varies a great deal. Even in developed countries, the approach to the investigation of renal biopsies is not uniform among the different renal pathology laboratories. The chapter is intended to serve as a general guide to the pathologists and in particular, nephropathologists, to arrive at the best diagnosis of renal diseases causing NS. In

* Address of Correspondence: Muhammed Mubarak, Histopathology Department, Sindh Institute of Urology and Transplantation (SIUT), Karachi, Pakistan, Email: drmubaraksiut@yahoo.com

addition, only the common lesions underlying NS will be discussed. Rare lesions will not be described in detail in the chapter due to the constraints of space.

Keywords: Electron microscopy, immunoflourescence, light microscopy, nephrotic syndrome, renal biopsy, renal pathology

1. Introduction

Nephrotic syndrome (NS) is the most common clinical presenting feature of the medical diseases of the kidney in most parts of the world. [1] It can occur at any age, from the intrauterine life to very elderly and affects both sexes. [2] The gender ratio is slightly skewed in favor of males throughout the world. NS is classified in a number of ways, including the age of onset of NS, therapeutic response to a 4-8 week trial of corticosteroids, and hereditary or acquired types. [3-5] One additional and very important way of classifying NS is as the primary or secondary NS. The latter is also important from the point of view of management of the condition. [6-8] It should be made clear from the outset of this discussion that NS is not a single disease entity; rather it is a clinical constellation of findings which is observed in a wide variety of both primary and secondary diseases of the kidney. [9-12]

Pathologically, among the four components of normal kidney parenchyma, NS is most commonly caused by the diseases affecting primarily the glomeruli, better termed glomerulopathies. This term is preferred to the often used term of glomerulonephritis (GN), which should be reserved for the inflammatory or proliferative diseases of the glomeruli. Only occasional instances of tubulointerstitial or vascular diseases lead to NS. Hence, glomerulocentric approach should be adopted in the assessment of renal biopsies in cases of NS. [13-15] The nephropathology laboratory should have all the necessary diagnostic armamentarium required for a complete investigation of the glomerulopathies. This includes the necessary expertise and equipment for the light microscopy (LM), immunoflourescence (IF), and electron microscopy (EM). [16-18] This requirement is easily fulfilled in developed countries, but remains an uphill task in many developing countries. In the latter situation, establishment of one major national reference nephropathology laboratory where the renal biopsy samples can be referred is a viable option. [19]

The detailed account of the biopsy indications, their procurement, handling and processing is beyond the scope of this chapter. Several excellent reviews on this topic are available elsewhere. [20-22] Detailed consensus guidelines have been published to standardize the approach to renal biopsy handling and processing in the pathology laboratories. [23] However, the actual practice does vary a lot, even in developed countries. [24] A note of caution is warranted here regarding procurement of the renal biopsy specimen. The renal biopsy procedure should be performed as a planned and elective procedure with a technologist from the histopathology laboratory present at the site of biopsy to handle the biopsy material and ensure adequacy of the biopsy sample. The details of this procedure are available in excellent review articles on this topic. [25-28] The point to emphasize here is that it is absolutely essential to do so. Otherwise, adequacy of renal biopsy cannot be guaranteed. The need for adequate renal biopsy material is all the more important for the diagnosis of NS, although, it is also disease-based to some extent. For example, in the case of MGN, the presence of just one glomerulus with the spikes on silver stain is enough to diagnose the condition. But, the diagnosis of the disease is not the sole objective of the biopsy, it also provides prognostic information. The accurate prognostic information can only be provided if there is sufficient cortex in the biopsy. [29] An optimal thickness and quality of staining of the renal biopsy sections is of paramount importance for an accurate diagnosis of the glomerulopathies underlying NS. The ideal thickness of sections is 2-3 um. This is readily achieved in most nephropathology laboratories in temperate climates. However, in tropical regions, attainment of this thickness may be a challenge for the technologists. [30]

2. Etiologic Diagnosis of Nephrotic Syndrome

Ideally, one should aim at the diagnosis of the underlying etiology of any disease, which provides a rational basis for the treatment and cure of the disease. However, this is not always possible and often an empiric approach is utilized for the management of diseases. NS is also no exception to the above general principle. In fact, NS is caused by a large number of both primary and secondary medical diseases of the kidney. [31-35] The common causes of NS in both adults and children are listed in Table 1. The pathologist needs to be familiar with this list and should follow an algorithmic approach for arriving at the best pathological diagnosis. He can render the pathological diagnosis only in the majority of cases. In some cases, the pathologist may be able to arrive at an etiological diagnosis of NS. For example, in cases of membranous GN, the biopsy diagnosis may be that of lupus nephritis (LN), class V. In other cases, the diagnosis of the etiological basis of NS can be further helped by clinical and laboratory investigations, which is the job of attending nephrologist. A close liaison between the pathologist and nephrologist will go a long way in accurately diagnosing the causes of NS in individual cases. [36]

Table 1. Common causes of nephrotic syndrome

Focal segmental glomerulosclerosis (all variants)
Membranous glomerulopathy
Minimal change glomerulopathy
Diabetic glomerulosclerosis
Type I membranoproliferative glomerulonephritis
Idiopathic mesangioproliferative glomerulonephritis
Amyloidosis
C1q nephropathy
Fibrillary glomerulonephritis
Monoclonal immunoglobulin deposition disease
Dense deposit disease (Type II membranoproliferative glomerulonephritis)
Immunotactoid glomerulopathy
Collagenofibrotic glomerulopathy

3. Approach to Renal Biopsy Interpretation

It should be emphasized from the beginning that the pathologist should examine the renal biopsy specimens with the general rule in mind that the common things are common. Our description in this chapter will also follow this principle and only common lesions will be described in detail. The prevalence of various diseases in renal biopsy specimens of nephrotic individuals depends upon the age of the patients biopsied, the part of the world and the local biopsy policies of the center or nephrologists. [37-40] To give an example, in adults with NS, three conditions are common. These are membranous glomerulonephritis (MGN), focal and segmental glomerulosclerosis (FSGS) and minimal change disease (MCD). It is widely known that the syndrome is commoner in developing countries than in developed countries; however, there are often no accurate data on the incidence and prevalence of the disorder in poor countries. [41]

The assessment of renal biopsy sections should be started with the low-power examination of the whole biopsy material available for the study. The presence of cortex and medulla should be noted. The total number of glomeruli should be counted and noted. An assessment of all the four components of the renal parenchyma (of which interstitium is normally just a potential space and not readily visible under the LM) should be made under the scanning objective lens. For NS biopsies, it may be better to start with the silver or PAS stains. Thereafter, high-power examination should focus on the glomeruli to identify the underlying pathological lesions. The focus in cases of NS should obviously be on looking for the glomerular pathology, as glomerulopathies are responsible for the vast preponderance of cases of NS. [42] All the above points should be detailed in the final report. Recently, consensus guidelines have been published for standardized reporting of non-tumor renal pathological lesions. [43, 44]

The common glomerular lesions seen on nephrotic renal biopsies can be broadly categorized into following types:

1. Minor glomerular changes
2. Non-proliferative glomerulopathies
3. Proliferative glomerulopathies or true glomerulonephritides
4. Glomerular infiltration/deposition diseases

Each of the above morphological categories will be described in detail. It is also pertinent to point out here that one disease may give rise to more than one morphological patterns, often in variable combination. This is the reason for the need for a correlative or integrative approach for the diagnosis of glomerular diseases on renal biopsy.

3.1. Minor Glomerular Changes

This term is commonly used synonymously with "minimal change disease", a practice which should be abandoned. The term "minimal change" is in use since the days when EM was not used routinely in the evaluation of renal biopsy specimens from patients with NS and is deeply rooted in nephrology and nephropathology literature. This pattern describes no significant changes in the glomerular appearance under LM (Figure 1) or only minor alterations, such as mild increase in mesangial hypercellularity, mild increase of mesangial matrix and/or focal glomerular basement membrane (GBM) alterations. [45] There is some controversy regarding the degree of mesangial hypercellularity that is allowed in minor glomerular changes, but most authors agree that upto 3 cells in some lobules are allowed (which is in fact upper limit of normal). [11] As noted previously, this glomerular appearance is not pathognomonic of any single disease.

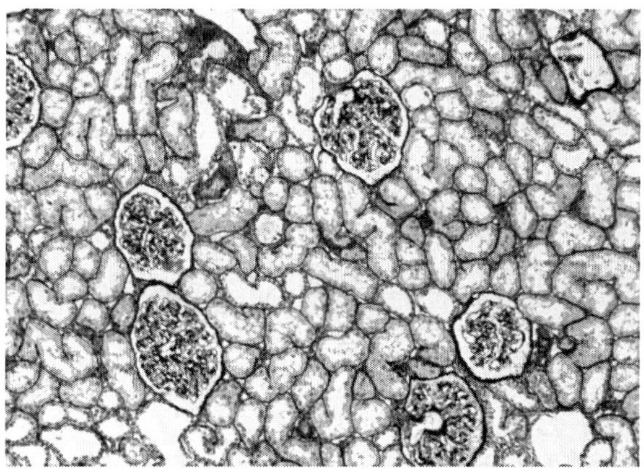

Figure 1. Low-power photomicrograph showing minor changes in all the four components of the renal parenchyma. All the glomeruli show minor changes. There is no tubular atrophy. There is no interstitial inflammation. Arterioles included are also unremarkable. This is a section from a biopsy in a child of 8 years with steroid dependant nephrotic syndrome and will qualify for minimal change disease, provided immunoflourescene is also negative. (Jones Metheneamine Silver, ×50).

Table 2. Causes of minor glomerular changes on light microscopy of renal biopsy

Minimal change disease
Early focal segmental glomerulosclerosis
IgM nephropathy
IgA nephropathy
Lupus nephritis
Alport's syndrome
Thin basement membrane nephropathy
Amyloidosis
Early stage I membranous glomerulopathy

On the contrary, many diseases with variable clinical expressions can give rise to this glomerular morphology (Table 2). Their definitive diagnosis requires, in addition to LM study, a recourse to clinical history, laboratory investigations including serology, IF and EM studies. [10, 11, 16] A listing of the definitive diagnostic tests for an accurate diagnosis of these conditions is also provided in Table 3. An example of a diagnostic approach in such glomerular appearance follows. As is obvious from table 2, MCD is the foremost condition causing this glomerular appearance on LM, especially in children with NS. However, to diagnose MCD on firm footing, there should be an absence of alterations in the other components of kidney, including blood vessels and the tubulointerstitial compartment. All the four components should be unremarkable in a patient with clinical NS before a diagnosis of MCD can be entertained.

Table 3. Common conditions and their diagnostic tests in cases of minor glomerular changes on light microscopy of renal biopsy

Disease	Diagnostic test
Minimal change disease	EM
Early focal segmental glomerulosclerosis	
IgM nephropathy	IF
IgA ncphropathy	IF
Lupus nephritis	Serology, IF, EM
Alport's syndrome	EM
Thin basement membrane nephropathy	EM
Amyloidosis	EM, IHC
Early stage I membranous glomerulopathy	IF, EM

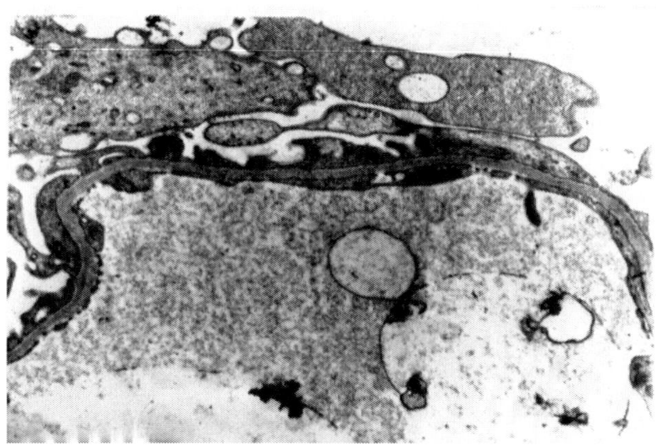

Figure 2. Electron micrograph showing almost diffuse effacement of foot processes. No electron-dense deposits are seen. Glomerular basement membrane structure is normal. (Uranyl acetate and Lead citrate, ×6000).

This diagnosis can be made more confidently in a child with NS and no atypical clinical or laboratory features and highly selective proteinuria and characteristic findings on EM (Figure 2). However, in adult patients with NS and this pattern of glomerulopathy, further investigation with IF and EM is warranted. [10, 11, 16, 46]

There are some other diseases which also commonly present this picture on renal biopsy at least in early stages, but their clinical presentation is different. [47]

3.2. Non-Proliferative Glomerulopathies

This morphological pattern is the one most commonly found on renal biopsies in patients with NS, especially in adults. [11, 48] This appearance describes no significant increase in the glomerular cellularity. However, there are significant changes in the glomerular structure, which are easily identified on LM, such as focal and segmental glomerulosclerosis or diffuse membranous thickening. There may be mild increase in the mesangial cellularity but a marked increase in cellularity of any component precludes this diagnosis. [11] Two broad categories of glomerular morphological changes are noted in this type.

1. Focal and segmental glomerular lesions.
2. Diffuse membranous thickening.

These are described below.

3.2.1. Focal and Segmental Glomerular Sclerosis

This is one of the non-proliferative glomerular patterns observed commonly in NS, the other being diffuse membranous thickening. This is a broad and heterogeneous category caused by a large number of both primary and secondary renal diseases. [49-54] This pattern is characterized by focal (involving some but not all; to be more specific, less than 50% of the glomeruli) and segmental (involving only part of an involved glomerulus) distribution of the pathological lesions. [11, 55] The lesions can be further categorized as proliferative, necrotizing and/or inflammatory or sclerosing in nature with frequent transitions and admixtures of these. Some authors, however, do not distinguish among these categories and use the term "focal glomerulonephritis" for the whole group of lesions. The reason for this is that it is not always possible to clearly distinguish among these categories, or the occurrence of transitional forms in the form of fibroinflammatory lesion. It is, however, always worthwhile to attempt to separate them as this has clinical and therapeutic significance. A correlation of the morphological features, clinical presentation, laboratory features and serology will help in distinguishing among these subtypes in the majority of cases. [56-60]

The clinical presentation of focal segmental glomerulopathies is equally varied ranging from acute nephritic syndrome to nephrotic syndrome to acute renal failure to chronic renal failure. Thus, the clinical presentation is not specific for this morphological pattern. [61]

The histological features of FSGS are also not specific and are seen in many other specific glomerular diseases such as membranous glomerulopathy, IgA nephropathy, Alport's syndrome, hypertension, and pyelonephritis. Hence, it is essential to adopt a correlate at the best clinicopathological diagnosis. [62-65]

From the NS point of view, the most important lesion in this category is that of FSGS, also known as focal segmental hyalinosis and sclerosis (FSHS). This morphological lesion is also heterogeneous with respect to etiology, pathogenesis, morphology, clinical presentation and prognosis. A listing of the common causes of FSGS is provided in Table 4. This lesion is characterized by involvement of some portions of some glomeruli and the involved glomeruli show segmental solidification, i.e., occlusion of capillary lumens by mesangial sclerosis/fibrosis. These tufts look solid on staining with silver and PAS stains with loss of capillary lumens, as shown in Figure 3.

It should be mentioned here that normal glomeruli have a sieve-like appearance resulting from the presence of numerous patent capillary lumens. [11, 61, 65] In FSGS, since these capillaries in some tufts are occluded, the affected glomerular tufts look solid on light microscopy (LM). The solidification is caused by the excess accumulation of mesangial matrix and GBM-like material in the intercapillary spaces with consequent encroachment and collapse of capillary lumens. In early stages, mesangial cell proliferation and hypercellularity may be found. In addition, hyaline deposits are commonly seen in the sclerosed parts of the glomeruli.

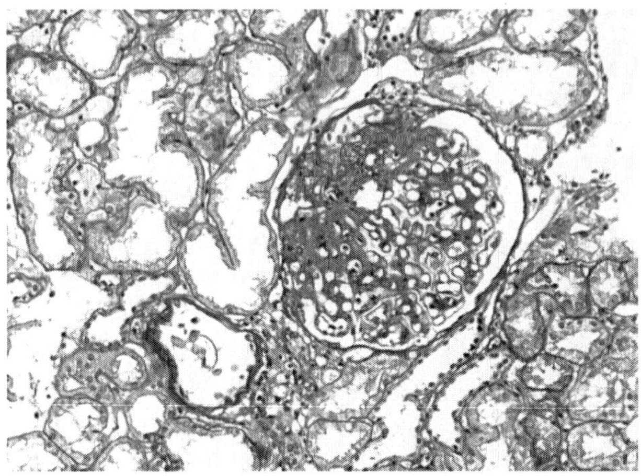

Figure 3. Medium-power view showing an area of segmental scarring and attachment with the Bowman's capsule. The lesion is in continuity of the vascular pole of the glomerulus. In the area of segmental scarring, capillary lumens are obliterated. (PAS, ×200).

Table 4. Causes of focal segmental glomerulosclerosis

Idiopathic or primary focal segmental glomerulosclerosis
Healed focal necrotizing glomerulonephritis
Heroin-associated nephropathy
HIV-associated nephropathy
Long-standing hypertension
Reflux nephropathy /chronic pyelonephritis
Reduced renal mass
Morbid obesity
Alport's syndrome
Sickle cell disease
IgA nephropathy
Membranous GN

These hyaline deposits are seen in the mesangium, in the capillary lumena and also in arterioles beside the glomeruli. The hyaline deposits of plasma proteins that have exuded into the capillary walls or in the interstitium. In many cases, lipid deposits also occur, either intracellularly in the endothelial or mesangial cells, giving rise to foam cells or extracellularly. The sclerosis and hyalinosis commonly occur together. However, the order of first appearance can vary. More commonly, sclerosis precedes the appearance of hyalinosis, however, occasionally hyalinosis may precede sclerosis. In some morphological variants of FSGS, there is expansion of capillary lumena with intracapillary hypercellularity. [11]

The disease process first involves the juxtamedullary glomeruli during the early stages of the disease. Hence, the need for the presence of corticomedullary junction in the biopsy sample to definitively rule out FSGS. In advanced stages, the disease process spreads centrifugally and involves more superficially located glomeruli in the cortex. Within the affected glomeruli, the disease typically starts at the vascular pole and usually on the side of afferent arteriole. Later on, it involves the peripheral lobules of the glomeruli. In advanced stages, the scarring process involves the whole of the glomerulus (global involvement). [56, 65]

The above mentioned segmental intracapillary alterations are often accompanied by alterations in the overlying visceral epithelial cells or podocytes. There can be both a decrease and an increase in the number of podocytes. The location and the quality of the intra- and extacapillary alterations are used to divide idiopathic FSGS into five hierarchical morphological types in Columbia classification. [11, 56] With disease progression, more and more glomeruli are involved in the sclerosing process and more and more of the glomeruli become globally sclerosed. When more than 80% of the glomeruli are involved with advanced glomerular sclerosis, the process is called diffuse chronic sclerosing glomerulonephritis. The glomerular changes described above are accompanied by changes in the tubulointerstitial compartment. Tubular atrophy is one of the early findings on renal biopsy and its presence on a biopsy should lead to a careful search for the lesions of FSGS in the glomeruli (Figure 4).

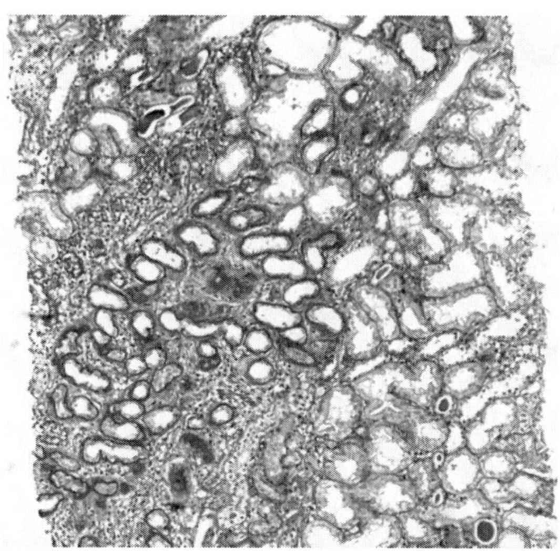

Figure 4. Periodic acid-Schiff (PAS) staining showing area of tubular atrophy, interstitial inflammation and fibrosis. Such features on a renal biopsy are not compatible with a diagnosis of minimal change disease. Instead, the finding of such changes should lead to a careful search for the diagnostic glomerular lesions. (PAS, ×100).

This may require examination of multiple serial sections and in some cases, cutting of the entire biopsy material. In fact, in the presence of tubular atrophy, the diagnosis of MCD is virtually excluded. The changes of interstitial inflammation and scarring parallel those of tubular atrophy. In late stages, vasculopathy also supervenes, culminating in the appearance of end-stage renal disease. [11] Although, FSGS is classified here under the category of non-proliferative glomerular lesions, in a significant number of FSGS cases, there may be mild to moderate mesangial proliferation, as in idiopathic mesangial proliferative glomerulonephritis. This additional feature has no specific clinical or prognostic significance. However, it helps to emphasize another point that in cases of mesangial proliferative glomerulonephritis, a careful search should always be made to rule out FSGS lesions. [11]

3.2.2. Diffuse Thickening of Glomerular Basement Membrane

In this category, all the glomeruli show diffuse thickening of the GBM on H&E staining. This alteration may or may not be accompanied by alterations in the other glomerular components, particularly, mesangial cells and matrix.

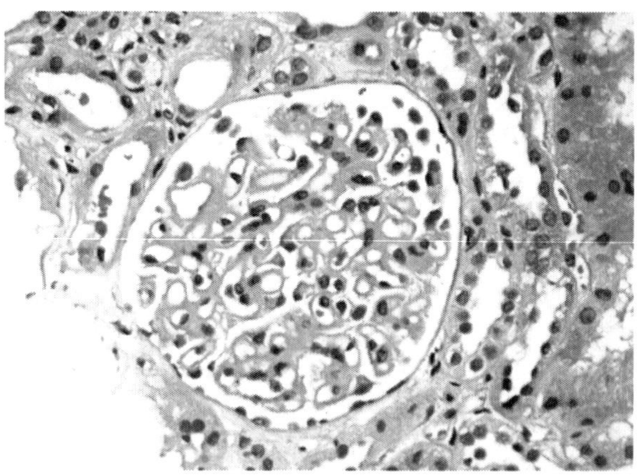

Figure 5. Hematoxylin and Eosin (H&E) staining showing diffuse thickening of glomerular basement membrane (GBM). Capillary walls appear refractile, rigid and taught. (H&E, ×200).

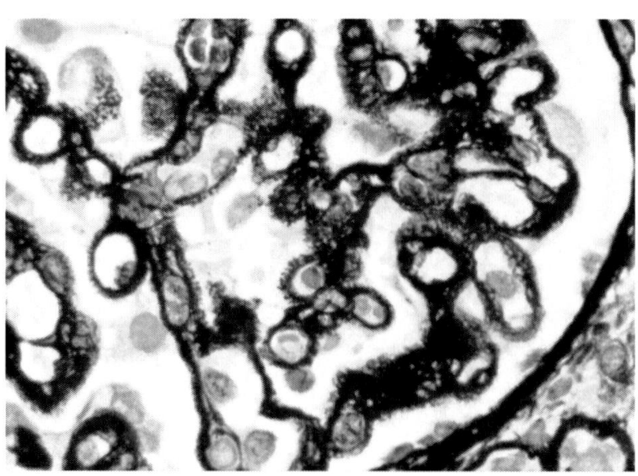

Figure 6. Silver staining showing numerous fine spikes extending outward from the glomerular basement membrane (GBM). These spikes represent extension of the GBM-like material in between the electron-dense deposits, which are not visualized with this stain. (Jones Methaneamine Silver, ×1000).

Table 5. Causes of diffuse glomerular basement membrane thickening

Idiopathic or secondary membranous glomerulopathy
Fibrillary glomerulonephritis
Diabetic glomerulosclerosis
Amyoloidosis
Monoclonal immunoglobulin deposition disease

Table 6. Causes of membranous glomerulopathy

Idiopathic or primary membranous glomerulopathy
Secondary membranous glomerulopathy
Infections
Hepatitis B viral infection
Hepatitis C viral infection
Syphilis
Parasitic infection
Hydatid disease
Drugs
Gold
Lithium
Penicillamine
Nonsteroidal anti-inflammatory drugs
Mercury
Immune disorders
Systemic lupus erythematosus
Rheumatoid arthritis
Sjogren's syndrome
Grave's disease
Mixed connective tissue disease
Neoplasms
Lymphomas and leukemias
Bladder neoplasms
Renal cell carcinoma
Melanoma
Seminoma
Lung cancer
Others
Allogenic hematopoietic stem cell transplantation
Diabetes
Polyarteritis nodosa
Sarcoidosis
Autosomal dominant polycystic kidney disease

This alteration is observed in a small number of renal diseases. [66-70] This alteration on H&E is not by itself diagnostic of membranous glomerulopathy (Figure 5). There are other causes of diffuse membranous thickening, as shown in Table 5. The diagnosis of MGN requires confirmation with silver stain, with the demonstration of spikes on the outer aspect of GBM (Figure 6). The spikes represent projections of GBM-like material outward from the GBM in between the electron-dense deposits. [71] The deposits themselves do not stain with the silver staining methods. The demonstration of the spikes on silver stains is the conclusive evidence in favor of MGN. As for the other patterns of glomerular injury, this membranous pattern may be caused by a number of different diseases, as shown in Table 6.

A pathologist can help in further classification of membranous pattern with the help of IF and EM. However, it should be noted that a pathological diagnosis of MGN is not the end diagnosis and the nephrologists should look for the underlying etiological factors by careful history, examination and laboratory investigations. [72-74]

MGN is the most common cause of diffuse GBM thickening. However, some cases may show focal thickening of the GBM, especially during early stages. In addition, early stages of MGN may not show conspicuous thickening of GBM on tinctorial stains. In such cases, taughtness of the GBM with rounding off of the peripheral capillary walls may provide a clue to the correct diagnosis. In addition, the use of IF and EM will prevent its misdiagnosis as MCD. This early stage is called pre-spike or stage I MGN. [71, 74] The vast majority of cases of MGN is diagnosed in stage II or spike stage. These stages are best diagnosed on EM. In majority of cases of MGN, the lesions involve the GBM, with little or no alteration in the mesangium. Sometimes, however, there may be mild to moderate mesangial proliferation, especially in cases of secondary MGN. Some cases of MGN also show additional glomerular lesions, especially, segmental and global glomerulosclerosis. The glomerular changes are accompanied by tubular atrophy and interstitial scarring as in other glomerulopathies. In advanced stages, the appearances resemble other chronic sclerosing glomerulopathies. [72]

3.3. Proliferative Glomerulopathies or True Glomerulonephritides

These lesions are characterized by focal to diffuse, and segmental to global proliferation of native glomerular cells including endothelial cells, mesangial cells, visceral and parietal epithelial cells. In addition, there can be swelling or enlargement of these cells and infiltration by circulating inflammatory cells. All these processes lead to narrowing or occlusion of capillary lumens and markedly hypercellular appearance of the glomeruli. [8, 10, 11] The proliferative glomerular lesions are usually divided into intracapillary and extracapillary proliferative lesions. Among these, the intracapillary lesions are commonly associated with nephrotic presentation. The extracapillary proliferative lesions or crescents only rarely lead to this presentation and will not be discussed further. The intracapillary proliferative glomerulopathies are divided into the following types:

- Mesangial proliferative GN
- Mesangiocapillary GN
- Acute diffuse proliferative and exudative GN.

Among these the latter subtype typically presents as nephritic syndrome and hence will not be discussed further. The first two conditions are described below:

3.3.1. Mesangial Proliferative GN

This intracapillary proliferative GN is characterized by the proliferation of the mesangial cells and matrix only. This is the milder form of all the proliferative glomerulopathies and usually manifests as proteinuria and/or hematuria. The capillary lumens in this condition remain patent (Figure 7). There is no encroachment of the expanded mesangium on to the capillary lumens. The peripheral capillary walls are not thickened. The degree of mesangial proliferation can be categorized into mild, moderate, or severe types. This pattern is one of the most common glomerular responses to different forms of injury. The most common causes of this reaction pattern are shown in Table 7. These can be further resolved into specific disease entities with the help of history, clinical features, laboratory investigations, serology, IF and EM studies. [11]

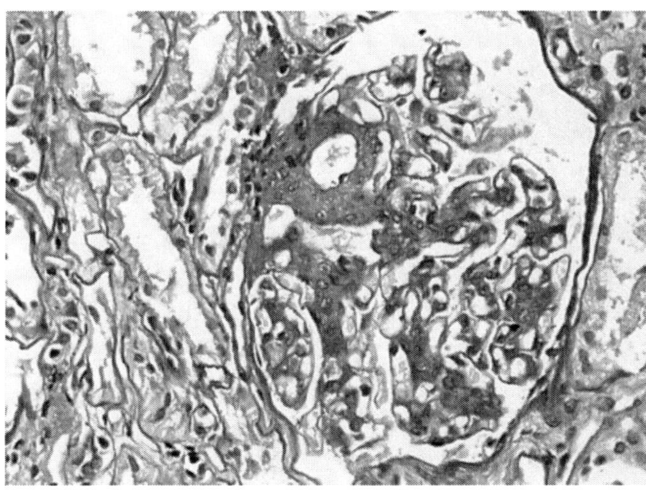

Figure 7. This glomerulus shows mild mesangial proliferation with upto 4-5 mesangial cells in many lobules. The capillary walls are thin and capillary lumens are patent. Bowman's space is empty. (PAS, ×400).

Table 7. Causes of mesangial proliferative glomerulonephritis (MesPGN)

Idiopathic MesPGN
IgA nephropathy
IgM nephropathy
Lupus nephritis, class II
Resolving postinfectious GN
Diffuse diabetic glomerulosclerosis.

3.3.2. Mesangiocapillary GN

This type of intracapillary proliferation is characterized by not only the proliferation of the mesangial structures (hence, mesangio-) but there is also involvement of the peripheral capillary walls (hence, -capillary) or GBMs (hence, clinical term of membranoproliferative GN). In fact this is the involvement of the later structures that distinguishes this pattern from the mesangial proliferative GN. [75-78] The mesangial proliferation is usually of moderate to severe degree. There is also prominence of the lobular architecture of the glomerular structure. [75] The peripheral capillary wall involvement consists of interpositioning of expanded mesangium into the peripheral capillary walls and formation of a neo-GBM like structure on the inside of the original GBM, producing tram-track appearance on PAS or silver staining (Figure 8).

This is because the interposed mesangial cells or their processes or electron-dense deposits do not stain with these stains but the original GBM and the newly formed basement membrane do stain, giving rise to double-countered appearance to the peripheral capillary walls. This also leads to narrowing of the capillary lumens or their occlusion. There is also frequently neutrophil exudation in the capillary lumens, further compromising the capillary lumens. [75-78]

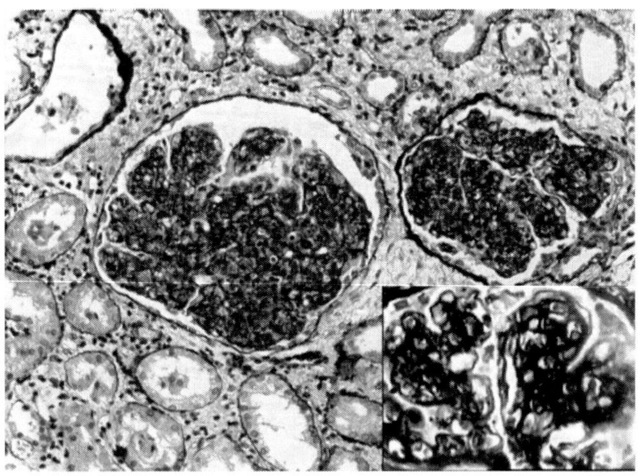

Figure 8. Two glomeruli showing severe and global hypercellularity. The hypercellularity mostly involves mesangial cells. The capillary lumens are obliterated. There is some lobular attenuation. Inset shows double contouring of the peripheral capillary walls. (Jones Methaneamine Silver, ×200).

Table 8. Causes of mesangiocapillary glomerulonephritis (MCGN)

Idiopathic or primary MCGN
Secondary MCGN
Infections
Hepatitis C virus infection
Hepatitis B virus infection
HIV infection
Brucellosis
Tuberculosis
Leprosy
Lyme disease
Malaria
Schistosomiasis
Hydatid disease

Rheumatological conditions
- Systemic lupus erythematosus
- Sjogren's syndrome
- Mixed cryoglobulinemia
- Rheumatoid arthritis
- Sarcoidosis

Neoplasms
- Lymphomas and leukemias
- Plasma cell dyscrasias
- Monoclonal immunoglobulin deposition disorders
- Epithelial tumors
- Melanoma

Chronic liver disease
- Chronic active hepatitis
- Cirrhosis
- Nodular regenerative hyperplasia

Hereditary or genetic
- Hereditary deficiencies of complement components
- Familial lecithin-cholesterol acyltransferase deficiency
- Alpha 1-antitrypsin deficiency
- X-linked
- Autosomal dominant
- Autosomal recessive MCGN type 1

Others
- Addison's disease
- Castleman's disease
- Celiac disease and sprue
- Cushing's disease

The mesangiocapillary pattern is also heterogeneous with respect to etiology, pathogenesis, pathology and clinical presentation. Etiologically, it can be idiopathic or secondary to a wide variety of disease processes, as shown in Table 8. Clinically, the majority of cases present as nephritic syndrome, but upto one third of cases present as NS. [79-81]

4. Mesangial and Membranous Infiltrative/Deposition Disorders

This morphological pattern is characterized by either excessive accumulation of native mesangial extracellular material or deposition of extraneous material in either the mesangium or the peripheral capillary walls, or both. The result is the expansion of the mesangial matrical areas with hypocellular material with variable tinctorial appearances. Although LM appearances of the various disorders in this category are fairly characteristic, further confirmation and definitive diagnosis can be achieved by correlation with history, clinical features, laboratory investigations, IF and EM studies. [82-86] This is the most heterogeneous of the morphological types of glomerular responses and the common causes are listed in Table 9.

Table 9. Glomerular deposition disorders

Amyloidosis
Cryoglobulinemia
Diabetic nephropathy
Monoclonal light chain deposition disease
Heavy chain deposition disease
Fibrillary glomerulopathy
Immunotactoid glomerulopathy

Among these disorders, the most prevalent type in developing countries is the amyloidosis. The other causes are less prevalent and will not be discussed further. Amyloidosis is a fibrillosis characterized by deposition of fine, non-branching fibrillar structures in the mesangium and capillary walls. These give a hyaline, acellular appearance to the glomerular mesangium. Congo red staining and examination under the polarizing microscopy shows characteristic apple-green birefringence. Further typing is done with the help of specific antibodies using immunohistochemistry.

Conclusion

In conclusion, renal biopsy plays a crucial role in the investigation of causes and pathology of the nephrotic syndrome. The pathological examination of renal biopsy is an integrative process, wherein the data obtained by light microscopy, immunoflourescence, and electron microscopy is integrated and correlated with clinical data, laboratory investigations, and serology to arrive at the best possible pathological diagnosis. An algorithmic approach for interpreting the renal biopsy is useful in arriving at the correct diagnosis and to avoid misdiagnosis.

References

[1] Madaio MP, Harrington JT. The diagnosis of glomerular disease. Acute glomerulonephritis and the nephrotic syndrome. *Arch. Intern. Med.* 2001;161:25-34.

[2] Floege J, Feehally J. Introduction to glomerular disease: clinical presentations. In: Floege J, Johnson RJ, Feehally J. editors. Comprehensive Clinical Nephrology. 4th ed. St. Louis, Missouri: Saunders; 2010. p.193-207.

[3] Olson JL. The nephrotic syndrome. In: Heptinstall RH, editor. Pathology of the kidney. 4th ed. Boston; Little, Brown; 1992. p.779-869.

[4] Sinha A, Bagga A. Nephrotic syndrome. *Indian J. Pediatr.* 2012;79:1045-1055.

[5] Brown EA. The nephrotic syndrome. *Postgrad. Med. J.* 1985;61:1057-1062.

[6] Cameron JS. The nephrotic syndrome and its complications. *Am. J. Kidney Dis.* 1987;10:157-171.
[7] Couser WG. Glomerulonephritis. *Lancet.* 1999;353:1509-1515.
[8] Falk RJ, Jennette JC, Nachman PH. Primary glomerular disease. In: Brenner BM, editor. Brenner and Rector's The kidney. 6th ed. Philadelphia: W. B. Saunders; 2000.p. 1263-1349.
[9] Schwartz MM. Nephrotic syndrome and proteinuria. In: Silva FG, D'Agati VD, Nadasdy T. editors. Renal biopsy interpretation. New York: Churchill Livingstone; 1996.p. 115-146.
[10] Lajoie J, Silva FG. Approach to the interpretation of renal biopsy. In: Silva FG, D'Agati VD, Nadasdy T. editors. Renal biopsy interpretation. New York: Churchill Livingstone; 1996.p. 31-70.
[11] Churg J, Bernstein J, Glassock RJ. Renal disease: Classification and atlas of glomerular disease. 2nd ed New York: Iqaku-Shoin; 1995. p. 1-359.
[12] Kumar V, Abbas AK, Fausto N. editors. The kidney. In: Robbins and Cotran Pathologic basis of disease. 7th ed. Philadelphia: W. B. Saunders; 2004.p. 955-1021.
[13] Liebeskind DS. Nephrotic syndrome. *Handb. Clin. Neurol.* 2014;119:405-415.
[14] Certikova-Chabova V, Tesar V. Recent insights into the pathogenesis of nephrotic syndrome. *Minerva Med.* 2013;104:333-347.
[15] Sinha A, Bagga A. Nephrotic syndrome. *Indian J. Pediatr.* 2012;79:1045-1055.
[16] Pirani CL. Evaluation of kidney biopsy specimens. In: Tisher CC, Brenner BM. editors. Renal pathology with clinical and functional correlation. 2nd ed. Philadelphia: JB Lippincott; 1994.p. 85-115.
[17] Bohle A, Aeikens B, Eenboom A, Fronholt L, Plate WR, Xiao JC, Greschniok A, Wehrmann M. Human glomerular structure under normal conditions and in isolated glomerular disease. *Kidney Int. Suppl.* 1998;67:S186-188.
[18] Agarwal SK, Sethi S, Dinda AK. Basics of kidney biopsy: A nephrologist's perspective. *Indian J. Nephrol.* 2013;23:243-252.
[19] Turner DR. Advances in understanding the morphology of glomerular disease. *J. Clin. Path.* 1981;34:1207-1213.
[20] Mubarak M, Kazi JI. Role of immunoflourescence and electron microscopy in the evaluation of renal biopsies in nephrotic syndrome in a developing country. *Ultrastruct Pathol.* 2009;33:260-264.
[21] Furness PN. Best Practice # 160. Renal Biopsy Specimen. *J. Clin. Pathol.* 2000; 53:433-438.
[22] Nelson CL, Mackinnon MWB, Charlesworth JA. Importance of renal biopsy. *Nephrology.* 2001;6:270-273.
[23] Walker PD. The renal biopsy. *Arch. Pathol. Lab. Med.* 2009;133:181-188.
[24] Walker PD, Cavallo T, Bonsib SM. The Ad Hoc Committee on renal biopsy guidelines of the Renal Pathology Society. Practice Guidelines for the renal biopsy. *Mod. Pathol.* 2004;17:1555-1563.
[25] Furness PN, Boyd S. Electron microscopy and immunocytochemistry in the assessment of renal biopsy specimens: actual and optimal practice. *J. Clin. Path.* 1996;49:233-237.
[26] Fogo AB. Approach to Renal Biopsy. *Am. J. Kidney Dis.* 2003;42: 826-836.
[27] Roberts IS, Davies DR. Handling of renal biopsies: different approaches reflect a lack of evidence for what constitutes "best practice". *J. Clin. Pathol.* 2001;54:413-414.

[28] Amann K, Haas CS. What you should know about the work-up of a renal biopsy. *Nephrol. Dial. Transplant.* 2006;21:1157-1161.
[29] Yong JL, Warren BA. A practical approach to the diagnosis of renal disease by biopsy. *Pathology.* 1994;26:370-396.
[30] Furness PN, Kazi JI. Laboratory investigation of renal biopsy specimen. *J. Nephrol. Urol. Transpl.* 1998;1:19-26.
[31] Orth SR, Ritz E. The nephrotic syndrome. *N. Engl. J. Med.* 1998;338:1202-1211.
[32] Eddy AA, Schnaper HW. The nephrotic syndrome: from the simple to the complex. *Semin. Nephrol.* 1998;18:304-316.
[33] Dorhout Mees EJ, Koomans HA. Understanding the nephrotic syndrome: what's new in a decade? *Nephron.* 1995;70:1-10.
[34] Carome MA, Moore J Jr. Nephrotic syndrome in adults. A diagnostic and management challenge. *Postgrad. Med.* 1992;92:209-215.
[35] Fogo A. Nephrotic syndrome: molecular and genetic basis. *Nephron.* 2000;85:8-13.
[36] Gibson IW, More IA. Glomerular pathology: recent advances. *J. Pathol.* 1998;184:123-129.
[37] Schena FP and the Italian Group of Renal Immunopathology. Survey of the Italian Registry of Renal Biopsies. Frequency of the renal diseases for 7 consecutive years. *Nephrol. Dial. Transplant.* 1997;12:418-426.
[38] Naumovic R, Pavlovic S, Stojkovic D, Basta-Jovanovic G, Nesic V. Renal biopsy registry from a single centre in Serbia: 20 years of experience. *Nephrol. Dial. Transplant.* 2009;24:877-885.
[39] Rivera F, Lopez-Gomez JM, Pérez-Garcia R. Frequency of renal pathology in Spain 1994-1999. *Nephrol. Dial. Transplant.* 2002;17:1594-1602.
[40] Mubarak M, Kazi JI, Naqvi R, Ahmed E, Akhter F, Naqvi SS A, Rizvi SA. Pattern of renal diseases observed in native renal biopsies in adults in a single centre in Pakistan. *Nephrology.* 2011;16: 87-92.
[41] Narasimhan B, Chacko B, John GT, Korula A, Kirubakaran MG, Jacob CK. Characterization of kidney lesions in Indian adults: towards a renal biopsy registry. *J. Nephrol.* 2006;19:205-210.
[42] Kashtan CE. Glomerular disease. *Semin Nephrol.* 1999;19:353-363.
[43] Chang A, Gibson IW, Cohen AH, Weening JW, Jennette JC, Fogo AB. A position paper on standardizing the nonneoplastic kidney biopsy report. *Hum. Pathol.* 2012;43:1192-1196.
[44] Chang A, Gibson IW, Cohen AH, Weening JJ, Jennette JC, Fogo AB. A position paper on standardizing the nonneoplastic kidney biopsy report. *Clin. J. Am. Soc. Nephrol.* 2012;7:1365-1368.
[45] Hogan J, Mohan P, Appel GB. Diagnostic tests and treatment options in glomerular disease: 2014 update. *Am. J. Kidney Dis.* 2014;63:656-666.
[46] Deegens JK, Wetzels JF. Diagnosis and treatment of primary glomerular diseases. Membranous nephropathy, focal segmental glomerulosclerosis and IgA nephropathy. *Minerva Urol. Nefrol.* 2005;57:211-36.
[47] Haas M. Alport syndrome and thin glomerular basement membrane nephropathy: a practical approach to diagnosis. *Arch. Pathol. Lab. Med.* 2009;133:224-232.
[48] Alexopoulos E. How important is renal biopsy in the management of patients with glomerular diseases? *Nephrol. Dial. Transplant.* 2001;16(suppl 6):83-85.

[49] Cameron JS. The enigma of focal segmental glomerulosclerosis. *Kidney Int.* 1996;50 (Suppl 57):S119-S131.
[50] D'Agati V. Pathologic classification of focal segmental glomerulosclerosis. *Semin. Nephrol.* 2003;23:117-134.
[51] Barisoni L, Schnaper HW, Kopp JB. A proposed taxonomy for the podocytopathies: a reassessment of the primary nephrotic diseases. *Clin. J. Am. Soc. Nephrol.* 2007;2:529-542.
[52] Thomas DB, Franceschini N, Hogan SL, Ten Holder S, Jennette CE, Falk RJ, Jennette JC. Clinical and pathologic characteristics of focal segmental glomerulosclerosis pathologic variants. *Kidney Int.* 2006;69:920-926.
[53] Shi SF, Wang SX, Zhang YK, Zhao MH, Zou WZ. Clinicopathologic study of different variants of focal segmental glomerulosclerosis. *Zhonghua Bing Li Xue Za Zhi.* 2007;36:11-14.
[54] Haas M, Spargo BH, Coventry S. Increasing incidence of focal segmental glomerulosclerosis among adult nephropathies: A 20-years renal biopsy study. A*m. J. Kidney Dis.* 1995;26:740-750.
[55] Howie AJ. Problems with 'focal segmental glomerulosclerosis'. *Pediatr. Nephrol.* 2011;26:1197-1205.
[56] Noël LH. Morphological features of primary focal and segmental glomerulosclerosis. *Nephrol. Dial. Transplant.* 1999;14 (Suppl 3):53-7.
[57] Daskalakis N, Winn MP. Focal and segmental glomerulosclerosis: varying biologic mechanisms underlie a final histopathologic end point. *Semin Nephrol.* 2006;26:89-94.
[58] Cameron JS. Focal segmental glomerulosclerosis in adults. *Nephrol. Dial. Transplant.* 2003;18 (Suppl 6):vi45-51.
[59] Ichikawa I, Fogo A. Focal segmental glomerulosclerosis. *Pediatr. Nephrol.* 1996;10:374-391.
[60] Diamond JR, Karnovsky MJ. Focal and segmental glomerulosclerosis: analogies to atherosclerosis. *Kidney Int.* 1988;33:917-924.
[61] Thomas DB. Focal segmental glomerulosclerosis: a morphologic diagnosis in evolution. *Arch. Pathol. Lab. Med.* 2009;133:217-223.
[62] Meyrier A. Focal and segmental glomerulosclerosis: multiple pathways are involved. *Semin. Nephrol.* 2011;31:326-332.
[63] D'Agati VD. The spectrum of focal segmental glomerulosclerosis: new insights. *Curr. Opin. Nephrol. Hypertens.* 2008;17:271-281.
[64] Daskalakis N, Winn MP. Focal and segmental glomerulosclerosis. *Cell. Mol. Life Sci.* 2006;63:2506-2511.
[65] Kanjanabuch T, Lewsuwan S, Kitiyakara C, Cheunsuchon B, Eiam-Ong S. Update in pathophysiology and histopathology of focal segmental glomerulosclerosis. *J. Med. Assoc. Thai.* 2006;89 (Suppl 2):S262-279.
[66] Glassock RJ. Secondary membranous glomerulonephritis. *Nephrol. Dial. Transplant.* 1992;7 (Suppl 1):64-71.
[67] Markowitz GS. Membranous glomerulopathy: emphasis on secondary forms and disease variants. *Adv. Anat. Pathol.* 2001;8:119-125.
[68] Cybulsky AV. Membranous nephropathy. *Contrib. Nephrol.* 2011;169:107-125.
[69] Ponticelli C. Membranous nephropathy. *J. Nephrol.* 2007;20:268-287.

[70] Glassock RJ. Diagnosis and natural course of membranous nephropathy. *Semin. Nephrol.* 2003;23:324-332.
[71] Wasserstein AG. Membranous glomerulonephritis. *J. Am. Soc. Nephrol.* 1997;8:664-674.
[72] Mathieson P. Renal disease. II. Membranous nephropathy. *J. R. Coll. Physicians Lond.* 1997;31:133-137.
[73] Honkanen E, Törnroth T, Grönhagen-Riska C. Natural history, clinical course and morphological evolution of membranous nephropathy. *Nephrol. Dial. Transplant.* 1992;7 (Suppl 1):35-41.
[74] Ponticelli C, Passerini P. The natural history and therapy of idiopathic membranous nephropathy. *Nephrol. Dial. Transplant.* 1990;5 (Suppl 1):37-41.
[75] Cattran DC. Idiopathic membranous glomerulonephritis. *Kidney Int.* 2001;59:1983-1994.
[76] D'Amico G, Ferrario F. Mesangiocapillary glomerulonephritis. *J. Am. Soc. Nephrol.* 1992;2(Suppl 10):S159-166.
[77] Nakopoulou L. Membranoproliferative glomerulonephritis. *Nephrol. Dial. Transplant.* 2001;16 (Suppl 6):71-73.
[78] Sethi S, Fervenza FC. Membranoproliferative glomerulonephritis: pathogenetic heterogeneity and proposal for a new classification. *Semin. Nephrol.* 2011;31:341-348.
[79] Alchi B, Jayne D. Membranoproliferative glomerulonephritis. *Pediatr. Nephrol.* 2010;25:1409-1418.
[80] Sethi S, Fervenza FC. Membranoproliferative glomerulonephritis-a new look at an old entity. *N. Engl. J. Med.* 2012;366:1119-1131.
[81] Smith KD, Alpers CE. Pathogenic mechanisms in membranoproliferative glomerulonephritis. *Curr. Opin. Nephrol. Hypertens.* 2005;14:396-403.
[82] Sen S, Sarsik B. A proposed histopathologic classification, scoring, and grading system for renal amyloidosis: standardization of renal amyloid biopsy report. *Arch. Pathol. Lab. Med.* 2010;134:532-544.
[83] Herrera GA, Turbat-Herrera EA. Renal diseases with organized deposits: an algorithmic approach to classification and clinicopathologic diagnosis. *Arch. Pathol. Lab. Med.* 2010;134:512-531.
[84] Iskandar SS, Herrera GA. Glomerulopathies with organized deposits. *Semin. Diagn. Pathol.* 2002;19:116-132.
[85] Joh K. Pathology of glomerular deposition diseases. *Pathol. Int.* 2007;57:551-565.
[86] Joh K. Pathology of glomerular deposition diseases and fibrillary glomerulopathies associated with paraproteinemia and haematopoietic disorder. *Nephrology* (Carlton). 2007;12 (Suppl 3):S21-24.

In: Nephrotic Syndrome: Etiology, Pathogenesis and Pathology ISBN: 978-1-63482-154-4
Editor: Muhammed Mubarak

Chapter 7

Pathology of Idiopathic Nephrotic Syndrome in Children

Shaheera Shakeel and Muhammed Mubarak*
Histopathology Department,
Sindh Institute of Urology and Transplantation (SIUT),
Karachi, Pakistan

Abstract

The nephrotic syndrome (NS) is a clinical complex, characterized by massive proteinuria (>3.5 g/24-hour in adults and in children it is defined as protein excretion of more than 40 $mg/m^2/h$ or a first-morning urine protein:creatinine ratio of 3.5 or greater), which is accompanied by hypoalbuminemia, hyperlipidemia, generalized edema, and lipiduria. Some of these manifestations are clinical while others are laboratory abnormalities. Thus, the diagnosis of NS is a clinicopathological one and the role of pathologists in the diagnosis and management of this condition is enormous. The vast preponderance of cases of NS is caused by glomerular diseases. Glomerular diseases underlying NS can be primary or secondary to systemic involvement of the kidney and are many. These also vary depending on a large number of factors, including the age of onset of NS, geographic location, biopsy policies and other factors. In this chapter, we will present the brief histopathology of the lesions underlying idiopathic NS (INS) in children. A brief account of clinical presentation, course and prognosis of the common entities will also be described.

Keywords: Children, nephrotic syndrome, proteinuria, renal biopsy, pathogenesis, pathology

* Address of Correspondence: Muhammed Mubarak. Histopathology Department, Sindh Institute of Urology and Transplantation (SIUT), Karachi, Pakistan. Email: drmubaraksiut@yahoo.com

1. Introduction

The nephrotic syndrome (NS) is a clinical complex, characterized by massive proteinuria (>3.5 g/24-hour in adults and in children it is defined as protein excretion of more than 40 $mg/m^2/h$ or a first-morning urine protein:creatinine ratio of 3.5 or greater), which is accompanied by hypoalbuminemia, hyperlipidemia, generalized edema, and lipiduria. [1-5] Some of these manifestations are clinical while others are laboratory abnormalities. So, in effect, the diagnosis of NS is a clinicopathological one. The clinical and laboratory manifestations of this syndrome are closely interrelated. The initiating point is mediated by the physicochemical alterations in the glomerular filtration barrier (GFB) leading to increased permeability of plasma proteins across the barrier in urine and hypoalbuminemia. [6-12] This hypoalbuminemia contributes to the development of edema, hypoproteinemia, and hyperlipidemia, the hallmarks of idiopathic NS (INS). [13-20]

Glomerular diseases underlying this clinicopathological syndrome can be primary or secondary to systemic involvement of the kidney. [21-24] The major pathological lesions underlying NS are listed in Table 1. The relative frequencies of different causes of NS vary according to age, geography and socioeconomic status of the affected population. [25-34] Although, these causes are numerous and varied, but only a relatively small number of disorders constitutes the bulk of conditions encountered in clinical nephrology practice. For instance, in children <17 years, NS is almost always caused by primary lesion of the kidney, whereas among adults, it is more frequently secondary to a systemic disease. [21-24, 35]

Table 1. Major causes of nephrotic syndrome in both children and adults

Primary Glomerular diseases
1-Minimal change disease
2-Focal and segmental Glomerulosclerosis
3-Membranous GN
4-Mesangioproliferative GN
5-IgM Nephropathy
6-Mesangiocapillary GN
Systemic Diseases
1-Systemic Lupus Erythematosus
2-Diabetes Mellitus
3-Amyloidosis
4-Malignant Diseases (carcinoma, lymphoma)
5-Light Chain deposition disease
6-Fibrillary GN
7-Immunotactoid GN
8-Miscellaneous (drugs, infections, allergies)

The clinical course and management of NS also vary according to age, treatment strategy of nephrology centers and, last but not the least, the histology on renal biopsies. [36-48] Renal biopsy indications and policies are different in different centers and different parts of the world. In general, renal biopsy is indicated in the evaluation of INS in adults, but in children, often the renal biopsy is deferred because of increased likelihood of response to steroid treatment and likelihood of minimal change disease (MCD) on histology. [49-52]

The histopathological spectrum underlying INS varies according to the age groups. [28, 32, 33, 49] We have previously published the histopathological spectrum observed on native renal biopsies in adults, children and adolescents presenting with INS. [28, 32-33] The relative frequencies of different histopathological lesions according to age groups are shown in Table 2.

Table 2. Relative frequencies of common histopathological entities underlying idiopathic nephrotic syndrome according to different age groups

Histopathological lesions	Children	Adolescents	Adults
Minimal change disease	43.8%	28.9%	14.82%
IgM nephropathy	13.6%	-----	2.9%
Focal segmental glomerulosclerosis	38.14%	36.4%	39.87%
Membranous GN	7.96%		26.58%
Mesangioproliferative GN	4.81%		4.11%
Mesangiocapillary GN	3.14%		4.3%

INS is categorized in a variety of ways. One common classification used in children divides it into five groups: 1. congenital NS, 2. infantile NS, 3. adolescent NS, 4. steroid dependant NS (SDNS), and 5. steroid resistant NS (SRNS). The first three categories are based on the age of onset of NS and the last two on the response to initial steroid treatment. [28, 53-56]

In this chapter, we would like to briefly describe the histopathological spectrum underlying INS in children. A brief description of the etiology, pathogenesis, pathology, clinical presentation and prognosis of common lesions will be presented in the following paragraphs.

2. Minimal Change Disease (MCD)

As mentioned earlier, MCD is the most common glomerulopathy observed in nephrotic children worldwide. However, its prevalence varies according to the clinical course and response to steroid treatment. The peak incidence is between 2 to 6 years.

MCD accounted for 58.7 % of cases presenting with SDNS and 23.2% of cases with SRNS at our center. [28] The most characteristic feature of the disease is the dramatic response to steroids which is remarkable in the majority of cases.

2.1. Etiopathogenesis

There are different hypotheses regarding the etiopathogenesis of MCD including infectious diseases, history of recent immunizations, drugs, allergies, some immune dysfunctions and genetic predisposition. [57-60] the later phenomenon may be related to increased prevalence of certain human leukocyte antigen (HLA) haplotypes or due to mutations in any glomerular protein including nephrin. [61-64] This mutation is responsible for the hereditary forms of congenital nephrotic syndrome (CNS) (Finnish type) with minimal changes in glomerular morphology. Another morphological lesion underlying CNS is the diffuse mesangial sclerosis (DMS).

2.2. Pathology

The morphological hallmark of this entity is the near-normal appearance of glomeruli on light microscopy (LM). Glomerular volume is absolutely normal with thin, delicate, undulating glomerular basement membranes (GBMs) and normal amount of mesangium with ≤3 mesangial cells /mesangial area. This morphologic feature has important impact on the prognosis and clinical course in comparison with mesangial proliferative lesion. [65, 66]

Immunoflourescence (IF) usually demonstrates no immunoglobulins (Igs) or complement deposits. However, IgM deposits can be appreciated in some of the cases with minimal changes on LM. Some authors consider presence of IgM deposits as an epiphenomenon, as IgM is the largest Ig molecule, and is trapped in the mesangial area of the glomeruli. [67, 68] Others consider it as a separate entity from MCD and label it as IgM nephropathy (IgMN). [69-72] Many studies have been conducted on the clinical presentation, course, response to treatment and prognosis of IgMN; however, the controversy surrounding this entity is still far from settled.

On electron microscopy (EM), the principal lesion is found in the visceral epithelial cells revealing uniform and diffuse effacement of foot processes. It is a characteristic finding of MCD on EM, but is not pathognomonic for the disease, as it can be found in any proteinuric state. Thus, the diagnosis of MCD can be considered as one of exclusion. It is therefore necessary to correlate both the IF and EM findings before making definitive diagnosis of MCD.

2.3. Clinical Course and Prognosis

As mentioned earlier, the clinical course and response to steroids is markedly different in MCD as compared with other primary glomerulopathies found in children. We have previously published a comparative study of MCD and IgMN and observed that among children who presented with SRNS, overall 90% in the MCD group and 75% in IgMN group showed response to calcineurin inhibitors (CNIs). [73]

The long-term prognosis of patients with MCD is usually excellent, especially in young children. [73]

Some authors have observed the morphologic transition in cases with a primary diagnosis of MCD. They have demonstrated on follow-up biopsies transitions from minor changes in glomeruli to variable degrees of mesangial proliferation with or without IgM deposits and eventually, full blown focal segmental glomerulosclerosis (FSGS) on histology. [74, 75] The initial description of this morphological transition in MCD was described by McGoven in 1964, who noted that of 39 biopsies with primary diagnosis of MCD, 9 showed FSGS on repeat biopsy. These observations led several authors to think that these three histological lesions, commonly found in pediatric nephrotic biopsies, may represent a continuum of single entity with variable morphological features rather than separate disease entities. [76] These speculations can not be further elaborated without additional insight into the detailed knowledge on the pathogenesis of each entity.

3. IgM Nephropathy (IgMN)

IgMN is one of the common lesions encountered in children presenting with INS. However, there is wide variation in the reported frequency of this lesion (2 to 18.5%) among the native renal biopsy series from around the world. [73, 77-79] The main reason behind this wide variation is that different groups have used different diagnostic criteria and definitions of the disease. We have previously published the largest series of IgMN in children presenting with INS, in which IgMN accounted for 18.5% of all INS cases. [80]

3.1. Etiopathogenesis

The definite etiology of this entity is still unknown. However, it can be a primary disease or IgM deposits can be observed in some systemic disorders, such as, diabetes mellitus (DM), systemic lupus erythematosus (SLE), etc. Before considering IgMN as the primary disease, all other systemic diseases should be excluded by clinical history and serology. Exact pathogenesis of the disease is not known well, despite suggestions from investigations that it could be mesangial response to any inciting immune complex mediated injury. [80-83] The antigens triggering this immune mechanism are not well characterized, but no abnormalities have been detected in IgM molecule itself.

3.2. Pathology

The LM findings of this relatively newly described but not yet fully established entity are diverse ranging from minor changes in the glomeruli to variable degrees of mesangial proliferation and FSGS. Some authors have also observed small cellular crescents or mesangiocapillary proliferation in cases of IgMN. [80-84] Our group has described the first case of IgMN presenting as full-blown crescentic glomerulonephritis. [85] Vasculopathy has been rarely reported in IgMN. Tubular atrophy is usually mild in these cases.

The characteristic IF finding in IgMN is the diffuse and global deposition of IgM in the mesangial and/or membranous areas of the glomeruli. This can be sole immunoreactant or it can be accompanied by subdominant deposits of other Igs or complement components. IgM deposits are not only important for making a diagnosis of IgMN, but their intensity has been shown to correlate with disease activity. [79, 80, 86, 87]

EM is not very helpful in the diagnosis of IgMN as it is entirely based on IF finding. However, small mesangial or paramesangial electron-dense deposits can be found in a variable proportion of cases. These are usually associated with fusion of foot processes and variable degree of mesangial proliferation. [81, 87, 88]

3.3. Clinical course and prognosis

The clinical course, response to steroids and CNIs in IgMN are highly variable. [80, 84, 87, 89] The reason behind the variability is the varying length of follow-up period as well as variable treatment protocols and varying definitions of IgMN employed in different studies. As described earlier, the response to steroids and CNIs is comparatively less favorable in IgMN as compared to MCD. However, some studies have reported 70 to 88% of response rate in children treated with CNIs. A few studies have been published analyzing the correlation of histopathological features with treatment response in IgMN. [80, 88] We have previously reported the comparative study of CNI responders and non-responders, which showed that the degree of mesangial proliferation, global glomerulosclerosis, tubular atrophy and interstitial fibrosis were significantly higher in non-responder group than in the responding group. [80] Smoyer et al. also observed similar findings. [90] The morphological transition of IgMN to full-blown FSGS on repeat biopsies is a well known complication of IgMN. [86, 87]

4. Mesangioproliferative Glomerulonephritis

Idiopathic mesangioproliferative glomerulonephritis (MesPGN) is also one of the common glomerulopathy among children with INS. Its reported frequency varied from 7.2 to 25% throughout the world, which could possibly be explained by the lack of IF or EM studies in some of these studies. [77, 91-92] Thick paraffin sections can also give an erroneous diagnosis of MesPGN. We have previously reported an overall frequency of 4.8% of MesPGN among 538 children with INS. [28]

4.1. Etiopathogensis

Idiopathic mesangioproliferative GN is histologically demonstrated by proliferation of mesangial cells, suggesting the role of several growth factors including platelet derived growth factors (PDGF), interleukin-6 and endothelin 1 (ET-1). [93-95] Reactive oxygen species (ROS) are also increasingly believed to be important intracellular signaling molecules in mitogenic pathways involved in the pathogenesis of mesangioproliferative glomerulonephritis. [96] A few studies have elaborated the pivotal role of ET-1 in pathophysiology of renal mesangioproliferative diseases. Mesangial cells release ET-1 in response to a variety of factors, many of which are elevated in glomerular injury. Mesangial cells also express ET receptors, activation of which leads to a complex signaling cascade with resultant stimulation of mesangial cell hypertrophy, proliferation, contraction, and extracellular matrix accumulation by increase synthesis of fibronectin, type I and type IV collagen by mesangial cells. [94] Some authors have suggested that proliferation of glomerular mesangial cells occurs in response to platelet-derived growth factor (PDGF), and these cells release PDGF and express PDGF A and B chain mRNAs. [93]

4.2. Pathology

The morphological hallmark of this lesion is indicated by the name of the condition, ie. the proliferation of the mesangial components, both the cells and the matrix. However, there is no involvement of peripheral capillary walls, which distinguishes it from mesangiocapillary GN. The capillary lumens are typically patent. There is no endothelial cell reaction or polymorph exudation. The peripheral capillary walls are thin, delicate and single-contoured. This morphological alteration is seen in many diseases, and it is important to exclude other causes of this glomerular appearance, before labeling a case as idiopathic MesPGN. IF, EM, serology and clinical correlation are essential to fulfill the above objective. [97, 98]

The IF study is typically negative in cases of idiopathic MesPGN. In fact, the negativity of immune deposits distinguishes the idiopathic form of this lesion from the more common causes of this lesion, i.e., IgMN, lupus nephritis (LN), IgA nephropathy (IgAN), etc. [97, 99]

The ultrastructural study in idiopathic MesPGN is unrewarding except for demonstrating the mesangial proliferation, which is also obvious on LM. However, it helps to exclude other causes of this pattern. Variable degree of foot process fusion is also noted in the disease, proportionate to the degree of proteinuria.

4.3. Clinical Course and Prognosis

The clinical presentation, clinical course and prognosis of patients with idiopathic MesPGN is variable. [100-107] It may present with either hematuria, asymptomatic proteinuria, or NS. The clinical course is usually self-limited in patients with isolated hematuria, and spontaneous resolution of recurrent episodes of macroscopic hematuria has been observed in some series. [104,105] For patients with asymptomatic proteinuria, a spontaneous decrease in proteinuria occurred and none of these patients developed a progressive course. The clinical course of patients with NS was more or less similar to that usually observed in children and adults with pure minimal change lesions. A complete remission of the NS occurred in most of these patients during treatment with prednisone and cyclophosphamide. Several other studies suggest that children with INS generally have a good prognosis despite of early steroid resistance. [104-106] Despite early resistance to both steroids and cytotoxic drugs, six of seven patients reported by White, Glasgow, and Mills ultimately recovered without evidence for INS. [101] Overall, the outcome and prognosis of patients with idiopathic MesPGN is self limiting and quite good.

5. Focal Segmental Glomerulosclerosis (FSGS)

FSGS is a clinicopathological syndrome characterized by nephrotic or non-nephrotic proteinuria. It has emerged as the leading cause of INS in adult patients worldwide. [33, 108, 109] Pediatric FSGS is also rising in incidence and represents a major cause of chronic kidney diseases. [28, 31, 111, 112] We have earlier reported a frequency of 38.1% of FSGS among 538 children presenting with INS, and it was the second most common lesion underlying NS in that study. [28]

There are several diseases which produce the morphological appearance of FSGS on renal biopsy, referred to as secondary FSGS (Table 3). Idiopathic FSGS is defined by the absence of any antecedent cause. It is now established that idiopathic FSGS is the leading cause of INS in adults and its frequency ranges upto 35% of all biopsies in NS.

It is one of those lesions, for which adequacy of renal biopsy sample is of paramount importance. The lesion can be missed if the number of glomeruli in the biopsy is less or if corticomedullary junction is not included in the biopsy. [113]

Table 3. Classification of FSGS

Primary (idiopathic) (According to Columbia classification)	Secondary FSGS
1-Classic (NOS)	1-Unilateral renal agenesis
2-Cellular	2-Reflux nephropathy
3-Tip	3-Renal ablation
4-Perihilar	4-HIV nephropathy
5-Collapsing	5-Heroin addiction
	6-Morbid obesity
	7-Sickle cell disease
	8-Cyanotic congenital heart disease
	9-Hypertensive nephropathy
	10- Healed focal proliferative or necrotizing GN
	11-Glycogen storage disease

5.1. Etiopathogenesis

The exact cause and the pathogenesis of idiopathic FSGS still remain largely unclear. It is not yet clear whether it represents a separate disease or an evolutionary phase in a subset of patients with MCD. The pathogenetic hallmark of FSGS is the characteristic degeneration and focal loss of podocytes (podocytopenia). The morphological appearances of hyalinosis and sclerosis represent entrapment of plasma proteins in extremely permeable foci with increased extracellular matrix deposition. [114]

As in MCD, discovery of genetic mutations has offered insights into the pathogenetic mechanisms of FSGS. The first gene enumerated in this scenario, *NPHS1*, is found on chromosome 19q13 and encodes the protein Nephrin, which appears to be a key component of the slit diaphragm. The second enlisted gene is *NPHS2*, located on chromosome 1q25-3, which encodes protein Podocin and it has also been localized to slit diaphragm. [115, 116]

5.2. Pathology

On LM, only some of the glomeruli (<50%) are involved and portions of affected glomeruli are abnormal. The sclerotic segments of glomeruli are comprised of collapsed glomerular capillaries, increase in mesangial matrix, adhesions between capillary tufts and Bowman's capsule and segmental insudation of plasma proteins along the capillary walls forming hyaline deposits. Other morphologic features which could be appreciated are segmental or global mesangial hypercellularity with endocapillary foam cells. The morphological features and topography may vary according to different morphologic variants of FSGS. [117]

According to the well known Columbia classification, solely based on hierarchical morphological features on LM, FSGS is divided into five distinct categories: 1-NOS, 2-Perihilar, 3-Cellular, 4-Tip and 5-Collapsing variants. [118-122] Many authors have acknowledged that these variants have different etiologies, pathogenetic mechanisms and diverse clinical behavior in terms of presentation, clinical course, progression of disease and therapeutic response in both adults and pediatric FSGS population. [123, 124] However, some studies have reported conflicting results regarding the predictive values of these variants. We have previously reported the frequency and some clinicopathological characteristics of histologic variants of FSGS in adults and children. [118] Despite of the fact that there were certain limitations in that cross sectional study, we concluded that there is remarkable variation in the prevalence of these variants among different studies from different parts of the world.

IgM and C3 may be found in mesangium or sclerotic areas; however, they do not have great diagnostic significance until and unless there is diffuse, strong mesangial positivity of IgM in mesangium reaching upto the diagnostic criteria of IgMN.

In addition to diffuse effacement of foot processes in both sclerotic and non sclerotic areas, there may be focal denudation of GBM with detachment of overlying visceral epithelial cells. [125]

5.3. Clinical Course and Prognosis

The clinical course of patients with primary FSGS is one of progressive renal dysfunction leading to end-stage renal disease (ESRD) over 5-10 years in more than 50% of cases and recurrence following transplantation has been reported in 15 to 20% of patients. [126] However, a *de novo* form of FSGS in transplanted kidneys has also been described. A major factor prompting the heightened interest in understanding the pathogenetic mechanisms underlying FSGS is the aggressive nature of the disease. Despite the valuable information provided by several studies, which have highlighted the impact of histologic variants on clinical outcome, still there are some controversies regarding definitive predictive value of this categorization.

Schwartz et al. and the South West Pediatric Nephrology study group demonstrated that the pathologic variants have no predictive value for renal dysfunction. In contrast, Douglas, Agati, and Howie et al., described that the type of histologic variant may have significant impact on the clinical outcome as the tip variant predicts a more benign course. Overall, NOS variant had most favorable prognosis, cellular variant portended favorable outcome; however, collapsing variant carried the most guarded prognosis. [127-131]

6. Membranous Nephropathy (MN)

MN is one of the most common causes of NS in adults accounting for 30 to 40% of cases. [132, 133] It is still the leading cause of NS in elderly nephrotics aged more than 60 years. [134] Similar to FSGS, it is a pathologic descriptive term which signifies a glomerular disease of diverse etiology and characterized by diffuse and uniform thickening of GBM due to the deposition of subepithelial immune complexes.

As in FSGS, MN can be associated with numerous systemic diseases like SLE, connective tissue diseases, primary biliary cirrhosis and a variety of identifiable etiologic agents and it is referred to as secondary MN. [135] These associations are enlisted in Table 4. However, the majority (upto 85%) cases of MN are idiopathic and are referred to as primary MN.

Among children with INS, there is relatively lower frequency of MN world wide ranging from 0.4 to 5.7%. [136] We have previously reported the prevalence of 7.9 % and it constituted third most common cause of INS among children despite of the fact that majority of cases of MN presented as adolescent NS followed by SRNS. [28]

6.1. Etiopathogenesis

MN, either primary or secondary, is a form of chronic immune complex-mediated disease. The basic pathogenetic mechanism leading to subepithelial deposition of immune complexes is not yet clearly understood.

It is also not yet clear whether these complexes are formed *in situ* or these are circulating immune complexes that become deposited in that location. Some specific antigens that are responsible for these antigen antibody complexes are recognized in secondary MN, for example: Hepatitis B surface antigen, and thyroglobulin, which is an endogenous antigen. However, antigens involved in primary MN are largely unknown. Some authors suggest that these antigen antibody complexes evoke activation of membrane attacking complex (MAC) comprising C5b-C9, which in turn leads to activation of glomerular epithelial and mesangial cells and release of proteases that are responsible for protein leakage and capillary wall injury. [137-139]

Table 4. Systemic diseases associated with secondary Membranous nephropathy

A-Infections
1-Hepatitis B and C
2-Syphilis
3-Schistosomiasis
4-Malaria
5-Filariasis
6-Hydatid disease
7-Brucellosis
8-Endocarditis

B-Neoplasms:
1-Carcinoma (lung, GIT, breast, kidney)
2-Melanoma
3-Seminoma
4-Lymphoma (NHL)
5-Leukemia

C-Immunologic disorders:
1-Systemic Lupus Erythematosus
2-Connective tissue disorder
3-Systemic Scleroderma
4-Reuhmatoid Arthritis
5-Myasthenia Gravis
6-Hashimoto's Thyroiditis
7-Graves disease
8-Primary Biliary Cirrhosis
9-Autoimmune enteropathy
10-Sarcoidosis
11-Bullous Pemphigoid

D-Drugs:
1-Nonsteroidal anti-inflammatory drugs
2-Penicillamine
3-Gold
4-Mercury
5-Captopril
6-Lithium
7-Diclofenic

E-Miscellaneous:
1-Denovo renal allograft
2-Diabetes Mellitus
3-Primary sclerosing cholangitis
4-Kimura's disease
5-Renal vein thrombosis
6-Anti-GBM disease
7-Cryoglobulinemia
8-Gullian Bare Syndrome

6.2. Pathology

The morphologic features of glomerular capillary walls have been used to describe four histopathologic stages of the disease. [140]

Stage I

The glomeruli appear normal by LM with no significant increase in thickness of the GBM, which could be easily mislabeled as MCD if no parallel IF and EM findings are incorporated to reach the final diagnosis. EM is quite important and helpful in this regard. At this morphologic stage of MN, relatively sparse, small homogenous or uniform immune complex deposits have been found between epithelial cells and lamina densa of the GBM with obliteration of overlying foot processes. Because these deposits are small and irregularly deposited, their visibility by LM is limited. Higher magnification may reveal small focal spikes on silver stain and small red subepithelial deposits with Trichrome stain. [141-143]

Stage II

In this histopathologic stage, the capillary walls are thickened and numerous subepithelial deposits are present with lateral extensions of basement membrane that occasionally bridge over the deposits and this basement membrane could be remarkably appreciated on silver stain (GMS) as capillary loops covered with spikes. These spikes are composed of collagenous and non-collagenous extracellular matrix, hence creating impression on silver impregnation. The immune deposits are not visualized; they are partially embedded within the substance of GBM. [142-144].

Stage III

With the advancement of disease, subepithelial deposits are completely surrounded by newly formed basement membrane leading to narrowing of the capillary lumens, in addition to laying down of newly formed GBM over these deposits. These deposits gradually sink deeper into GBM and become intramembranous deposits. Gartener [145] divided these intramembranous deposits into the electron dense stage and the second in which these deposits loose their electron density and can no longer be identified in their lacunae. Correspondingly, due to loss of electron density, the Heidenhain and Trichrome stains do not stain these deposits well or at all. In fact, the majority of cases of MN present a mixed appearance and the morphologic classification requires careful judgment as to the dominant pattern.

Stage IV

As it was originally described by Ehrenreich and Churg, that stage III MN leads to stage IV with irregular thickening of GBM that contains neither electron dense deposits nor lacunae. [146, 147] The exact morphologic definition of stage IV is a major point of contention. According to some authors, stage IV is morphologically equivalent to progression of disease into ESRD.

Ehrenreich and Churg have also described stage V characterized by capillary collapse, adhesions, focal mesangial hypercellularity, crescents and sclerosis. [146, 147] At this stage of disease, the diagnosis of MN is possible only in the presence of focal classic areas of stage II, III or IV MN.

6.3. Clinical Course and Prognosis

MN is classically very slowly progressive disease. [148] Secondary MN may have relatively protracted course if underlying disease is treated. Segmental sclerosis, crescents, and prominent tubular atrophy associated with interstitial fibrosis are the morphologic indicators of unfavorable prognosis. MN may be complicated by collapsing variant of FSGS, also in HIV negative patients. [149] Among the clinical features, a high blood pressure, and very high and persistent proteinuria, portend rapidly progressive disease.

Other factors influencing progression of disease are numerous including age, renal function at presentation and interaction between gene polymorphisms, such as those of the renin-angiotensin system (RAS) and nitric oxide (NO) synthase. [133, 150] Further detailed insight into the molecular factors by molecular biologic techniques may help in further subclassification as well as more accurate prediction of prognosis.

However, in children the prognosis seems relatively better than adults; some authors have even described excellent prognosis in children. [151]

7. Membranoproliferative Glomerulonephritis (MPGN)

MPGN and mesangiocapillary GN (MCGN) are synonymous terminologies used to designate a glomerular lesion characterized by combination of alterations in the peripheral capillary walls, mesangial proliferation and leukocyte infiltration. MPGN accounts for 10 to 20% of cases of NS in children and young adults. [33, 112, 152] However, some of the patients present with non-nephrotic range proteinuria or hematuria and some may present with combined nephrotic and nephritic picture. Like many other glomerulopathies, MPGN may be idiopathic (primary) or associated with other systemic disorders.

The frequency of MPGN varies widely throughout the world with markedly high rates reported from Turkey, Thailand and New Zealand. We have previously reported the frequency of 3.14% of MPGN among children with INS at our center. [112] Primary MPGN is classified into type I and type II MPGN based on characteristic ultrastructural, IMF and pathologic findings. [154, 156, 157] Some authors further classify MPGN into very uncommon and controversial variant, type III MPGN.

7.1. Etiopathogenesis

In type I MPGN, there is evidence of immune complex deposition in the glomeruli and activation of both the classic and the alternative complement pathways; in type II, there is activation of the alternative complement pathway. [157-161]

7.1.1. Type I MPGN

Although type I MPGN has been recorded in patients of all ages, it is most commonly described in children. [162] As mentioned earlier, its clinical presentation is variable. In addition to the above mentioned presenting features, hypertension is commonly present at the time of clinical onset but usually of mild degree. Hypocomplementemia is also observed including the serum concentrations of early (C1q, C4 and C2) and terminal (C5-C9) components of classic pathway as well as some factors of alternative pathway. [156, 159]

7.1.1.1. Pathology

On LM, glomeruli show characteristic uniform and usually global increase in glomerular capillary tuft cellularity within each glomerular lobule creating an accentuation of the lobular configuration. It has been suggested that the severity of the mesangial lesions relates to the duration of renal disease and with the progression of the disease, cellularity tends to diminish, being replaced by mesangial sclerosis. Approximately one fourth of cases show exudative form with marked polymorphonuclear infiltration. Some studies have observed that largest number of monocytes were noted in biopsies with glomerular hypercellularity and largest number of subendothelial and subepithelial deposits. [163] There is lobular prominence in the glomeruli resulting from circumferential interpositioning of the mesangium into the peripheral capillary walls and marked diffuse thickening of glomerular capillary walls which can be best appreciated on silver stains. [142] The thickened capillary walls often have two basement membranes with nonargyrophilic region between them. This imparts double contour appearance which is sometimes termed as splitting, tram tracking or duplication of the GBM. [164]

Other morphologic features which may also be observed in MPGN type I include crescent formation, which may be found in approximately 10% of cases. [165] In several studies of crescentic GN in children, many cases stem from underlying MPGN type I and crescents are often indicative of poor prognosis. [166] A few reports have been published describing focal or segmental MPGN I, that is, only some glomeruli show lesion, while others do not. [166] However, there are observations that focal MPGN may progress to classic MPGN or classic MPGN may regress to focal MPGN, indicating the heterogeneity of the process. [153, 154]

In patients with nephrotic-range proteinuria, molecular alterations of slit diaphragm followed by podocyte detachment, hypertrophy and even death are also observed if early damage is not recovered.

The predominant pattern observed on IF in MPGN type I is intense, diffuse, positivity of IgG and C3 along peripheral capillary walls. In C3, mesangial positivity may also be observed, but it is nonspecific and inconsistent finding. [167] Other immunoglobulins including IgM and IgA may also show positivity in the mesangium.

EM remains cornerstone in the diagnosis and classification of MPGN. In type I, there is increase in the mesangial matrix and cellularity with large discrete, electron dense subendothelial deposits. [168]

7.1.1.2. Clinical Course and Prognosis

The clinical course is quite variable but often progressive and overall prognosis is poor. ESRD results in a significant number of patients. No major differences have been found in clinical outcome between children and adults with slight variation among survival rates. [161] Among clinical parameters, the presence of NS at presentation, initial deranged renal functions and hypertension were reported by some authors as indicators of poor prognosis. [167] However, there is some disagreement regarding these findings. Morphologic indicators of poor renal prognosis are also not absolute. Crescents, glomerulosclerosis and finding of tubulointerstitial injury have been thought to signal dismal prognosis. [165] As mentioned earlier, focal MPGN may progress to diffuse MPGN; however, Watson et al., suggested that patients with focal duplication of GBM had favorable outcome as compared to those with more diffuse disease. [169]

7.1.2. MPGN Type II (Dense Deposit Disease)

It is a distinct entity from type I, only resembling type I on LM. It is less common than type I and type III accounting for 5 to 33% of total cases of MPGN. [161] The majority of cases are reported in adults but children younger than 5 years have also been described. The clinical presentation is quite similar to type I, hence, it is impossible to distinguish it from type I on clinical grounds alone. Hypocomplementemia (low C3) is observed in many cases but in contrast to type I, C4 and C1q are usually normal. [170]

7.1.2.1. Pathology

The LM findings in type II are variable with an inconsistent degree of mesangial hypercellularity. At one extreme, the glomeruli appear almost normal on LM with mild hypercellularity and some capillary wall thickening and on the other hand marked hypercellularity and diffuse proliferative pattern may be observed. The GBMs are thickened and highly refractile and eosinophilic giving appearance of string of sausages. The deposits give ribbon like fuschinophilic staining along all of the capillary walls on trichrome stain corresponding to deposits seen by EM. [170] Similar deposits could be identified along proximal and distal tubular basement membranes. With progression of the disease, the glomeruli undergo sclerosis and tubulointerstitial atrophy with interstitial fibrosis also develops with advancement of the disease. [170, 171]

On IF study, intense, diffuse, global staining of C3 is noted in the mesangium as rings as well as pseudolinear or ribbon like (rail road tracks) positivity along glomerular capillary walls. Some authors have described that these rail road tracks and mesangial rings represent deposition of C3 along margins but not within central portions of large intramembranous or mesangial deposits suggesting the view that the complement system was activated at the edge of intramembranous deposits rather than within the deposits. This staining pattern is not found in type I MPGN. [167]

The hallmark ultrastructural feature of this disease is the presence of dense osmiophilic transformation of the GBM, basal lamina of the Bowman's capsule, tubular basement membranes and the mesangium. Hence the disease is labeled as dense deposit disease (DDD). Its confirmation requires EM, although suspicion can be made on the basis of LM and IF findings. These deposits appear as large, discrete subepithelial humps/deposits in addition to dense intramembranous deposits with effacement of overlying foot processes. [172]

7.1.2.2. Clinical Course and Prognosis

The long-term prognosis of patients with DDD is overall poor with gradual progression to ESRD. [161, 173] In several reported series among children with DDD, most patients developed ESRD over a varying time period. The clinical features that are suggestive of poor renal prognosis are absence of remission during the course of the disease, the presence of gross hematuria and the presence of NS. The histologic indicators include glomerulosclerosis, degree of mesangial hypercellularity with lobulation, mesangial sclerosis and presence of mesangial deposits. The overall prognosis of DDD is not significantly different from type I MPGN. [174]

7.1.3. MPGN Type III

It is a very uncommon and a controversial variant of MPGN, of which two morphologic subtype variants have been described. [175, 176] First subtype described by Burkholder et al., is a mixed membranous and proliferative GN. In this pattern, some features of typical MPGN type I, such as double contours, mesangial interpositioning and subendothelial deposits are observed in addition to silver positive spikes along the outer GBM and Trichrome positive subepithelial humps such as found in stage II MN. Ultrastructural studies confirm the presence of glomerular electron dense deposits. [177] Many renal pathologists consider it to be a variant of MPGN type I with an extreme degree of glomerular subepithelial immune complex deposition. Another form of type III MPGN is often called MPGN type III of Strife is characterized by distinctive pattern of GBM disruption observed by EM. [178]

7.1.3.1. Pathology

LM findings include varying degree of mesangial hypercellularity, more diffuse thickening of the peripheral capillary walls than type I and DDD. [176] There are some similarities in comparative morphologic analysis of type I, II and III. Some authors noted less pronounced mesangial hypercellularity and enlargement in type III as compared to type I, while others observed greater cellularity as compared to type II. Subepithelial spikes were more commonly found in type III as compared to other types.

On IF, C3 is found in a finely granular pattern along capillaries as well as in the mesangium. C4 is rarely present (but is usually present in type I). [167]

On ultrastructural study, in MPGN type III of Burkholder, the deposits are electron dense like those of MPGN type I or MN. In MPGN type III of Strife, the deposits have a washed out electron lucent appearance. The complex lesion of GBM unique to type III, appears to arise from several generations of subepithelial and subendothelial deposits in addition to several interruptions of the lamina densa.

In contrast to type III of Burkholder, spikes and subepithelial deposits are less common in type III of Strife. The remnant GBM is quite argyrophilic but contains numerous large and sometimes confluent deposits leading to complex disruptions of the lamina densa. [179, 180]

7.1.3.2. Clinical Course and Prognosis

Most of the patients present clinically with incidental finding of hematuria and non-nephrotic proteinuria in otherwise healthy individuals which suggests that onset remains subclinical for some time; however, NS is also common presenting feature.

Several authors have observed that a presentation with NS, hypertension or impaired renal functions at the time of biopsy, is harbinger of poor prognosis. [169] Survival analysis reveals more guarded prognosis for long-term renal survival in patients with type III as compared to type II. [181-183] No study has been published comparing the clinical course, prognosis and outcome among two subtypes of type III MPGN.

Conclusion

In conclusion, the pathology of NS in children is quite varied. However, a handful of lesions account for the majority of the lesions underlying INS in children. An integrated approach can be helpful in correctly diagnosing the underlying pathology of INS in children.

References

[1] Neverov NI, Srinivas KV. Nephrotic hyperlipidemia and its clinical significance. *Ter. Arkh.* 1990;62:150-153.

[2] Thabet MA, Salcedo JR, Chan JC. Hyperlipidemia in childhood nephrotic syndrome. *Pediatr. Nephrol.* 1993;7:559-566.

[3] Wheeler DC, Bernard DB. Lipid abnormalities in the nephrotic syndrome: causes, consequences, and treatment. *Am. J. Kidney Dis.* 1994;23:331-346.

[4] Davin JC, Rutjes NW. Nephrotic Syndrome in Children: From Bench to Treatment. *Int. J. Nephrol.* 2011:372304.

[5] Egli F. Nephrotic syndrome in childhood. *Ther. Umsch.* 1983;40:402-410.

[6] Sharma A, Gupta R, Bagga A, Dinda AK. Glomerular filtration barrier in pediatric idiopathic nephrotic syndrome. *Saudi J. Kidney Dis. Transpl.* 2013;24:286-291.

[7] Siddall EC, Radhakrishnan J. The pathophysiology of edema formation in the nephrotic syndrome. *Kidney Int.* 2012;82:635-642.

[8] Sahali D, Sendeyo K, Mangier M, Audard V, Zhang SY, Lang P, Ollero M, Pawlak A. Immunopathogenesis of idiopathic nephrotic syndrome with relapse. *Semin. Immunopathol.* 2014;36:421-429.

[9] Tsuruya K. Pathogenesis and management of minimal change nephrotic syndrome. *Nihon. Naika. Gakkai. Zasshi.* 2013;102:1105-1113.

[10] Certikova-Chabova V, Tesar V. Recent insights into the pathogenesis of nephrotic syndrome. *Minerva Med.* 2013;104:333-347.

[11] Kruger D. The pathophysiology, diagnosis, and management of proteinuria. *JAAPA.* 2012;25:32-37.

[12] Rondon-Berrios H. New insights into the pathophysiology of oedema in nephrotic syndrome. *Nefrologia.* 2011;31:148-154.

[13] Kashtan CE, Segal Y. Glomerular basement membrane disorders in experimental models for renal diseases: impact on understanding pathogenesis and improving diagnosis. *Contrib. Nephrol.* 2011;169:175-182.

[14] Zhang Sy, Audard V, Fan Q, Pawlak A, Lang P, Sahali D. Immunopathogenesis of idiopathic nephrotic syndrome. *Contrib. Nephrol.* 2011;169:94-106.

[15] Ducloux D. Physiopathology and treatment of nephrotic syndrome complications. *Nephrol. Ther.* 2011;7:52-57.

[16] Audard V, Ory V, Zhang SY, Candelier M, Pawlak A, Lang P, Sahali D. Recent advances in the pathophysiology of idiopathic nephrotic syndrome. *Arch. Pediatr.* 2009;16:793-795.

[17] Bruneau S, Dantal J. New insights into the pathophysiology of idiopathic nephrotic syndrome. *Clin. Immunol.* 2009;133:13-21.

[18] Kawachi H, Suzuki K, Miyauchi N, Hashimoto T, Otaki Y, Shimizu F. Slit diaphragm dysfunction in proteinuric states: identification of novel therapeutic targets for nephrotic syndrome. *Clin. Exp. Nephrol.* 2009;13:275-280.

[19] Zacchia M, Trepiccione F, Morelli F, Pani A, Capasso G. Nephrotic syndrome: new concepts in the pathophysiology of sodium retention. *J. Nephrol.* 2008;21:836-842.

[20] Tesar V, Zima T. Recent progress in the pathogenesis of nephrotic proteinuria. *Crit. Rev. Clin. Lab. Sci.* 2008;45:139-220.

[21] Fukuoka K, Nakabayashi K. Secondary nephrotic syndrome due to collagen disease and vasculitis. *Nihon. Rinsho.* 2004;62:1898-1906.

[22] Ozkok A, Yildiz A. Hepatitis C virus associated glomerulopathies. *World J. Gastroenterol.* 2014;20:7544-7554.

[23] Philipneri M, Bastani B. Kidney disease in patients with chronic hepatitis C. *Curr. Gastroenterol. Rep.* 2001;3:79-83.

[24] Yoshida A, Morozumi K, Takeda A, Koyama K. Nephropathy in patients with mixed connective tissue disease. *Ryumachi.* 1994;34:976-980.

[25] Ingulli E, Tejani A. Racial differences in the incidence and renal outcome of idiopathic focal segmental glomerulosclerosis in children. *Pediatr. Nephrol.* 1991;5:393-397.

[26] Habib R, Kleinknecht C. The primary nephrotic syndrome of childhood: Classification and clinicopathologic study of 406 cases. *Pathol. Annu.* 1971;6:417-474.

[27] McKinney PA, Feltbower RG, Brocklebank JT, Fitzpatrick MM.Time trends and ethnic patterns of childhood nephrotic syndrome in Yorkshire, UK. *Pediatr. Nephrol.* 2001; 16:1040-1044.

[28] Mubarak M, Kazi JI, Shakeel S, Lanewala Ali, Hashmi S. The Spectrum of Histopathological Lesions in Children Presenting with Steroid-Resistant Nephrotic Syndrome at a Single Center in Pakistan. *ScientificWorldJournal.* 2012;2012:681802.

[29] Olowu WA, Adelusola KA, Adefehinti O. Childhood idiopathic steroid resistant nephrotic syndrome in Southwestern Nigeria. *Saudi J. Kidney Dis. Transpl.* 2010; 21:979-990.

[30] Kari JA, Halawani M, Mokhtar G, Jalalah SM, Anshasi W. Pattern of steroid resistant nephrotic syndrome in children living in the kingdom of Saudi Arabia: a single center study. *Saudi J. Kidney Dis. Transpl.* 2009;20:854-857.

[31] Ali A, Ali MU, Akhtar SZ. Histological pattern of paediatric renal diseases in northern Pakistan. *J. Pak. Med. Assoc.* 2011;61:653-658.

[32] Shakeel S, Mubarak M, Kazi JI. Frequency and clinicopathological correlations of histopathological variants of idiopathic focal segmental glomerulosclerosis in nephrotic adolescents. *J. Pak. Med. Assoc.* 2014;64:322-326.

[33] Kazi JI, Mubarak M, Ahmed E, Akhter F, Naqvi SA, Rizvi SA. Spectrum of glomerulonephritides in adults with nephrotic syndrome in Pakistan. *Clin. Exp. Nephrol.* 2009;13:38-43.

[34] Mundi I, D'Cruz S, Punia RP, Kaur R, Sachdev A. Clinico-pathological study of glomerular diseases in patients with significant proteinuria in North India. *Saudi J. Kidney Dis. Transpl.* 2014;25:443-449.

[35] Skrzypczyk P, Panczyk-Tomaszewska M, Roszkowska-Blaim M, Wawer Z, Bienias B, Zajgzkowska M, Kilis-Pstrusinska K, Jakubowska A, Szczepaniak M, Pawlak-Bratkowska M, Tkaczyk M. Long-term outcomes in idiopathic nephrotic syndrome: from childhood to adulthood. *Clin. Nephrol.* 2014;81:166-173.

[36] Horvatic I, Tisljar M, Bulimbasic S, Bozic B, Galesic Ljubanovic D, Galesic K. Epidemiologic data of adult native biopsy-proven renal diseases in Croatia. *Int. Urol. Nephrol.* 2013;45:1577-1587.

[37] Stanković N, Vlahović P, Savić V. Histomorphological and clinical study of primary and secondary glomerulopathies in Southeast Serbia (20-year period of analysis). *Vojnosanit. Pregl.* 2013;70:1085-1090.

[38] Barnett HL, Edelmann CM, Greifer I. The primary nephrotic syndrome in children. Identification of patients with minimal change nephrotic syndrome from initial response to prednisone. A report of the international study of kidney disease in children. *J. Pediatr.* 1981;98:561-564.

[39] Ladapo TA, Esezobor CI, Lesi FE. Pediatric kidney diseases in an African country: prevalence, spectrum and outcome. *Saudi J. Kidney Dis. Transpl.* 2014;25:1110-1116.

[40] Paul SK, Muinuddin G, Jahan S, Begum A, Rahman MH, Hossain MM. Long versus standard initial prednisolone therapy in children with idiopathic nephrotic syndrome. *Mymensingh Med. J.* 2014;23:261-267.

[41] Kamei K, Okada M, Miyazono A, Sato M, Fujimaru T, Ogura M, Ito S. Long-term prognosis of patients with steroid-dependent nephrotic syndrome treated with rituximab. *Nihon. Jinzo. Gakkai. Shi.* 2013;55:947-55.

[42] Straatmann C, Ayoob R, Gbadegesin R, Gibson K, Rheault MN, Srivastava T, Tran CL, Gipson DS, Greenbaum LA, Smoyer WE, Vehaskari VM. Treatment outcome of late steroid-resistant nephrotic syndrome: a study by the Midwest Pediatric Nephrology Consortium. *Pediatr. Nephrol.* 2013;28:1235-1241.

[43] Bock ME, Cohn RA, Ali FN. Treatment of childhood nephrotic syndrome with long-term, low-dose tacrolimus. *Clin. Nephrol.* 2013;79:432-438.

[44] Nakanishi K, Iijima K, Ishikura K, Hataya H, Nakazato H, Sasaki S, Honda M, Yoshikawa N. Two-year outcome of the ISKDC regimen and frequent-relapsing risk in children with idiopathic nephrotic syndrome. Japanese Study Group of Renal Disease in Children. *Clin. J. Am. Soc. Nephrol.* 2013;8:756-762.

[45] Tellier S, Brochard K, Garnier A, Bandin F, Llanas B, Guigonis V, Cailliez M, Pietrement C, Dunand O, Nathanson S, Bertholet-Thomas A, Ichay L, Decramer S. Long-term outcome of children treated with rituximab for idiopathic nephrotic syndrome. *Pediatr. Nephrol.* 2013;28:911-918.

[46] Wong W, Morris MC, Kara T. Congenital nephrotic syndrome with prolonged renal survival without renal replacement therapy. *Pediatr. Nephrol.* 2013;28:2313-2321.

[47] Kronbichler A, König P, Busch M, Wolf G, Mayer G, Rudnicki M. Rituximab in adult patients with multi-relapsing/steroid-dependent minimal change disease and focal segmental glomerulosclerosis: A report of 5 cases. *Wien. Klin. Wochenschr.* 2013;125:328-333.

[48] Bruchfeld A, Benedek S, Hilderman M, Medin C, Snaedal-Jonsdottir S, Korkeila M. Rituximab for minimal change disease in adults: long-term follow-up. *Nephrol. Dial. Transplant.* 2014;29:851-856.

[49] Horvatic I, Tisljar M, Bulimbasic S, Bozic B, Galesic Ljubanovic D, Galesic K. Epidemiologic data of adult native biopsy-proven renal diseases in Croatia. *Int. Urol. Nephrol.* 2013;45:1577-1587.

[50] Insalaco M, Zamboli P, Floccari F, Marrocco F, Andrulli S, Logias F, Di Lullo L, Fiorini F, Granata A. Indication to renal biopsy in DM2 patients: potential role of intrarenal resistive index. *Arch. Ital. Urol. Androl.* 2012;84:283-286.

[51] Sabir S, Mubarak M, Ul-Haq I, Bibi A.J. Pattern of biopsy proven renal diseases at PNS SHIFA, Karachi: A cross-sectional survey. *J. Renal Inj. Prev.* 2013;2:133-137.

[52] Verde E, Quiroga B, Rivera F, López-Gómez JM. Renal biopsy in very elderly patients: data from the Spanish Registry of Glomerulonephritis. *Am. J. Nephrol.* 2012;35:230-237.

[53] Paripović D, Kostić M, Kruščić D, Spasojević B, Lomić G, Marković-Lipkovski J, Basta-Jovanović G, Smoljanić Ž, Peco-Antić A. Indications and results of renal biopsy in children: a 10-year review from a single center in Serbia. *J. Nephrol.* 2012;25:1054-1059.

[54] Norio R, Rapola J. Congenital and infantile nephrotic syndromes. *Prog. Clin. Biol. Res.* 1989;305:179-192.

[55] Habib R. Nephrotic syndrome in the 1st year of life. *Pediatr. Nephrol.* 1993;7:347-353.

[56] Habib R, Kleinknecht C, Royer P. Primary nephrotic syndrome in children. Classification and anatomoclinical study of 406 cases. *Arch. Fr. Pediatr.* 1971;28:277-319.

[57] Ohl K, Eberhardt C, Spink C, Zahn K, Wagner N, Eggermann T, Kemper MJ, Querfeld U, Hoppe B, Harendza S, Tenbrock K. CTLA4 polymorphisms in minimal change nephrotic syndrome in children: a case-control study. *Am. J. Kidney Dis.* 2014;63:1074-1075.

[58] Pan Q, Wu J, Tao J, Chen Y, Li L, Deng Z, Liu W, Liu H. Role of basophils in the pathogenesis of minimal change nephrotic syndrome: A literature review. *Exp. Ther. Med.* 2014;8:1027-1031.

[59] Audard V, Lang P, Sahali D. Minimal change nephrotic syndrome: new insights into disease pathogenesis. *Med. Sci* (Paris). 2008;24:853-858.

[60] Audard V, Grimbert P, Valanciuté A, Lang P, Guellaën G, Sahali D. Recent approaches to the pathogenesis of minimal change nephrotic syndrome. *Nephrologie.* 2002;23:367-369.

[61] Hinkes BG, Mucha B, Vlangos CN, Gbadegesin R, Liu J, Hasselbacher K, Hangan D, Ozaltin F, Zenker M, Hildebrandt F. Nephrotic syndrome in the first year of life: two thirds of cases are caused by mutations in 4 genes (NPHS1, NPHS2, WT1, and LAMB2). *Pediatrics.* 2007;119:e907-e919.

[62] Machuca E, Benoit G, Antignac C. Genetics of nephrotic syndrome: connecting molecular genetics to podocyte physiology. *Hum. Mol. Genet.* 1978;13:159-165.

[63] Lahdenkari AT, Kestilä M, Holmberg C, Koskimies O, Jalanko H. Nephrin gene (NPHS1) in patients with minimal change nephrotic syndrome (MCNS). *Kidney Int.* 2004;65:1856-1863.

[64] Hingorani SR, Finn LS, Kowalewska J, McDonald RA, Eddy AA. Expression of nephrin in acquired forms of nephrotic syndrome in childhood. *Pediatr. Nephrol.* 2004;19:300-305.
[65] Waldherr R, Gubler MC, Levy M, Broyer M, Habib R. Thignificance of pure diffuse mesangial proliferation in idiopathic nephrotic syndrome. *Clin. Nephrol.* 1978;10:171-179.
[66] Allen WR, Travis LB, Cavallo T, Brouhard BH, Cunningham RJ. Immune deposits and mesangial hypercellularity in minimal change nephrotic syndrome: clinical relevance. *J. Pediatr.* 1982;100:188-191.
[67] Ji-Yun Y, Melvin T, Sibley R, Michael AF. No evidence for a specific role of IgM in mesangial proliferation of idiopathic nephrotic syndrome. *Kidney Int.* 1984;25:100-106.
[68] Joh K, Matsuyama N, Kanetsuna Y, Usui N, Hattori M, Yumura W, Aizawa S. Nephrotic syndrome associated with diffuse mesangial hypercellularity: is it a heterogeneous disease entity? *Am. J. Nephrol.* 1998;18:214-220.
[69] Bhuyan UN, Srivastava RN. Incidence and significance of IgM mesangial deposits in relapsing idiopathic nephrotic syndrome of childhood. *Indian J. Med. Res.* 1987;86:53-60.
[70] Mubarak M, Kazi JI, Shakeel S, Lanewala A, Hashmi S, Akhter F. Clinicopathologic characteristics and steroid response of IgM nephropathy in children presenting with idiopathic nephrotic syndrome. *APMIS.* 2011;119:180-186.
[71] Mubarak M. IgM nephropathy; time to act. *J. Nephropathol.* 2014;3:22-25.
[72] Mubarak M, Naqvi R, Kazi J, Shakeel S. Immunoglobulin M nephropathy in adults: a clinicopathological study. *Iran J. Kidney Dis.* 2013;7:214-219.
[73] Shakeel S, Mubarak M, Kazi JI, Lanewala A. The prevalence and clinicopathological profile of IgM nephropathy in children with steroid-resistant nephrotic syndrome at a single centre in Pakistan. *J. Clin. Pathol.* 2012;65:1072-1076.
[74] Andal A, Saxena S, Chellani HK, Sharma S. Pure mesangial proliferative glomerulonephritis. A clinicomorphologic analysis and its possible role in morphologic transition of minimal change lesion. *Nephron.* 1989;51:314-319.
[75] Hirszel P, Yamase HT, Carney WR, Galen MA, Graeber CW, Johnson KJ, Kennedy TL, Lapkin RA, McLean RH, Rosenworcel E. Mesangial proliferative glomerulonephritis with IgM deposits. Clinicopathologic analysis and evidence for morphologic transitions. *Nephron.* 1984;38:100-108.
[76] Mampaso F, Gonzalo A, Teruel J, Losada M, Gallego N, Ortuno J, Bellas C. Mesangial deposits of IgM in patients with the nephrotic syndrome. *Clin. Nephrol.* 1981;16:230-234.
[77] Lawler W, Williams G, Tarpey P, Mallick NP. IgM associated primary diffuse mesangial proliferative glomerulonephritis. *J. Clin. Pathol.* 1980;33:1029-1038.
[78] Vanikar AV, Kanodia KV, Patel RD, Suthar KS, Patel HV, Gumber MR, Trivedi HL. IgM nephropathy in India: a single centre experience. *Indian J. Pediatr.* 2012;79:1025-1027.
[79] Myllymäki J, Saha H, Helin H, Pasternack A, Mustonen J. IgM nephropathy. *Duodecim.* 2004;120:1563-1568.
[80] Mubarak M, Kazi JI, Malik S, Lanewala A, Hashmi S. Clinicopathologic characteristics and steroid response of IgM nephropathy in children presenting with idiopathic nephrotic syndrome. *APMIS.* 2011;119:180-186.

[81] Hsu HC, Chen WY, Lin GJ, Chen L, Kao S-L, Huang C-C, Lin CY. Clinical and immunopathologic study of mesangial IgM nephropathy: report of 41 cases. *Histopathology.* 1984;8:435-446.

[82] Disciullo SO, Abeulo JG, Moalli K, Pezzullo JC. Circulating heavy IgM in IgM nephropathy. *Clin. Exp. Immunol.* 1988;73:395-400.

[83] Border WA. Distinguishing minimal change disease from mesangial disorders. *Kidney Int.* 1988;34:419-424.

[84] Arias LF, Prada MC, Vélez-Echeverri C, Serna-Higuita LM, Serrano-Gayubo AK, Ochoa CL, Vanegas-Ruiz JJ. IgM nephropathy in children: clinicopathologic analysis. *Nefrologia.* 2013;33:532-538.

[85] Kazi J, Mubarak M. IgM nephropathy presenting as full blown crescentic glomerulonephritis: first report in the literature. *Nefrologia.* 2014;34:423-424.

[86] Zeis PS, Kavazarakis E, Nakopoulou L, Moustaki M, Messaritaki A, Zeis MP, Nicolaidou P. Glomerulopathy with mesangial IgM deposits: long-term follow up of 64 children. *Pediatr. Int.* 2001;43:287-292.

[87] Myllymäki J, Saha H, Mustonen J, Helin H, Pasternack A. IgM nephropathy: clinical picture and long-term prognosis. *Am. J. Kidney Dis.* 2003;41:343-350.

[88] Al Eisa A, Carner JE, Lirenman DS, Magil AB. Childhood IgM nephropathy: comparison with minimal change disease. *Nephron.*1996;72:37-43.

[89] O'Donoghue DJ, Lawler W, Hunt LP, Acheson EJ, Mallick NP. IgM associated primary diffuse mesangial proliferative glomerulonephritis: natural history and prognostic indicators. *Q. Med. J.* 1991;79:333-350.

[90] Smoyer WE, Gregory MJ, Bajwa RS, Johnson KJ, Bunchman TE. Quantitative morphometry of renal biopsies prior to cyclosporine in nephrotic syndrome. *Pediatr. Nephrol.* 1998;12:737-743.

[91] Polito MG, de Moura LA, Kirsztajn GM. An overview on frequency of renal biopsy diagnosis in Brazil: clinical and pathological patterns based on 9,617 native kidney biopsies. *Nephrol. Dial. Transplant.* 2010;25:490-496.

[92] Abdelraheem MB, Ali el-TM, Mohamed RM, Hassan EG, Abdalla OA, Mekki SO, Yousif BM, Watson AR. Pattern of glomerular diseases in Sudanese children: a clinico-pathological study. *Saudi J. Kidney Dis. Transpl.* 2010;21:778-783.

[93] Gesualdo L, Pinzani M, Floriano JJ, Hassan MO, Nagy NU, Schena FP, Emancipator SN, Abboud HE. Platelet-derived growth factor expression in mesangial proliferative glomerulonephritis. *Lab. Invest.* 1991;65:160-167.

[94] A Sorokin, DE Kohan. Physiology and pathology of endothelin-1 in renal mesangium. *Am. J. Physiol. Renal Physiol.* 2003;285:579-589.

[95] Horii Y, Iwano M, Hirata E, Shiiki M, Fujii Y, Dohi K, Ishikawa H. Role of interleukin-6 in the progression of mesangial proliferative glomerulonephritis. *Kidney Int. Suppl.* 1993;39:71-75.

[96] Budisavljevic MN, Hodge L, Barber K, Fulmer JR, Durazo-Arvizu RA, Self SE, Kuhlmann M, Raymond JR, Greene EL. Oxidative stress in the pathogenesis of experimental mesangial proliferative glomerulonephritis. *Am. J. Physiol. Renal Physiol.* 2003;285:1138-1148.

[97] Tabassum S, Rahman KM, Mamun KZ, Ahmed AN, Islam KM, Rahman H. Immunofluorescent microscopic findings in glomerulonephritis. *Bangladesh Med. Res. Counc. Bull.* 1997;23:77-81.

[98] Kurihara S, Sakurai Y, Takeuchi M, Yoneshima H, Matsunobu S, Hayama N, Iino Y, Kitamura H, Shimizu A, Yamanaka N. A case of mesangioproliferative glomerulonephritis (GN) associated with unique lesions of juxtaglomerular apparatus (JGA) and interstitium. *Nihon. Jinzo. Gakkai. Shi.* 1993;35:869-873.

[99] Abbas K, Mubarak M, Kazi JI, Muzaffar R. Pattern of morphology in renal biopsies of nephrotic syndrome patients. Correlation with immunoglobulin and complement deposition and serology. *J. Pak. Med. Assoc.* 2009;59:540-543.

[100] Churg J, Habib R, White RH. Pathology of the nephritic syndrome in children. *Lancet.* 1970;760:1299-1302.

[101] White RH, Glasgow EF, Mills RJ. Clinicopathological study of nephrotic syndrome in childhood. *Lancet.* 1970;7661:1353-1359.

[102] Bhasin HK, Abuelo JG, Nayak R, Esparza AR. Mesangial proliferative glomerulonephritis. *Lab. Invest.* 1978;39:21-29.

[103] Murphy WM, Jukkola AF, Roy S. Nephrotic syndrome with mesangial cell proliferation in children-a distinct entity? *Am. J. Clin. Pathol.* 1979;72:42-47.

[104] Brown EA, Upadhyaya K, Hayslett JP, Kashgarian M, Siegel NJ. The clinical course of mesangial proliferative glomerulonephritis. *Medicine.* 1979;58:295-303.

[105] Papadopoulou ZL, Jenis EH, Tina LU, Novello AC, Jose PA, Calcagno PL. Chronic relapsing minimal change nephrotic syndrome with or without mesangial deposits: long term follow-up. *Int. J. Pediatr. Nephrol.* 1982;3:179-186.

[106] Siegel NJ, Gaudio KM, Krassner LS, McDonald BM, Anderson FP, Kashgarian M. Steroid-dependent nephrotic syndrome in children: histopathology and relapses after cyclophosphamide treatment. *Kidney Int.* 1981;19:454-459.

[107] Brown EA, Upadhyaya K, Hayslett JP, Kashgarian M, Siegel NJ. The clinical course of mesangial proliferative glomerulonephritis. *Medicine* (Baltimore). 1979;58:295-303.

[108] Golay V, Trivedi M, Kurien AA, Sarkar D, Roychowdhary A, Pandey R. Spectrum of nephrotic syndrome in adults: clinicopathological study from a single center in India. *Ren. Fail.* 2013;35:487-491.

[109] Nawaz Z, Mushtaq F, Mousa D, Rehman E, Sulaiman M, Aslam N, Khawaja N. Pattern of glomerular disease in the Saudi population: a single-center, five-year retrospective study. *Saudi J. Kidney Dis. Transpl.* 2013;24:1265-1270.

[110] The changing spectrum of primary glomerular diseases within 15 years: a survey of 3331 patients in a single Chinese centre.Zhou FD, Zhao MH, Zou WZ, Liu G, Wang H. *Nephrol. Dial. Transplant.* 2009;24:870-876.

[111] Tizki S, Lasry F, Khalifa HH, Itri M. Primary focal segmental glomerular sclerosis in children: epidemiology and prognosis. *Nephrol. Ther.* 2013;9:433-437.

[112] Mubarak M, Lanewala A, Kazi JI, Akhter F, Sher A, Fayyaz A, Bhatti S. Histopathological spectrum of childhood nephrotic syndrome in Pakistan. *Clin. Exp. Nephrol.* 2009;13:589-593.

[113] Gilani SM, Ockner D, Qu H. Role of on-site microscopic evaluation of kidney biopsy for adequacy and allocation of glomeruli: comparison of renal biopsies with and without on-site microscopic evaluation. *Pathologica.* 2013;105:342-345.

[114] Jefferson JA, Shankland SJ. The pathogenesis of focal segmental glomerulosclerosis. *Adv. Chronic Kidney Dis.* 2014;21:408-416.

[115] Basiratnia M, Yavarian M, Torabinezhad S, Erjaee A. NPHS2 gene in steroid-resistant nephrotic syndrome: prevalence, clinical course, and mutational spectrum in South-West Iranian children. *Iran J. Kidney Dis.* 2013;7:357-362.

[116] Bouchireb K, Boyer O, Gribouval O, Nevo F, Huynh-Cong E, Morinière V, Campait R, Ars E, Brackman D, Dantal J, Eckart P, Gigante M, Lipska BS, Liutkus A, Megarbane A, Mohsin N, Ozaltin F, Saleem MA, Schaefer F, Soulami K, Torra R, Garcelon N, Mollet G, Dahan K, Antignac C. NPHS2 mutations in steroid-resistant nephrotic syndrome: a mutation update and the associated phenotypic spectrum. *Hum. Mutat.* 2014;35:178-186.

[117] Taneda S, Honda K, Uchida K, Nitta K, Yumura W, Oda H, Nagata M. Histological heterogeneity of glomerular segmental lesions in focal segmental glomerulosclerosis. *Int. Urol. Nephrol.* 2012;44:183-196.

[118] Shakeel S, Mubarak M, I Kazi J, Jafry N, Ahmed E. Frequency and clinicopathological characteristics of variants of primary focal segmental glomerulosclerosis in adults presenting with nephrotic syndrome. *J. Nephropathol.* 2013;2:28-35.

[119] D'Agati V. Pathologic classification of focal segmental glomerulosclerosis. *Semin. Nephrol.* 2003;23:117-134.

[120] Arias LF, Jiménez CA, Arroyave MJ. Histologic variants of primary focal segmental glomerulosclerosis: presentation and outcome. *J. Bras. Nefrol.* 2013;35:112-119.

[121] Choi MJ. Histologic classification of FSGS: does form delineate function? *Clin. J. Am. Soc. Nephrol.* 2013;8:344-346.

[122] Deegens JK, Steenbergen EJ, Borm GF, Wetzels JF. Pathological variants of focal segmental glomerulosclerosis in an adult Dutch population-epidemiology and outcome. *Nephrol. Dial. Transplant.* 2008;23:186-192.

[123] Silverstein DM, Craver R. Presenting features and short-term outcome according to pathologic variant in childhood primary focal segmental glomerulosclerosis. *Clin. J. Am. Soc. Nephrol.* 2007;2:700-707.

[124] D'Agati VD, Alster JM, Jennette JC, Thomas DB, Pullman J, Savino DA, Cohen AH, Gipson DS, Gassman JJ, Radeva MK, Moxey-Mims MM, Friedman AL, Kaskel FJ, Trachtman H, Alpers CE, Fogo AB, Greene TH, Nast CC. Association of histologic variants in FSGS clinical trial with presenting features and outcomes. *Clin. J. Am. Soc. Nephrol.* 2013;8:399-406.

[125] Ben-Bassat M, Braslavsky D, Lotan D, Eisenstein B, Davidovitz M, Stark H. Ultrastructural changes suggestive of focal segmental glomerulosclerosis in atypical minimal change nephrotic syndrome. *Ultrastruct. Pathol.* 1988;12:1-16.

[126] Paik KH, Lee BH, Cho HY, Kang HG, Ha IS, Cheong HI, Jin DK, Moon KC, Choi Y. Primary focal segmental glomerular sclerosis in children: clinical course and prognosis. *Pediatr. Nephrol.* 2007;22:389-395.

[127] Thomas DB, Franceschini N, Hogan SL, Ten Holder S, Jennette CE, Falk RJ, Jennette JC. Clinical and pathologic characteristics of focal segmental glomerulosclerosis pathologic variants. *Kidney Int.* 2006;69:920-926.

[128] Stokes MB, D'Agati VD. Morphologic variants of focal segmental glomerulosclerosis and their significance. *Adv. Chronic Kidney Dis.* 2014;21:400-407.

[129] Stokes MB, Markowitz GS, Lin J, Valeri AM, D'Agati VD. Glomerular tip lesion: a distinct entity within the minimal change disease/focal segmental glomerulosclerosis spectrum. *Kidney Int.* 2004;65:1690-1702.

[130] Schwartz MM, Lewis EJ. Focal segmental glomerular sclerosis: the cellular lesion. *Kidney Int.* 1985;28:968-974.

[131] Das P, Sharma A, Gupta R, Agarwal SK, Bagga A, Dinda AK. Histomorphological classification of focal segmental glomerulosclerosis: a critical evaluation of clinical, histologic and morphometric features. *Saudi J. Kidney Dis. Transpl.* 2012;23:1008-1016.

[132] McGrogan A, Franssen CF, de Vries CS. The incidence of primary glomerulonephritis worldwide: a systematic review of the literature. *Nephrol. Dial. Transplant.* 2011;26:414-430.

[133] Yamaguchi M, Ando M, Yamamoto R, Akiyama S, Kato S, Katsuno T, Kosugi T, Sato W, Tsuboi N, Yasuda Y, Mizuno M, Ito Y, Matsuo S, Maruyama S. Patient age and the prognosis of idiopathic membranous nephropathy. *PLoS One.* 2014;9:e110376.

[134] Deegens JK, Wetzels JF. Membranous nephropathy in the older adult: epidemiology, diagnosis and management. *Drugs Aging.* 2007;24:717-732.

[135] Ronco P, Debiec H. Idiopathic and secondary membranous nephropathies. *Presse. Med.* 2012;41:290-297.

[136] Lee BH, Cho HY, Kang HG, Ha IS, Cheong HI, Moon KC, Lim IS, Choi Y. Idiopathic membranous nephropathy in children. *Pediatr. Nephrol.* 2006;21:1707-1715.

[137] Kwatra IS, Prasher PK. Pathogenesis of membranous nephropathy: update. *J. Assoc. Physicians India.* 2013;61:807-810.

[138] Santos FR. Membranous glomerulonephritis: new insights in pathophysiology and therapeutic approach. *J. Bras. Nefrol.* 2014;36:59-62.

[139] Glassock RJ. Pathogenesis of membranous nephropathy: a new paradigm in evolution. *Contrib. Nephrol.* 2013;181:131-142.

[140] Paraskevakou H, Kavantzas N, Pavlopoulos PM, Voudiklari S, Zerefos N, Papagalanis N, Davaris P. Membranous glomerulonephritis: a morphometric study. *Pathol. Res. Pract.* 2000;196:141-144.

[141] Yokoyama H, Yoshimoto K, Wada T, Furuichi K, Goshima S, Kida H, Kobayashi K. Electron-dense deposition patterns and the outcomes of idiopathic membranous nephropathy in Japanese. *Med. Electron Microsc.* 2002;35:81-86.

[142] Sato S, Ishizaki M, Shimizu A, Ghazizadeh M, Kitamura H, Adachi A, Sasaki Y, Dai W, Wakamatsu K, Sugisaki Y. Identification of an electron densification of the glomerular basement membrane in renal biopsy specimens. *Med. Electron Microsc.* 2003;36:106-111.

[143] Zhou GY. Ultrastructure and immunologic pathology of membranous glomerulonephritis of 91 cases. *Zhonghua Bing. Li. Xue. Za. Zhi.* 1989;18:182-184.

[144] Dowling JP, Mathews DC. Silver methenamine impregnation: a useful adjunct to renal electron microscopy. *Pathology.* 1987;19:410-414.

[145] Gärtner HV. Membranous (peri-, epi-, extramembranous) glomerulonephritis. Prototype of an immune complex glomerulonephritis. A clinical morphological study. *Veroff. Pathol.* 1980;113:1-136.

[146] Churg J, Ehrenreich T. Membranous nephropathy. *Perspect. Nephrol. Hypertens.* 1973;1:443-448.

[147] Ehrenreich T, Yunis SL, Churg J. Membranous nephropathy following exposure to volatile hydrocarbons. *Environ. Res.* 1977;14:35-45.

[148] Zuo K, Wu Y, Li SJ, Xu F, Zeng CH, Liu ZH. Long-term outcome and prognostic factors of idiopathic membranous nephropathy in the Chinese population. *Clin. Nephrol.* 2013;79:445-453.
[149] Gupta R, Sharma A, Mahanta PJ, Jacob TG, Agarwal SK, Roy TS, Dinda AK. Focal segmental glomerulosclerosis in idiopathic membranous glomerulonephritis: a clinico-pathological and stereological study. *Nephrol. Dial. Transplant.* 2010;25:444-449.
[150] Dumoulin A, Hill GS, Montseny JJ, Meyrier A. Clinical and morphological prognostic factors in membranous nephropathy: significance of focal segmental glomerulosclerosis. *Am. J. Kidney Dis.* 2003;41:38-48.
[151] Roberti I, Vyas S. Long-term outcome of children with steroid-resistant nephrotic syndrome treated with tacrolimus. *Pediatr. Nephrol.* 2010;25:1117-1124.
[152] Severgina LO, Varshavskiĭ VA, Serov VV. Clinico-morphologic correlations in various types of mesangiocapillary glomerulonephritis. *Arkh. Patol.* 1993;55:28-33.
[153] D'Amico G, Ferrario F. Mesangiocapillary glomerulonephritis. *J. Am. Soc. Nephrol.* 1992;2:159-166.
[154] Severgina LO. Comparative characteristics of morphologic types of mesangiocapillary glomerulonephritis (morphologic correlation analysis). *Arkh. Patol.* 1994;56:63-65.
[155] Plotkin VI. Clinico-morphologic comparisons in mesangiocapillary glomerulonephritis. *Vrach. Delo.* 1989;10:43-46.
[156] West CD, McAdams AJ. Glomerular paramesangial deposits: association with hypocomplementemia in membranoproliferative glomerulonephritis types I and III. *Am. J. Kidney Dis.* 1998;31:427-434.
[157] Sethi S, Fervenza FC. Membranoproliferative glomerulonephritis: pathogenetic heterogeneity and proposal for a new classification. *Semin. Nephrol.* 2011;31:341-348.
[158] Hattori M, Kim Y, Steffes MW, Mauer SM. Structural-functional relationships in type I mesangiocapillary glomerulonephritis. *Kidney Int.* 1993;43:381-386.
[159] Mirapeix E, Yagüe J, Vives J, Revert L. Studies of complement, nephritic factor, and circulating immune complexes in chronic mesangiocapillary glomerulonephritis types I and II. *Med. Clin* (Barc). 1981;77:21-26.
[160] Rashid HU, Biswas CK, Morley AR, Kerr DN. Mesangiocapillary glomerulonephritis type I associated with immunoglobulin deficiency. *Br. Med. J.* 1981;283:407-408.
[161] Sakaguchi H, Hazikano H, Hasegawa O, Ito H. Histological subtype of mesangiocapillary glomerulonephritis (MPGN type 1). *Nihon. Jinzo. Gakkai. Shi.* 1984;26:671-689.
[162] Cameron JS, Turner DR, Heaton J, Williams DG, Ogg CS, Chantler C, Haycock GB, Hicks J. Idiopathic mesangiocapillary glomerulonephritis. Comparison of types I and II in children and adults and long-term prognosis. *Am. J. Med.* 1983;74:175-192.
[163] Laohapand T, Cattell V, Gabriel JR. Monocyte infiltration in human glomerulonephritis: alpha-1-antitrypsin as a marker for mononuclear phagocytes in renal biopsies. *Clin. Nephrol.* 1983;19:309-316.
[164] Nast CC. Renal pathology: Current approach to classification of membranoproliferative glomerulonephritis. *Pathology.* 2014;46:S41.
[165] Sharma A, Gupta R, Lal C, Agarwal SK, Dinda AK . Crescentic glomerulonephritis developing in the course of idiopathic membranoproliferative glomerulonephritis. *Saudi J. Kidney Dis. Transpl.* 2013;24:333-337.

[166] Yoshikawa N, Yoshiara S, Yoshiya K, Matsuo T, Matsuyama S, Okada S. Focal and diffuse membranoproliferative glomerulonephritis in children. *Am. J. Nephrol.* 1988;8:102-107.

[167] di Belgiojoso B, Tarantino A, Colasanti G, Bazzi C, Guerra L, Durante A. The prognostic value of some clinical and histological parameters in membranoproliferative glomerulonephritis (MPGN): report of 112 cases. *Nephron.* 1977;19:250-258.

[168] Dische FE, Parsons V. Experience in the diagnosis of glomerulonephritis using combined light microscopical, ultrastructural and immunofluorescence techniques--an analysis of 134 cases. *Histopathology.* 1977;1:331-362.

[169] Watson AR, Poucell S, Thorner P, Arbus GS, Rance CP, Baumal R. Membranoproliferative glomerulonephritis type I in children: correlation of clinical features with pathologic subtypes. *Am. J. Kidney Dis.* 1984;4:141-146.

[170] Sato H. Ultrastructural study on membranoproliferative glomerulonephritis with special reference to subepithelial deposits. *Nihon. Jinzo. Gakkai. Shi.* 1990;32:973-983.

[171] Cansick JC, Lennon R, Cummins CL, Howie AJ, McGraw ME, Saleem MA, Tizard EJ, Hulton SA, Milford DV, Taylor CM. Prognosis, treatment and outcome of childhood mesangiocapillary (membranoproliferative) glomerulonephritis. *Nephrol. Dial. Transplant.* 2004;19:2769-2777.

[172] Liu JC, Yang JY, Xiao HJ, Huang JP, Yao Y, Li X, Wang SX. Clinical and pathological characteristics of children with dense deposit disease. *Zhonghua. Er. Ke. Za. Zhi.* 2009;47:593-597.

[173] Taranta-Janusz K, Wasilewska A, Szynaka B. Childhood-onset dense deposit disease: a rare cause of proteinuria. *Ir. J. Med. Sci.* 2014;183:455-459.

[174] Muda AO, Barsotti P, Marinozzi V. Ultrastructural histochemical investigations of "dense deposit disease". Pathogenetic approach to a special type of mesangiocapillary glomerulonephritis. *Virchows Arch. A. Pathol. Anat. Histopathol.* 1988;413:529-537.

[175] Iitaka K, Nakamura S, Moriya S, Koshino H, Iwasaki N, Motoyama O, Sakai T. Long-term follow-up of type II membranoproliferative glomerulonephritis in two children. *Clin. Exp. Nephrol.* 2003;7:58-62.

[176] Bennett WM, Fassett RG, Walker RG, Fairley KF, d'Apice AJ, Kincaid-Smith P. Mesangiocapillary glomerulonephritis type II (dense-deposit disease): clinical features of progressive disease. *Am. J. Kidney Dis.* 1989;13:469-476.

[177] Trinn C, Nagy J, Deák G, Burger T. Mesangiocapillary glomerulonephritis, type 3. *Morphol. Igazsagugyi. Orv. Sz.* 1989;29:1-7.

[178] Khokhlov SE, Borovoĭ SG, Vorob'eva OA, Borisova EA, Kardanova ZhZh, Nevorotin AI. Type 3 membranoproliferative glomerulonephritis: an unusual variety of well-known pathology. *Arkh. Patol.* 2009;71:32-35.

[179] Fujigaki Y, Ohashi N, Yonemura K, Fujimoto T, Fukasawa H, Togawa A, Suzuki H, Yasuda H, Yamamoto T, Hishida A. A mechanism for the development of subepithelial deposits in a patient with type III membranoproliferative glomerulonephritis. *Nephrology* (Carlton). 2003;8:280-284.

[180] Strife CF, Jackson EC, McAdams AJ. Type III membranoproliferative glomerulonephritis: long-term clinical and morphologic evaluation. *Clin. Nephrol.* 1984;21:323-334.

[181] Anders D, Thoenes W. Basement membrane-changes in membranoproliferative glomerulonephritis: a light and electron microscopic study. *Virchows Arch. A. Pathol. Anat. Histol.* 1975;369:87-109.

[182] Iitaka K, Moriya S, Nakamura S, Tomonaga K, Sakai T. Long-term follow-up of type III membranoproliferative glomerulonephritis in children. *Pediatr. Nephrol.* 2002;17:373-378.

[183] Abreo K, Moorthy AV. Type 3 membranoproliferative glomerulonephritis: clinicopathologic correlations and long-term follow-up in nine patients. *Arch. Pathol. Lab. Med.* 1982;106:413-417.

In: Nephrotic Syndrome: Etiology, Pathogenesis and Pathology ISBN: 978-1-63482-154-4
Editor: Muhammed Mubarak

Chapter 8

Pathology of Nephrotic Syndrome in Adults

Lavleen Singh, Geetika Singh and Amit Dinda*
Department of Pathology, All India Institute of Medical Sciences,
New Delhi, India

Abstract

Nephrotic syndrome (NS) is a clinicopathological complex that constitutes an important presenting syndrome of various renal diseases of both primary and secondary nature. An accurate diagnosis of the underlying pathological disease process is imperative for proper management and prognostication of the individual patient. Renal biopsy constitutes one of the most important diagnostic tools for this purpose. A variety of lesions may be found on renal biopsy in cases of NS in adults. This chapter describes the main or common diseases, both primary as well as secondary, which present clinically as NS in adults. Rare or exotic diseases are beyond the scope of this chapter.

Keywords: Adults, glomerulonephritis, immunoflourescence, nephrotic syndrome, proteinuria, renal biopsy

1. Introduction

The four basic structural components of kidney are: glomeruli, tubules, interstitium, and blood vessels. The renal dysfunction can arise from the affliction of one or more of these compartments. The nephrotic-range proteinuria arises mainly due to glomerular injury.

In this chapter, we will discuss various disorders leading to nephrotic-range proteinuria in adults. The total protein excretion in a normal adult is <150 mg/day with albuminuria of <30

* Address of Correspondence: Dr. AK Dinda, Professor, Department of Pathology, All India Institute of Medical Sciences, Ansari Nagar, New Delhi, 110029, Email: dindaaiims@gmail.com

mg/day. The total protein in a normal individual comprises of filtered proteins like albumin (less than 30 mg/day), beta-2 microglobulin, proprotein enzymes, peptide hormones and proteins secreted by the tubules (Tamm-Horsfall, IgA, and urokinase).

The pathological proteinuria occurs either due to loss of size and charge selective filtration barrier or when there is excessive production of abnormal protein that overwhelms the tubular reabsorption capacity. A total daily protein excretion of more than 3.5 g is called nephrotic-range proteinuria and when this is associated with hypoalbuminemia, hyperlipidemia, and edema; the constellation of the features is known as nephrotic syndrome (NS). In NS, hypoalbuminemia occurs due to excessive urinary losses and increased proximal tubule catabolism of filtered albumin. Edema occurs due to excessive renal sodium retention and reduced plasma oncotic pressure. The decrease in effective intravascular volume, leads to activation of renin-angiotensin system, stimulation of antidiuretic hormone (ADH), and activation of the sympathetic nervous system that promote continued salt and water reabsorption and progressive edema. NS also leads to hypercoagulable state due to urinary losses of antithrombin III, reduced serum levels of proteins S and C, hyperfibrinogenemia, and enhanced platelet aggregation. Hypercholesterolemia results from increased hepatic lipoprotein synthesis.

The various primary glomerular disorders leading to NS in adults include focal segmental glomerulosclerosis (FSGS), membranous nephropathy (MN), minimal change disease (MCD), membranoproliferative glomerulonephritis (MPGN) and C3 glomerulopathy (Dense Deposit Disease and C3 glomerulonephritis). The secondary glomerular disorders leading to nephrotic-range proteinuria include diabetic nephropathy (DN), hypertensive nephropathy, amyloidosis, systemic lupus erythematosus (SLE), cryoglobulinemia, light chain deposition disease, fibrillary and immunotactoid glomerulopathy. Various infectious agents leading to nephrotic-range proteinuria include human immunodeficiency virus (HIV), hepatitis B, hepatitis C, malaria, leprosy, schistosomiasis and syphilis.

A brief description of individual glomerular diseases leading to NS is provided below:

2. Minimal Change Disease (MCD)

MCD, or nil lesion, is responsible for 70% to 90% of NS in childhood and 10% to15% of NS in adults. MCD is usually primary but can be associated with several other conditions, like, Hodgkin's lymphoma, allergies, or use of non-steroidal anti-inflammatory agents (NSAIDs). The exact pathogenesis of MCD remains elusive; however, loss of glomerular charge has been implicated for proteinuria. The association of MCD with conditions like atopy, hypersensitivity, food allergies and Hodgkin's lymphoma suggests that altered immune response nay have etiological role. The structural or functional alteration of various slit diaphragm (SD) proteins may be responsible for a fraction of cases.

2.1. Clinical Features

MCD presents clinically with edema and NS. The urinary sediments are mostly acellular. The other clinical features include hypertension (30% in children, 50% in adults), microscopic hematuria (20% in children, 33% in adults), atopy or allergic symptoms (40% in children, 30% in a adults), and decreased renal function (<5% in children, 30% in adults). [1] There may be acute renal failure (ARF) in adults which is often attributed to low serum albumin and intrarenal edema. In MCD, the urinary protein loss comprises principally of albumin with minimal amounts of higher-molecular-weight proteins, thus there is selective proteinuria.

2.2. Light Microscopy

In MCD, on light microscopy, the glomeruli are either absolutely normal or show minimal changes. [Figure 1] No endocapillary proliferation, basement membrane thickening or tuft necrosis is seen. In a minority of MCD cases, segmental or diffuse increase in mesangial cellularity can be present. These patients are more prone to hematuria. [2, 3]

The tubulointerstitial and vascular compartments are generally unremarkable. Hyaline droplets and clear vacuoles may be seen in proximal tubular epithelial cells due to proteinuria and lipiduria respectively. Interstitial edema may be seen in few patients of MCD.

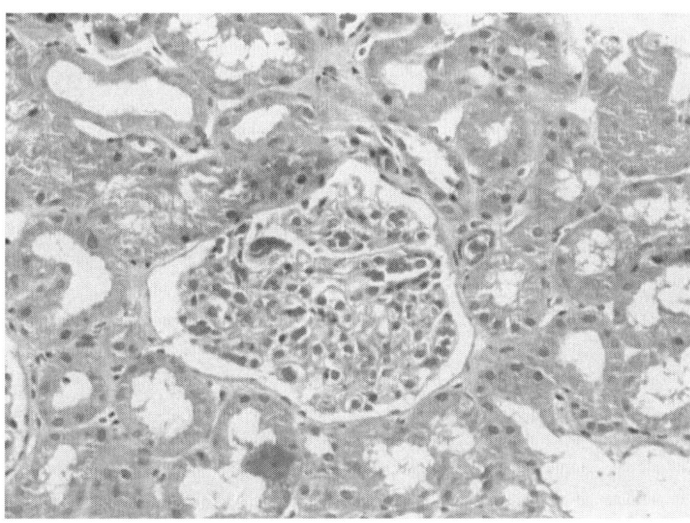

Figure 1. Minimal change disease (MCD). The glomerulus is normal on light microscopy. There is no tubulointerstitial fibrosis. [H&E, ×200]

2.3. Immunofluorescence (IF)

Immunofluorescent (IF) studies are unremarkable as no identifiable glomerular lesion or immune complex deposition is noted. In a minority of cases, focal IgM or C3 deposition is noted in the mesangium. A glomerular pathology with histological features of MCD and bright mesangial deposition of IgM is labelled as IgM nephropathy (IgMN) when there are mesangial electron dense deposits. [4]

2.4. Electron Microscopy

The electron microscopy demonstrates diffuse effacement of the podocyte foot processes, vacuolization of podocyte cytoplasm and microvillous transformation of podocytes. [Figure 2]

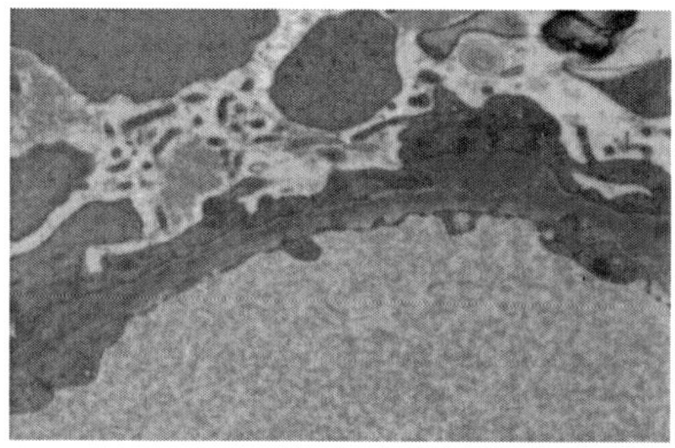

Figure 2. Minimal change disease (MCD). There is diffuse effacement of podocyte foot processes with microvillous transformation. [TEM, ×2000].

3. Focal Segmental Glomerulosclerosis (FSGS)

The incidence of FSGS is increasing, and it is now the commonest cause of NS in adults especially in African Americans. [5-8] An array of etiological factors may lead to FSGS, thus all the secondary causes have to be ruled out before making the diagnosis of primary FSGS. [Table 1]

3.1. Clinical Features

The patients present with NS. The average age of presentation is more than MCD and patients are more likely to show hematuria, hypertension, renal insufficiency, non- selective proteinuria and steroid resistance. [9]

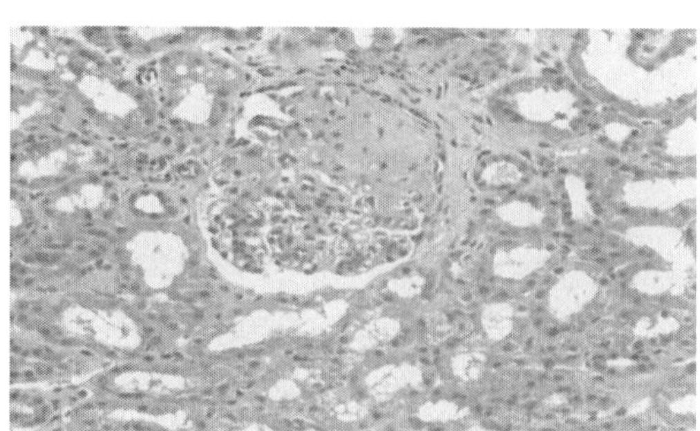

Figure 3. Focal segmental glomerulosclerosis (FSGS). There is segmental sclerosis of the glomerular tuft with obliteration of capillary lumina. [H&E, ×200].

Table 1. The main causes of focal segmental glomerulosclerosis

- Primary focal segmental glomerulosclerosis
- Secondary focal segmental glomerulosclerosis
- Due to podocyte injury
- Viruses: HIV/Hepatitis B/Parvovirus
- Drugs: pamidronate, lithium, interferons, heroin, analgesics
- Secondary to structural or functional adaptations of podocytes
    - Unilateral renal agenesis
    - Oligomeganephronia and segmental hypoplasia
    - Renal dysplasia
    - Polycystic kidney disease, adult type
    - Reflux nephropathy
    - Renal transplantation
    - Increased muscle mass
    - Chronic interstitial nephritis and pyelonephritis
    - Partial cortical necrosis
    - Papillary necrosis
    - Sickle cell disease
    - Nephrectomy or extensive surgical ablation
    - Cholesterol atheroembolization
    - Hypertension
    - Morbid obesity
    - Cyanotic congenital heart disease
    - Diabetic nephropathy
    - Glycogen storage diseases
    - Familial dysautonomia
    - Acromegaly
- Parasites: Loa Loa Filariasis, Schistosomiasis
- Secondary to genetic defects
    - Autosomal recessive FSGS
        - NPHS1 mutations: Nephrin
        - NPHS2 mutations : Podocin
    - Autosomal dominant FSGS
        - ACTN4 mutations
        - CD2AP mutations
    - Syndromic FSGS
        - WT1 mutations
        - Diffuse mesangial sclerosis
        - Denys-Drash syndrome
        - Frasier syndrome
        - Nail-patella syndrome
        - Alport's syndrome
        - Galloway Mowat syndrome
        - Autosomal dominant progressive nephropathy with FSGS and sensorineural deafness
        - Autosomal recessive FSGS with neurologic findings
        - Mitochondrial DNA mutations
        - MELAS syndrome
- Secondary to focal proliferative glomerulonephritides
    - Pauci-immune glomerulonephritis
    - Lupus nephritis class III

3.2. Light Microscopy

FSGS is characterized by glomerular scars which are focal (involvement of some but not all glomeruli) and segmental (part of involved glomerulus) in distribution. The uninvolved segment appears normal on light microscopy. The sclerosis occurs due to accumulation of extracellular matrix. Areas of hyalinosis, which occurs due to insudation of plasma proteins, may be superimposed on the areas of sclerosis. The hyalinosis frequently occurs in FSGS associated with hypertension especially in parahilar location. Even a single glomerulus with segmental sclerosis is sufficient to make the diagnosis of FSGS. The diagnosis may be missed in small needle biopsy due to focal nature of the lesion and multiple step cuts must be examined as lesions are segmental. Thus, focal and segmental nature of the lesion may lead to misdiagnosis of MCD in small biopsies. The chance of missing a focal lesion is of order of 35% if 10 glomeruli are sampled and probability of missing drops to 12% if 20 glomeruli are sampled. [10] The pathologic changes of FSGS are most prominent in glomeruli located at the corticomedullary junction [Figure 3], so if the renal biopsy specimen is from the superficial tissue, the lesions can be missed.

Recently, FSGS has been classified into 5 variants. [11] These include:

1. FSGS, not otherwise specified (NOS). Segmental glomerular sclerosis without features of other specific forms; most common variant. [Figure 3]
2. Perihilar variant. The segmental sclerosis is localized next to the vascular pole; common in some forms of secondary FSGS, such as in obesity-related FSGS. [Figure 4]
3. Cellular variant. Segmental sclerosis with intracapillary hypercellularity with or without foam cells and karyorrhexis; least common variant, somewhat controversial. [Figure 5]
4. Tip variant. Segmental sclerosis localized to the origin of the proximal tubule. Controversial to classify as FSGS; many patients respond to steroids and behave as minimal change NS (MCNS) clinically (see previous section on MCNS). [Figure 6]
5. Collapsing variant. Glomerular capillary collapse with overlying hypertrophic glomerular epithelial cells. [Figure 7]

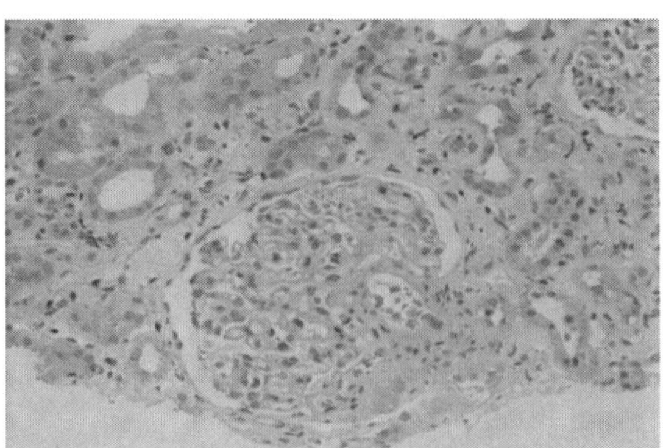

Figure 4. Perihilar focal segmental glomerulosclerosis. The segmental sclerosis is localized next to the vascular pole. [H&E, ×200].

3.3. Immunofluorescence

Idiopathic FSGS is non-immune mediated, so no immunoglobulins or C3 is deposited. Non-specific adsorption of C3 and IgM may occur in sclerotic areas.

Immunoglobulins and other serum proteins may appear in resorption droplets in tubular epithelial cells.

3.4. Electron Microscopy

The major ultrastructural finding in a case of FSGS is podocyte foot process effacement. There may be other features of podocyte damage as presence of resorption droplets, microvillus transformation and condensation of actin cytoskeleton in parallel to basal lamina in affected podocyte. The foot process effacement is characteristically more diffuse in cases of primary FSGS as compared to the secondary FSGS. An arbitrary cut off of 50% has been found useful to differentiate between primary and secondary FSGS ultrastructurally, where the case with more than 50% effacement of foot process is considered primary FSGS and those with less than 50% effacement are consired secondary FSGS.

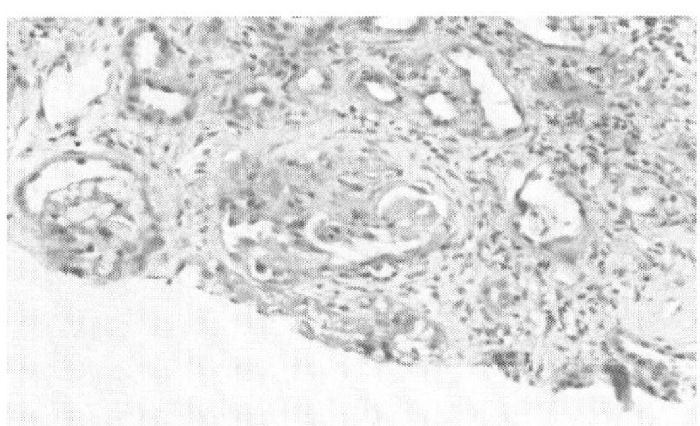

Figure 5. Cellular focal segmental glomerulosclerosis. There is segmental sclerosis with intracapillary hypercellularity. [H&E, ×200].

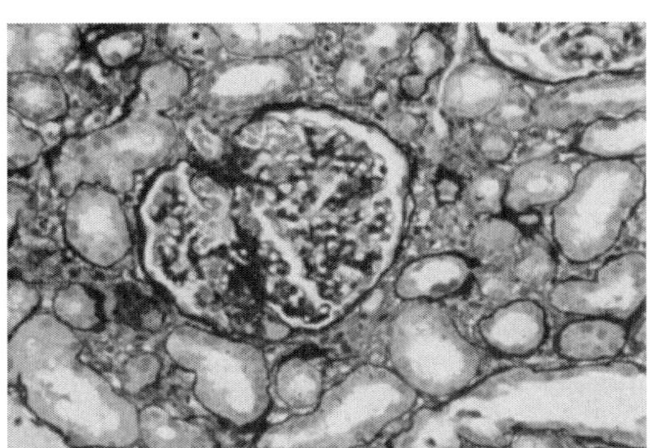

Figure 6. Focal segmental glomerulosclerosis, tip variant. There is segmental sclerosis localized to the origin of the proximal tubule. [SM, ×200].

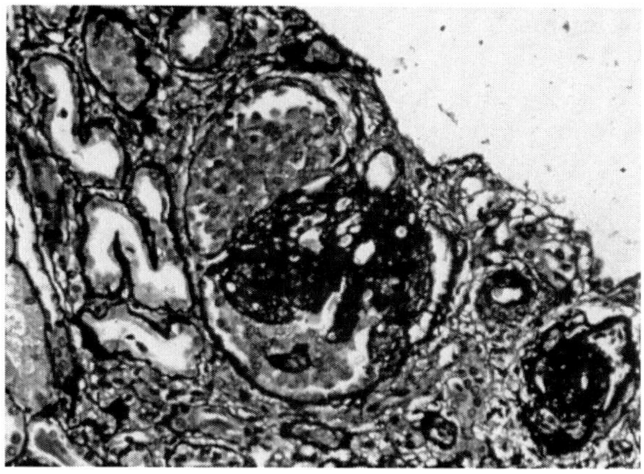

Figure 7. Focal segmental glomerulosclerosis, collapsing variant. There is collapse of glomerular capillary with overlying hypertrophic glomerular epithelial cells. [SM, ×200].

4. Membranous Nephropathy (MN)

MN accounts for approximately 30% of cases of NS in adults, with a peak incidence between 30 to 50 years of age and a male to female ratio of 2:1. [12] It was the commonest cause of NS in adults but recently has been surpassed by FSGS. [12] In approximately one third of cases, MN is secondary to malignancy (solid tumors of the breast, lung, colon), infection (hepatitis B, malaria, schistosomiasis), or rheumatologic disorders like SLE or rarely rheumatoid arthritis (Table 2).

Table 2. The main causes of membranous glomerulonephritis

Primary/idiopathic membranous glomerulonephritis
Secondary membranous glomerulonephritis
Infections:
Hepatitis B, Hepatitis C, syphilis, leprosy, filariasis, hydatid, malaria, schistosomiasis
Neoplasms:
Bladder, Breast, carcinoid, seminoma, colon, lung, stomach, kidney, esophagus, neuroblastoma
Drugs:
Gold, captopril, formaldehyde,mercury, penicillamine, nonsteroidal anti-inflammatory agents, probenecid
Autoimmune diseases:
Systemic lupus erythematosus, rheumatoid arthritis, primary biliary cirrhosis, ANCA- associated glomerulonephritis, auto-immune enteropathy, anti-GBM disease

Most of the cases of primary MN have been found to be caused by antibodies to phospholipase A2 receptor (PLA2R). The presence of segmental sclerosis in cases of MN is associated with worse prognosis.

4.1. Light Microscopy

On light microscopy, there is diffuse thickening of GBMs with little variation between glomeruli. Uniform thickening of the basement membranes along the peripheral capillary loops is seen by light microscopy on renal biopsy [Figure 8]; in the early stages, the glomerular capillaries appear rounded and stiff. In the later stages as disease progresses, the glomerular capillary walls become thicker and appear intensely eosinophilic and refractile in hematoxylin and eosin (H&E) stained sections.

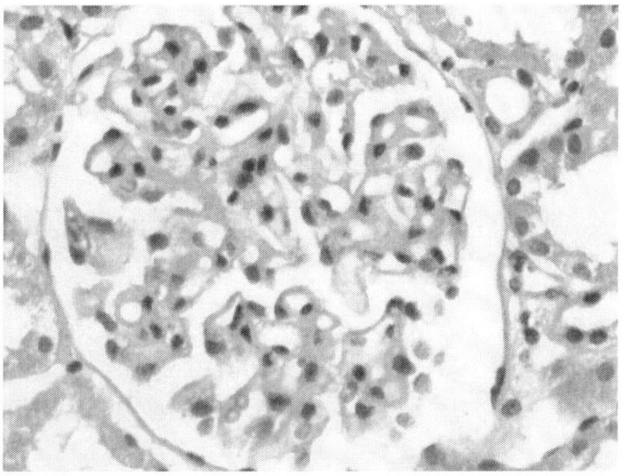

Figure 8. Membranous nephropathy (MN). There is stiffening and rounding of capillary lumina with diffuse thickening of the glomerular capillary wall. [H&E, ×400].

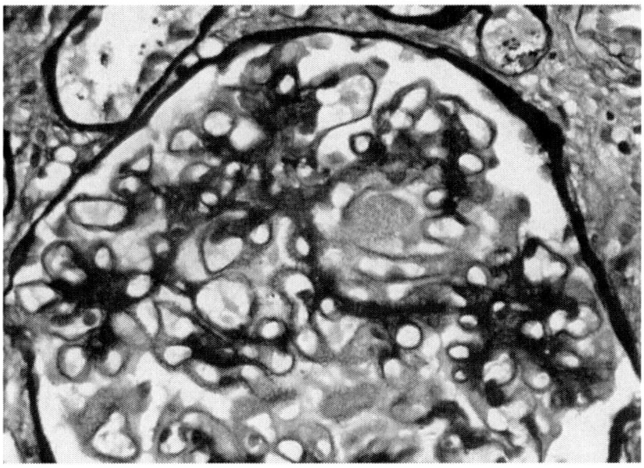

Figure 9. Membranous nephropathy (MN). There are fine spike like projections arising from the capillary wall. These are basement membrane reaction to subepithelial deposits. [SM, ×400].

In advanced stages, thickening of the GBM leads to mesangial matrix expansion and eventually segmental scarring and global sclerosis. The glomerular capillary wall changes in MN are better appreciated on silver methenamine stain. The earliest change in silver stained sections is mottling of the GBM.

This appearance results from alterations in the GBM caused by the subepithelial deposits, but they are not specific for MN. The non-specific mottling in the outer aspect of the GBM eventually resolves into small projections (spikes) of silver-positive material, [Figure 9] composed of type IV collagen and noncollagenous extracellular matrix proteins including laminin, heparan sulfate proteoglycans, and vitronectin. [13-15]

4.2. Immunofluorescence

IF shows finely granular capillary wall deposition of immune reactants in early stages and coarsely granular deposition in more advanced stages. The principal immune reactant in MN is IgG [Figure 10], other immunoglobulins or complements if present are of weaker intensity. The mesangial deposition in addition to capillary wall deposition is indicative of secondary MN. When IgA, IgM and C1q deposition is also present in addition to IgG and C3 deposition, the MN secondary to SLE nephritis should be considered. [16].

The immune deposits in idiopathic MN contain a preponderance of the IgG-4 subgroup, which fixes complement poorly; this explains why the C3 deposits are weak and variable, despite the large amounts of IgG. [17-19] Hass noted that IgG-3 was the predominant subclass in SLE MN whereas IgG-4 was predominant in idiopathic MN. [20] Hass suggested that the pattern of subclass staining might be useful in the differential diagnosis of cases in which the clinical diagnosis of SLE is equivocal.

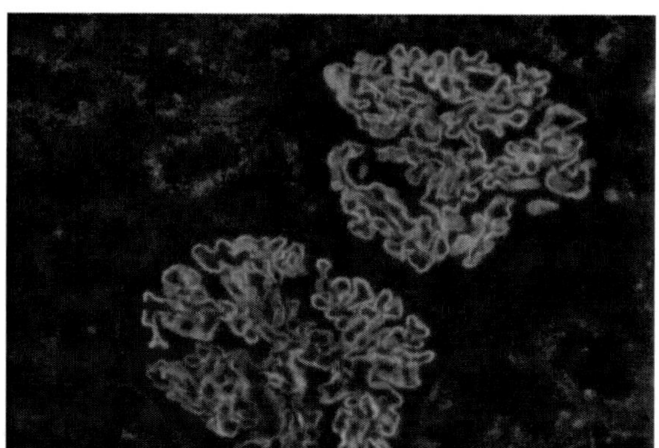

Figure 10. Membranous nephropathy (MN). There are fine granular capillary wall immune deposits corresponding to evenly distributed subepithelial deposits. Deposits in idiopathic MGN stain predominantly with IgG. [Anti IgG immunofluorescence, ×200].

4.3. Electron Microscopy

In electron microscopy based on the amount and texture of deposits, 4 stages of MN are identified. In early stage I MN, deposits may be extremely small and inconspicuous with no surrounding GBM reaction, corresponding to presence of non-specific mottling and absence of spikes on electron microscopy. In stage II MN, well formed spikes are present. In stage III, the deposits are encircled by GBM reaction. [Figure 11] In stage IV, the deposits are reabsorbed leaving behind lucent areas.

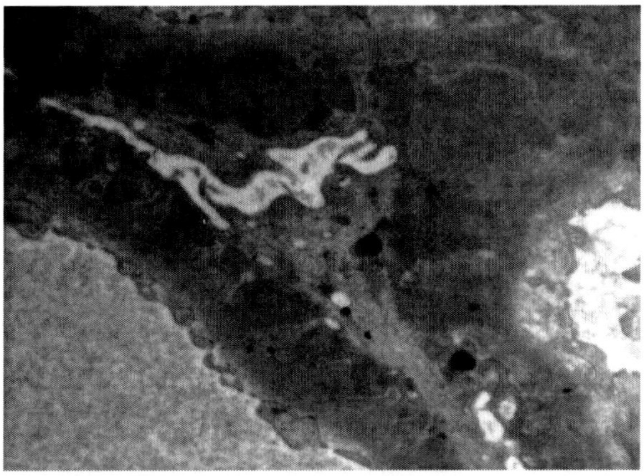

Figure 11. Membranous nephropathy (MN). There are large subepithelial electron dense deposits. [TEM, ×5000].

The secondary foot process effacement is often noted. If along with subepithelial electron dense deposits, the mesangial deposits are also noted, a possibility of secondary MN should be considered. The presence of endothelial tubuloreticular aggregates or accompanying sub endothelial deposits indicates MN secondary to lupus nephritis (LN).

5. Membranoproliferative Glomerulonephritis (MPGN)

The MPGN is a pattern of injury that can arise due to variety of insults mediated by immunoglobulins and/or complements. Previously, it was subclassified in to 3 subgroups: MPGN type 1, MPGN type 2 and MPGN type 3, on the basis of immune complex localization on electron microscopy. Recently, a new classification system has been developed based on IF where predominant or sole complement (C3) deposition is labelled as C-MPGN or C3 glomerulopathy and the cases with both immunoglobulins and complement deposition are known as immune complex mediated MPGN (IC-MPGN). [21] The IC-MPGN roughly corresponds to MPGN type 1 of the older classification.

5.1. Immune Complex-Mediated Membranoproliferative Glomerulonephritis

It occurs predominantly in the pediatric patients and young adults and presents with nephrotic and/or nephritic syndrome. This pattern of injury is caused predominantly by factors which lead to chronic antigenemia. The IC-MPGN is slowly progressive but overall renal outcome is dismal. The rate of recurrence in transplanted kidney is less as compared to C-MPGN but it is as high as 30%.

5.1.1. Light microscopy

On light microscopy, membranoproliferative pattern of injury is characterized by mesangial matrix expansion, increase in mesangial cellularity, infiltration of mononuclear inflammatory cells, and remodelling and thickening of the glomerular capillary walls. These changes result in an exaggeration of the lobular pattern of the glomerulus, hence the older designation of lobular glomerulonephritis for this lesion. [Figure 12 A]

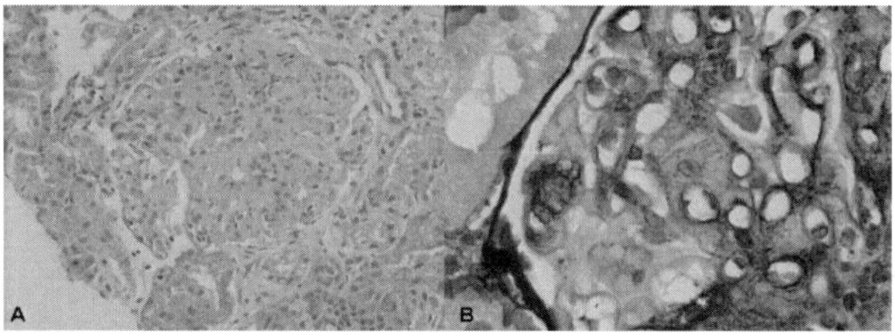

Figure 12. Membranoproliferative glomerulonephritis (MPGN). A. There is lobular accentuation with mesangial matrix expansion, hypercellularity and endocapillary proliferation. [H&E, ×200]. B. Note the remodeling and splitting of glomerular capillary wall. [SM, ×400].

The thickening and remodelling of the peripheral capillary wall can be segmental rather than global and diffuse in nature. On silver methenamine staining, thickened capillary loops display splitting or basement membrane reduplication. This appearance is known as tram track appearance. [Figure 12 B] This appearance occurs due to mesangial cell interposition into the peripheral capillary walls.

5.1.2. Immunofluorescence

There are large, granular, sometimes confluent, glomerular capillary wall and mesangial deposits of IgG with C3 of equal or less intensity. [Figure 13 A and B] Occasionally, other immunoreactants, like IgA and C1q, with less intense fluorescence are noted.

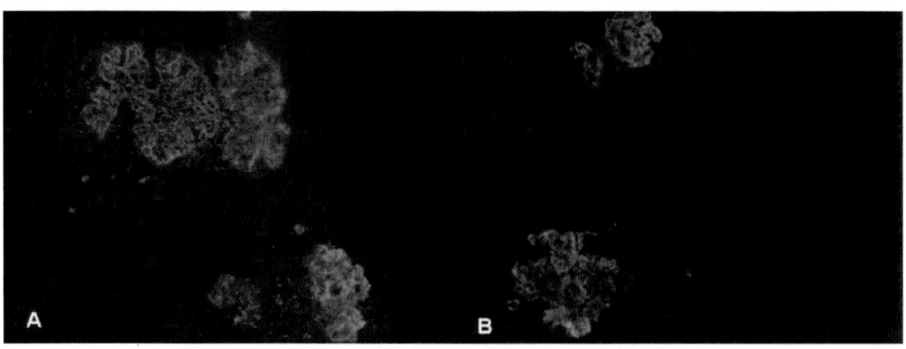

Figure 13. Immune complex-mediated membranoproliferative glomerulonephritis (IC-MPGN). A. There is irregular coarse capillary wall granular deposition of IgG with rounded outer counters corresponding to the subendothelial deposition [Anti IgG immunofluorescence, ×200]. B. In addition to IgG similar deposition of C3 is also noted. [Anti C3 immunofluorescence, ×200].

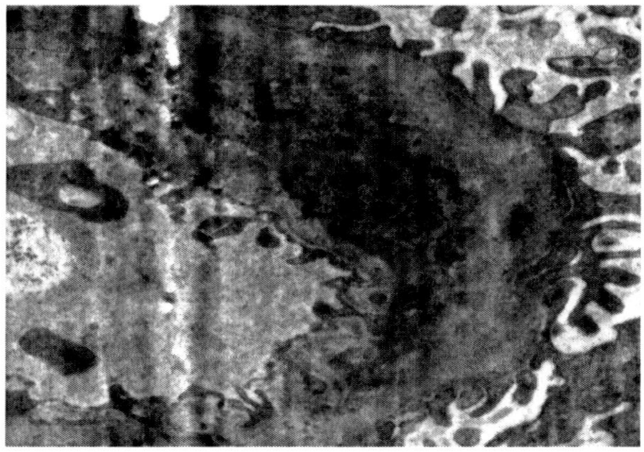

Figure 14. Immune complex-mediated membranoproliferative glomerulonephritis (IC-MPGN). There is massive subendothelial deposition in the capillary loop with secondary podocyte effacement. [TEM, ×10,000].

5.1.3. Electron Microscopy

The ultrastructural study shows wide-spread electron-dense, glomerular subendothelial deposits of varying sizes. (Figure 14] Marked mesangial hypercellularity with mesangial cell interpositioning are also noted. The electron-dense deposits are found in mesangial areas along with the classical subendothelial location in this type of MPGN.

5.2. C3 Glomerulopathy

It includes the group of glomerular disorders with sole or predominant C3 deposition. On the basis of ultrastructural study, it is subdivided in to 2 subgroups, i.e., dense deposit disease (DDD) and C3 glomerulonephritis. [22] The C3 glomerulopathies are caused by fluid phase dysregulation of alternate complement pathway. This dysregulation may be mediated either by mutation of alternative pathway complement regulatory proteins , their receptors or by presence of antibodies like C3 nephritic factor (C3Nef) , anti-factor H, or anti factor I, which interfere with functioning of complement regulatory proteins.

The patients present with nephrotic and/or nephritic syndrome. The DDD patients often have visual impairment and partial lipodystrophy. The disease progression is fast such that most patients have end-stage renal disease (ESRD) by adolescence. The recurrence rate following transplantation is almost 100% in DDD and variable in C3 glomerulonephritis.

5.2.1. Light Microscopy

The classical membranoproliferative pattern of glomerular injury is found in approximately 25% of patients with C3 glomerulopathy. Walker et al. described five histological patterns of DDD which include mesangial proliferative (45%), membranoproliferative (25%), crescentic (18%) and acute proliferative/exudative pattern (12%) mimicking a post infectious glomerulonephritis. Two cases were deemed unclassified. Unclassified DDD showed intermediately electron-dense transformation of the GBMs and mesangial regions. [23] Fervenza et al. reported a case of C3 glomerulonephritis with light microscopic picture of segmental necrotizing GN simulating pauci-immune GN. This case had a novel factor H mutation. [24] Thus, on light microscopy, the C3 glomerulopathy can show a variety of patterns of glomerular injury.

5.2.2. Immunofluorescence

C3 glomerulopathy characteristically shows staining for only complement C3 in glomeruli. [Figure 15 A and B] The extent of immunoglobulins in the case of C3 glomerulopathy remains debatable. According to new guidelines, dominant C3 of more than or equal to 2 orders of magnitude of intensity by IF (using a scale of 0 to 3, including 0, trace, 1+ , 2+ , 3+) than any other immunoreactant can be a useful cut off in cases of C3 glomerulopathy. [23]

5.2.3. Electron Microscopy

The DDD is characterized by large, dense, intramembranous deposits in the GBM. [Figure 16] There may be similar deposits in the nearby mesangial regions. The Bowman's capsule and the tubular basement membranes (TBMs) may also show intramembranous deposits. Similar deposits are noted in the basement membranes of other organs, such as the liver, spleen, and eye. The C3 glomerulonephritis does not show characteristic dense intramembranous deposits pathognomonic of DDD. The ultrastructural examination in these cases shows glomerular subendothelial, subepithelial, and transmembranous deposits of varying intensity. [Figure 17]

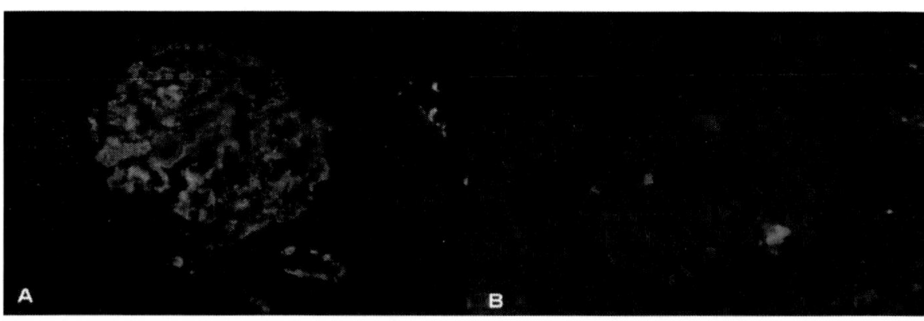

Figure 15. Complement-mediated membranoproliferative glomerulonephritis (C-MPGN). A. There is coarse granular capillary wall deposition of C3. [Anti C3 immunofluorescence ×200]. B. There is no IgG deposition in the glomerulus. [Anti IgG immunofluorescence, ×200].

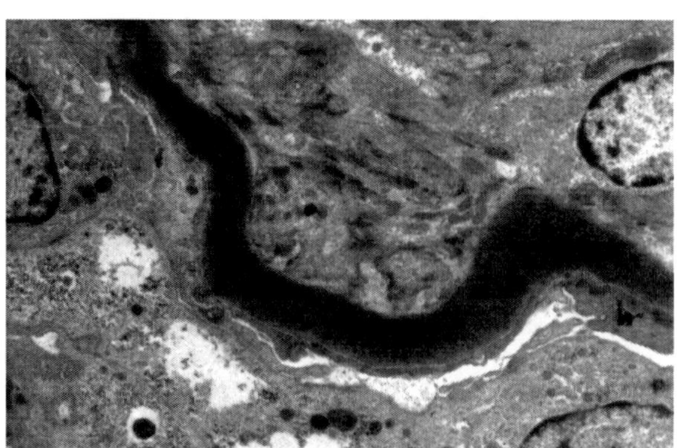

Figure 16. Dense Deposit Disease (DDD). There is dense transformation of glomerular basement membrane. [TEM ×5000].

6. Diabetic Nephropathy (DN)

DN is the single most common cause of chronic renal failure in the United States, accounting for 45% of patients receiving renal replacement therapy, and is a rapidly growing problem worldwide. [25]

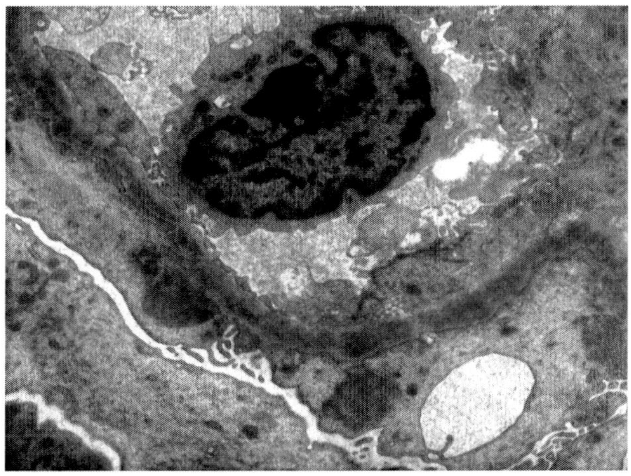

Figure 17. C3 glomerulonephritis (C3GN).There is intermediately dense transformation of glomerular basement membrane along with subepithelial and mesangial electron dense deposits. [TEM, ×5000].

Table 3. The classification of diabetic nephropathy

Class	Description	Inclusion criteria
1	GBM thickening	Biopsy not showing criteria for class II, III or IV GBM thickness exceeding 395 nm in females and 430 nm in males with age≥ 9 years.
2a	Mild mesangial expansion (mesangial area less than capillary lumen)	Mild mesangial expansion in > 25% of observed mesangium.
2b	Severe mesangial expansion (mesangial area more than capillary lumen)	Severe mesangial expansion in > 25% of observed mesangium.
3	Nodular sclerosis (Kimmelsteil-Wilson lesion)	Presence of KW lesion
4	Advanced diabetic glomerulosclerosis	At least one convincing KW lesion and global glomerulosclerosis in >50% of glomeruli.

Microalbuminuria is the first warning sign of renal disease in patients with DM. [26] With time, proteinuria becomes more and more severe and less selective. Most patients with DN experience nephrotic-range proteinuria and renal failure. Diabetes mellitus (DM) is the commonest cause of nephrotic-range proteinuria in adults. DN usually shows good correlation with fundus changes, particularly in type 1 DM. More than 90% of type 1 DM patients with DN already have diabetic retinopathy. Thus, in a patient of type 1 DM, a diagnosis other than DN should be considered if there is no diabetic retinopathy. This correlation is not very good in type 2 DM and only 60% patients of DM type 2 with DN have diabetic retinopathy. The indications of kidney biopsy in a diabetic patient are absence of retinal changes or an atypical clinical course.

6.1. Light Microscopy

The light microscopic features of type 1 and 2 DM are the same. [27, 28] The earliest morphological change is glomerulomegaly. The characteristic lesions of DN include: diffuse glomerulosclerosis (diffuse thickening of the GBM and diffuse increase in mesangial matrix), nodular glomerulosclerosis (Kimmelstiel-Wilson mesangial nodules), insudative changes (fibrin caps, capsular drops) and arteriolar hyalinosis involving both the afferent and efferent arterioles. The diffuse diabetic glomerulosclerosis is identified by diffuse thickening of basement membranes and diffuse increase in mesangial matrix. This pattern of glomerular change may be seen in non-diabetic hypertensive patients as well. It was in 1936 that nodular diabetic glomerulosclerosis was described first by Kimmelstiel and Wilson, hence it is called Kimmelstiel-Wilson (KW) nodule. There are sclerotic nodules located in the intercapillary or mesangial regions of the glomerular tuft (Figure 18). The KW nodules are acellular, have the same staining tinctorial staining properties as mesangial matrix and GBM. The KW nodule is often surrounded by dilated glomerular capillary loops (microaneurysms). Nodular glomerulosclerosis is almost always superimposed on pre-existing diffuse diabetic glomerulosclerosis. The number of KW nodules tends to increase with the duration of DN.

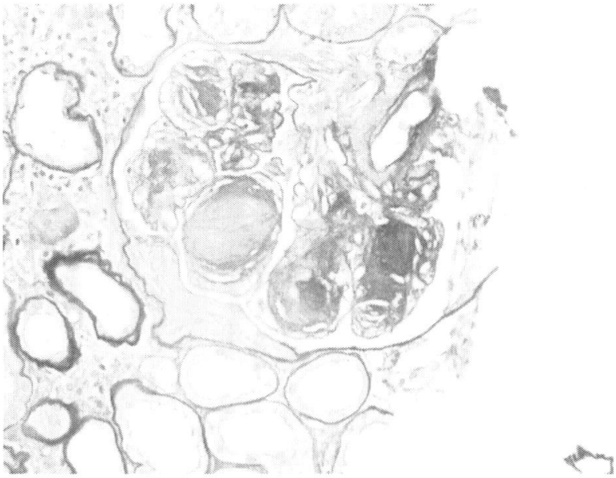

Figure 18. Diabetic Nephropathy (DN). There is diffuse basement membrane thickening, mesangial matrix expansion and nodular glomerulosclerosis. In nodular glomerulosclerosis, there are multiple asymmetric nodules of mesangial matrix surrounded by intact capillary lumina. [PAS, ×200].

The insudative lesions of DN include fibrin caps and capsular drops [Figure 19]. These insudative lesions are the result of accumulation of plasma proteins in the walls of blood vessels. In fibrin caps, this accumulation is seen between endothelium and GBM, while in capsular drops, the accumulation is between parietal epithelial cells and the basement membrane. These insudative lesions are not diagnostic of DN but are more often seen in later stages.

Recently a schema has been proposed to grade the severity of DN based on the morphological features (Table 3). The arteriolar hyalinosis is frequently seen in DN. The hyalinosis of both afferent and efferent arterioles is considered to be pathognomonic of DN. Superimposed non-diabetic kidney disease is not uncommon in the setting of DN. The post infectious glomerulonephritis is a common association, more commonly in patients with infected leg ulcers. [29]

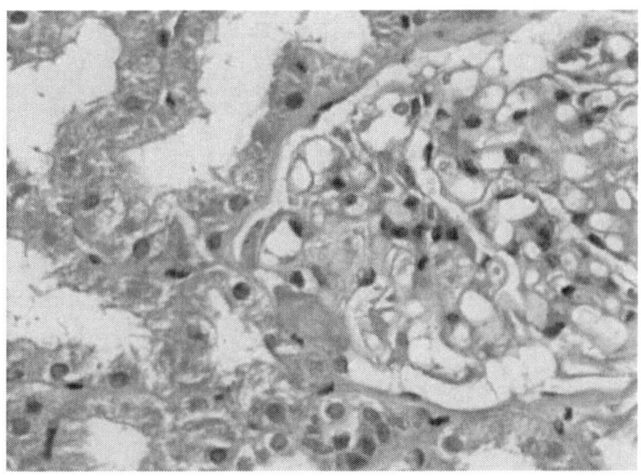

Figure 19. Diabetic Nephropathy (DN). There is diffuse basement membrane thickening and mesangial matrix expansion. A capsular drop is seen at the Bowman's capsule. [H&E, ×400].

MN is another glomerular disease that is commonly superimposed on DN. The association of MN with DM is believed to be coincidental, because MN is the most common form of GN in the elderly, the population most often affected by type 2 DM. IgA nephropathy (IgAN) and obesity-related hilar FSGS are other common associations.

6.2. Immunofluorescence

The typical finding in DN is the linear staining along the glomerular capillary walls with immunoglobulin G (IgG) [Figure 20]. [30] The linear staining of capillary walls has also been reported with IgM, C3, fibrinogen and albumin. [31] Hyalinosis usually stains brightly with IgM and C3, as in FSGS or pyelonephritis.

Linear staining for IgG and albumin has also been reported along TBMs and Bowman's capsule in patients with advanced diabetic glomerulosclerosis. [32] The linear staining of GBM is thought to reflect structural changes; it is now thought that advanced glycosylation end products may bind to the basement membranes and change their properties. [33]

Figure 20. Diabetic Nephropathy (DN). There is often accentuation of glomerular and tubular basement membranes in IgG immunostaining. [Anti IgG immunofluorescence, ×200]

6.3. Electron Microscopy

On ultrastructural examination, the thickening of the GBM and mesangial volume increase, are the earliest detectable changes; they become more prominent with disease progression. The KW nodules show a fibrillary substructure (diabetic fibrillosis) and need to be differentiated from amyloidosis or fibrillary GN. Discrete "immune-type," electron-dense deposits are not seen; if present, they are suggestive of a superimposed immune complex-mediated glomerulonephritis.

7. Glomerular Deposition Diseases

Plasma cell dyscrasias producing excess of monoclonal immunoglobulins or their fragments may lead to the formation of glomerular and tubular deposits that lead to heavy proteinuria and renal failure; the similar mechanism leads to the accumulation of serum amyloid A protein fragments seen in several chronic inflammatory diseases. This subgroup of proteinuric patients has glomerular deposition disease.

7.1. Light Chain Deposition Disease (LCDD)

This is the second most common plasma cell dyscrasia-related renal disease after primary amyloidosis. The disease generally occurs in adults and elderly. The LCDD patients generally produce kappa light chains. These light chains do not have the biochemical features necessary to form amyloid fibrils. The kappa chains tend to self-aggregate and form granular deposits along the glomerular capillary walls and mesangium, TBMs, and Bowman's capsule. When the deposits are predominantly in the glomerulus the clinical presentation is of NS. The factors leading to deposition include self-aggregating properties at neutral pH, and abnormal metabolism. The cases of light chain as well as light and heavy chain are reported. [34]

7.1.1. Light Microscopy

The most characteristic lesion of LCDD is nodular glomerulosclerosis. Light-chain deposits are not fibrillar and do not stain with Congo red, but they are easily discernible on IF showing light chain restriction and granular deposits on electron microscopy. Other glomerular injury patterns such as membranoproliferative or other intracapillary or extracapillary proliferative patterns may be seen. [35, 36]. Another important clue to the morphological diagnosis of LCDD is the homogeneous, glassy thickening of the basement membranes of non-atrophic tubules. The most important light microscopic differential is DN; however, the nodular glomerulosclerosis of LCDD is more diffuse and other lesions suggestive of DN such as fibrin caps, capsular drops, glomerular capillary wall thickening and severe arteriolar hyalinosis are absent. Treatment for LCDD is treatment of the primary disease. As so many patients with LCDD progress to renal failure, the overall prognosis is grim.

7.1.2. Immunofluorescence

There is light chain restriction, with predominance of kappa chains in most of the cases. [Figure 21 A and B] The deposits consist of only one light chain but rarely there is deposition of heavy chains as well or there may be heavy chains only. The fluorescence staining is usually in a linear fashion along glomerular capillaries and TBMs. This staining is most often restricted to only kappa chains. The mesangium is also positive.

7.1.3. Electron Microscopy

On electron microscopy, finely granular, electron-dense, deposits are noted along the subendothelial aspect of the GBM in mostly continuous manner. (Figure 23) These electron-dense, powdery deposits may be present in the mesangial matrix and, along the outer aspect of the TBMs; the deposits may be found in the interstitium as well. At times, the characteristic powdery deposits are not visible despite the characteristic IF. The immune electron microscopy in these cases shows deposition of either kappa or lambda light chains.

The reason behind absence of powdery deposits is the alteration in the density of deposits, such that they are not differentiated from basement membrane material. Rarely, the deposits show fibrillary appearance focally.

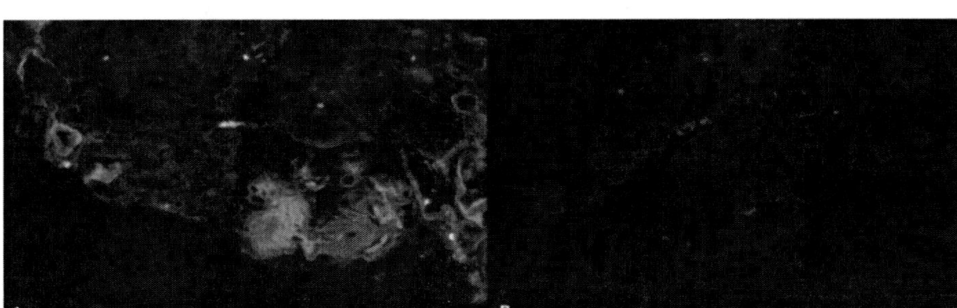

Figure 21. Light Chain Deposition Disease (LCDD). There is kappa light chain restriction demonstrated by bright kappa light chain immunostaining in the glomerulus. [Fig 21 A, Anti kappa immunofluorescence, ×200], while there is no deposition of lambda light chains [Fig 21 B, Anti Lambda immunofluorescence, ×200].

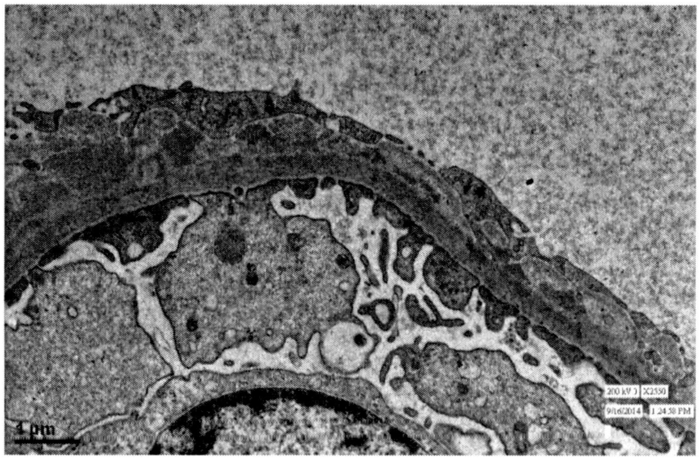

Figure 22. Light Chain Deposition Disease (LCDD). There is thin granular line of deposition in early LCDD. The diagnosis has to be confirmed on immunofluorescence. [TEM, ×2550].

7.2. Renal Amyloidosis

Amyloidosis is a unique group of protein-folding disorders with different etiology in which deposits of abnormally folded proteins share unique staining properties and ultrastructural appearance. [37]

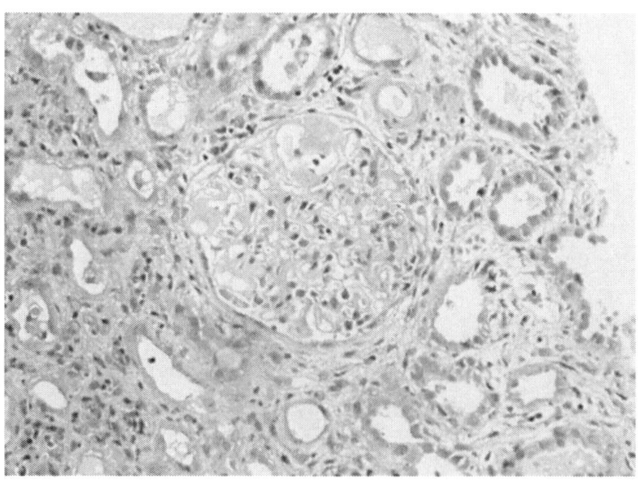

Figure 23. Amyloidosis. There is deposition of amorphous, eosinophilic, hyaline material in the mesangium. [H&E, ×200].

Amyloidosis is a rare disorder, with prevalence of approximately 1 per 60,000. [4] It accounts for 1% to 5% cases of NS in adults but is extremely rare in children. [38, 39].

Most cases of renal amyloidosis can be divided in to two broad subgroups, one due to deposition of monoclonal light chains (mostly lambda) or rarely heavy chains and other due to deposition of serum amyloid A (SAA) protein in patients with chronic inflammatory diseases. The former is called primary and the latter as secondary amyloidosis. These two subgroups are etiologically different but share the same clinicopathophysiological features. Amyloid infiltrates the liver, heart, peripheral nerves, carpal tunnel, upper pharynx, spleen and kidney. Only 10 to 20 % patients with primary amyloidosis have overt myeloma, the rest have serum and/or urine monoclonal spikes. In the developed nations, the amyloidosis is primary and occurs in elderly, but in countries where tuberculosis and leprosy are endemic, secondary amyloidosis outnumbers primary amyloidosis.

7.2.1. Light Microscopy

The histological features and staining characteristics of amyloid are the same irrespective of the type of amyloid. In H&E stained sections, amyloid appears as eosinophilic, amorphous, hyaline material (Figure 24). The deposition of amyloid can occur in any renal compartment but begins in the mesangium replacing the normal mesangial matrix and later extends into the peripheral capillary walls. The other common site of amyloid deposition is the renal vasculature. Interstitial deposition especially adjacent to the renal vasculature may be seen in the later stages.

The amyloid has a characteristic salmon pink or pale pink colour on Congo red staining. The Congo red stained amyloid gives a characteristic apple-green birefringence on polarised microscopy, which is considered diagnostic. Thick sections, with an optimum thickness of 9 or 10 μm, are recommended to demonstrate amyloid satisfactorily, instead of the customary 4 μm sections. [1] Thioflavin T fluorescence is much more sensitive than Congophilia in the detection of small amounts of amyloid. [40] The thioflavin T is the most sensitive while apple-green birefringence on Congo red stained slides is the most specific method for the detection of amyloid.

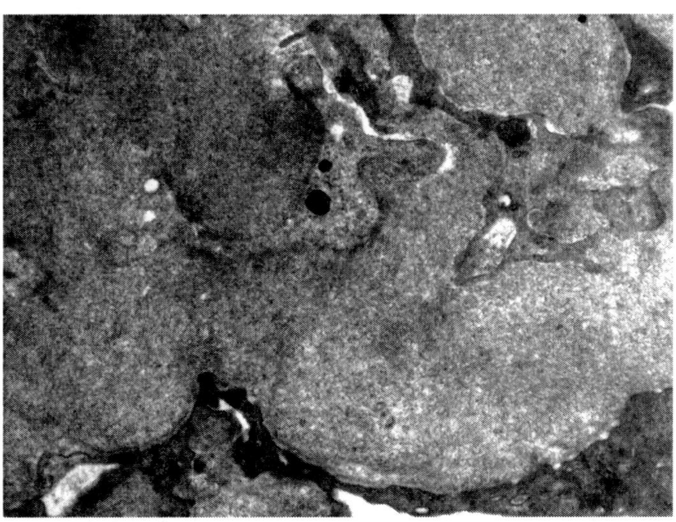

Figure 24. Amyloidosis. Amyloid appears as randomly oriented fibrils of indeterminate length and measuring approximately 10 nm in diameter. [TEM, ×20000].

7.2.2. Immunofluorescence

IF is better than the immunoperoxidase method in the detection of light chain restriction in primary amyloidosis. The lambda light chain restriction is much common in primary amyloidosis as compared to kappa chain restriction. The non-specific staining of amyloid is not uncommon owing to its sticky characteristic. Thioflavin T staining of paraffin sections will give a bright green fluorescence, but this is not considered an IF method because thioflavin T is not an antibody.

7.2.3. Electron Microscopy

Randomly arranged, rigid, non-branching 8- to 10-nm fibrils are virtually diagnostic of amyloidosis (Figure 24).

7.3. Fibrillary-Immunotactoid Glomerulopathy

Fibrillary glomerulonephritis is a non-amyloid fibrillary disease with deposition of fibrils, 12–24 nm in diameter, in the glomeruli. Fibrillary glomerulonephritis is a rare disease of adults. It is more common in whites than in blacks. [41] The patient presents frequently with nephrotic-range proteinuria. Microscopic hematuria, hypertension, and renal insufficiency are also common.

7.3.1. Light Microscopy

It may present with wide variety of histologic lesions, including mesangioproliferative glomerulonephritis, diffuse proliferative and exudative glomerulonephritis, MPGN or MN. The crescents may be present in 15 to 20% of cases. [41] The most frequently encountered glomerular lesion however is mesangial expansion with glomerular capillary wall thickening. The deposited material is mostly methenamine silver negative, but it is admixed with silver-positive glomerular extracellular matrix. The Congo red staining is negative.

7.3.2. Immunofluorescence

On IF, there is strong, diffuse, smudgy mesangial and glomerular capillary wall deposition of IgG. In fibrillary GN, kappa fluorescence may be stronger than lambda fluorescence. C3 is frequently present. The deposited IgG is mainly of the IgG-4 subtype. [42]

7.3.3. Electron microscopy

Randomly arranged, rigid fibrils, 12 to 24 nm in diameter, are seen. The glomerulopathy with presence of fibrils thicker than 24 nm (microtubules, mostly 40 to 60 nm) is referred as immunotactoid glomerulopathy by some authors. The other group of investigators defies the need of this distinction. [41, 42] This debate continues.

8. Basement Membrane Syndromes

The podocyte foot processes rest on the GBM. The GBM is composed of collagen IV interweaved with laminins and sulphated proteoglycans and is organized in the inner and outer layers of lamina rara interna, lamina rara externa and the middle layer of lamina densa. The collagen type IV is a trimeric molecule comprising of any 3 of 6 alpha chains (α1-α6).

Early in the human development all the basement membranes of epithelia are composed of collagen type IV (α1α1α3 type).

Later due to increased requirement of the tensile strength there is a switch-over in various organs. In the kidney GBM, lung, testis, cochlea, and eye, this switch replaces α1α1α3 collagen type IV with α3α4α5 collagen type IV while an α5α5α 6 (IV) switch occurs in skin, smooth muscle, esophagus and Bowman's capsule in the kidney. The structural disorganisation of GBM may lead to the syndrome of isolated hematuria and proteinuria in later stages.

The basement membrane syndromes include Alport's syndrome, thin basement membrane disease and nail-patella syndrome (LAMB2 mutation).

8.1. Alport's Syndrome

Classical Alport's syndrome shows X-linked inheritance, and accounts for 85% of Alport's cases. The rest of the cases are caused by autosomal recessive mutations; exceptionally, autosomal dominant mutations may also be present. The genetic defect in Alport's syndrome consists of absence of α3, α4 or α5 chains of collagen IV heterotrimer.

In X-linked forms, only males are affected; the females may be affected if there is unfavourable lyonization.

The initial presentation is microscopic hematuria, later in the course of disease, nephrotic-range proteinuria may occur due to secondary FSGS. Female carriers of X-linked Alport's syndrome usually have hematuria as the only abnormality. The extrarenal manifestations of Alport's syndrome include sensorineural hearing deficit, ocular defects (anterior lenticonus), diffuse leiomyomatosis, and hematologic abnormalities (e.g., giant platelets, granulocyte abnormalities), etc.

The patients of Alport's syndrome present with hematuria and mild proteinuria (<1–2 g/24-hour), which appears late in the course. The non-renal manifestations include sensorineural deafness, anterior lenticonus, "dot and fleck" retinopathy, and rarely, mental retardation or leiomyomatosis.

Approximately 85% of patients with Alport's syndrome have an X-linked inheritance with mutations in the α5 chain of collagen type IV, on chromosome Xq22–24. Female carriers are generally asymptomatic; however, some may show hematuria and proteinuria of variable degree due to unfavourable mosaicism created by X inactivation. Rest of the patients have autosomal recessive mutations of the α3 (IV) or α4 (IV) chains on chromosome 2q35–37. The autosomal dominant pattern of inheritance of α3 (IV) or α4 (IV) chains' mutation may also occur very rarely.

8.1.1. Light Microscopy

In the early stages, the glomeruli are unremarkable; eventually segmental glomerulosclerosis develops in some patients. Accompanying interstitial fibrosis with tubular atrophy is seen in such cases. The presence of interstitial foam cells in the absence of nephrotic-range proteinuria is characteristic (but not specific) of Alport's syndrome.

8.1.2. Immunofluorescence

On IF, no immune deposits are noted. Monoclonal antibody staining for α 3, α4 and α5 chains in the skin and renal biopsies may be diagnostic. The type IV collagen is a heterotrimer composed of various combinations of alpha 1-6 collagen chains. The epidermal basement membrane contains α1, α2, α5 and α6 chains of collagen type IV and does not contain α3 or α4 chains. Thus, in X-linked Alport's syndrome, the skin biopsy shows absence of staining of α5 chain.

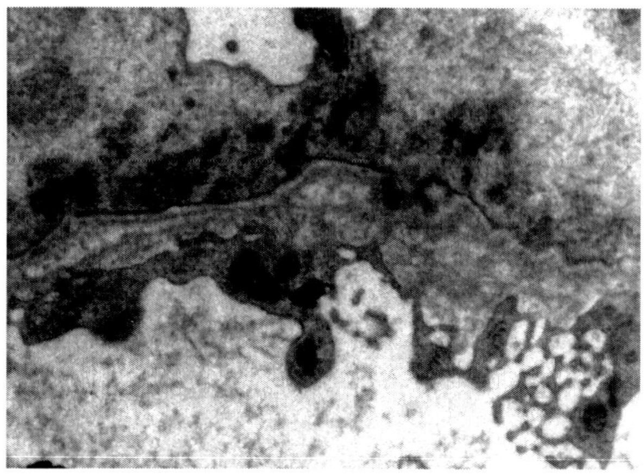

Figure 25. Alport's syndrome. There is alternate thickening and thinning of glomerular basement membrane with loose basket-weave appearance. The overlying foot processes show effacement. [TEM, ×5000].

In kidney, the GBM type IV collagen comprises of α3, α4 and α5 chains. While the Bowman's capsule and distal TBM contain α1, 1, 2 and α5, 5, 6 heterotrimers. In kidney, in X-linked Alport's syndrome, there is absence of α5 staining in TBMs and Bowman's capsule. There is absence of α3 and α4 as well in the GBM because the absence of α5 chain leads to the defective incorporation of α3 and α4 in the GBM. In autosomal recessive Alport's syndrome, there is absence of all the α3, α4 and α5 in the GBM but there will be presence of α5 chain in Bowman's capsule, distal TBMs and skin biopsy.

As α3 and α4 are normally absent in the epidermal basement membrane, the skin biopsy alone cannot diagnose autosomal recessive Alport's syndrome.

8.1.3. Electron Microscopy

Ultrastructural examination shows diffuse splintering, splitting, and lamellation of the lamina densa (Figure 25). [43, 44] The diagnostic changes in the basement membrane may be focal, the exact percentage of glomerular capillaries showing these changes is unclear, but some authors suggest that at least 50% of glomerular capillaries must show such changes.

9. Glomerular-Vascular Syndromes

In this section, diseases which lead to glomerular vascular injury secondary to vasculitis, endothelial injury/dysfunction, thrombosis, and ischemia are discussed.

9.1. Hypertensive Nephrosclerosis

The hypertensive nephrosclerosis is the second most common cause of ESRD in adults after DN.

9.1.1. Clinical Features

In an adult, hypertension is usually defined as systolic blood pressure consistently greater than 140/90 mm Hg. When the diastolic blood pressure is below 120 mm Hg, the hypertension is called “benign.” The first sign of hypertensive nephrosclerosis is decreased glomerular filtration rate (GFR) reflected by an increased serum creatinine level. Proteinuria develops in later stages and is frequently subnephrotic range but can be nephrotic range as well.

9.1.2. Light Microscopy

The vascular changes seen are arterial intimal fibroplasia and lamination of the lamina elastica interna (intimal fibroelastosis). There is hyalinization of the afferent arterioles and small interlobular arteries (hyaline arteriolosclerosis). The arteriolar hyalinosis occurs due to insudation of plasma proteins into the vessel walls. These vascular changes are virtually omnipresent in autopsied kidneys from older patients but are found most prominently in kidneys from patients with hypertension, DM or chronic calcineurin inhibitor (CNI) toxicity.

There are no characteristic glomerular lesions, but due to vascular changes, there may be secondary ischemic changes in the glomeruli with wrinkling and thickening of glomerular capillary walls and secondary global sclerosis. The global sclerosis is either obsolescent type (glomerular tuft sclerosed and Bowman’s space filled with collagenous material) or solidified type (global solidification of tuft without collagenous material within Bowman’s space). Another glomerular lesion seen frequently in later stages is secondary FSGS, often with GBM wrinkling, periglomerular fibrosis and subtotal secondary podocyte effacement.

There is tubular atrophy/ interstitial fibrosis of variable degree secondary to vascular compromise and ischemia. Glomeruli with segmental or global sclerosis and/or hyalinosis in the absence of idiopathic FSGS are indicators of glomerular hyperfiltration injury. These glomerular changes occur later in the course of hypertension and occur more commonly with an accelerated phase of hypertension and are associated with increasing degrees of proteinuria. This constellation of changes has been called decompensated benign nephrosclerosis by Fahr and later by Bohle et al. [45].

9.2. Systemic Lupus Erythematosus (SLE)

Systemic lupus erythematosus (SLE) is an autoimmune disease affecting multiple organ systems. The disease frequently involves the kidney and all the four components may be involved.

9.2.1. Clinical Features

The involvement of renal system by SLE is called LN and it poses greatest mortality and morbidity risk from this multisystem disorder.

The LN may appear at any time during the course of SLE and its manifestations may range from microscopic hematuria and minimal proteinuria to nephrotic- range proteinuria and rapidly progressive renal failure. The course of LN is complicated by repeated exacerbations and remissions.

9.2.2. Light Microscopy

The LN may involve any or all the four renal compartments i.e., glomeruli, tubules, interstitium, and blood vessels. Owing to this complexity of LN, various classification systems have been devised.

The first classification system was given by World Health Organization (WHO) in 1974. [46] The WHO classification was modified in 1982, [47] and later in 1995, [48] by the International Study of Kidney Disease in Children (ISKDC). A third classification was formulated in 2004 through a large consensus conference of renal pathologists, nephrologists, and rheumatologists, organized by the International Society of Nephrology (ISN) and the Renal Pathology Society (RPS).

The 2004 ISN/RPS classification is summarized below:

1. Class I (Minimal mesangial lupus nephritis): The kidney is normal by light microscopy. IF and electron microscopy reveal mesangial immune complex deposition.
2. Class II (Mesangial proliferative LN): Mesangial proliferative lupus nephritis (ISN/RPS). In addition to mesangial deposits by IF and electron microscopy, light microscopy reveals pure mesangial hypercellularity with patent glomerular capillaries.
3. Class III (Focal LN): There is focal (less than 50% glomeruli) segmental, and/or global endocapillary and/or extracapillary glomerulonephritis. There is subendothelial immune deposits, with or without mesangial deposition on IF and electron microscopy.

III (A): purely active lesions: focal proliferative LN
III (A/C): active and chronic lesions: focal proliferative and sclerosing LN
III (C): chronic inactive with glomerular scars: focal sclerosing LN

4. Class IV (Diffuse LN): There is diffuse (more than 50% glomeruli), segmental, and/or global endocapillary and/or extracapillary glomerulonephritis. IF shows peripheral capillary wall immune deposition with diffuse subendothelial and mesangial immune deposits on electron microscopy. This class is divided into diffuse segmental (IV-S) when >50% of the involved glomeruli have segmental lesions and diffuse global (IV-G) when >50% of the involved glomeruli have global lesions.

IV-S (A) or IV-G (A): purely active lesions: diffuse segmental or global proliferative LN

IV-S (A/C) or IV-G (A/C): active and chronic lesions: diffuse segmental or global proliferative and sclerosing LN

IV-S (C) or IV-G (C): inactive with glomerular scars: diffuse segmental or global sclerosing LN

5. Class V(Membranous LN): The light microscopic picture is similar to idiopathic MGN. There is frequently accompanying mesangial hypercellularity. The light microscopy shows peripheral capillary wall thickening, while IF shows peripheral capillary wall and mesangial immune deposition while electron microscopy shows predominantly subepithelial immune deposition.

Class VI (Advanced sclerosing LN): More than 90% glomeruli showing global glomerular sclerosis.

The renal biopsy is important in establishing the diagnosis of LN especially in cases where LN precedes the development of extrarenal manifestations. The ideal time of renal biopsy is debated; some nephrologists believe that a baseline renal biopsy should be performed in all the cases of newly diagnosed SLE while most nephrologists believe that indication of renal biopsy should be the appearance of features like hematuria and proteinuria or deranged renal functions which suggest renal involvement in the course of SLE. A repeat biopsy is performed if there is sudden change in renal parameters. The tubulointerstitial changes in patients of LN may be secondary to NS or due to active inflammation and edema. The former is common in class III, IV and V LN.

These changes include presence of fat resorption droplets or protein resorption droplets (hyaline degeneration). The intratubular oval fat bodies which comprise of desquamated fat laden tubular epithelial cells are found in setting of heavy proteinuria especially in class V LN. The active tubulointerstitial inflammation and edema is common in class III and IV LN. The tubulointerstitial immune deposition is also noted most frequently with class IV LN.

The vascular lesions in LN are varied and include:

1. Arteriosclerosis and arteriolosclerosis.
2. Uncomplicated vascular immune deposits: It is the most common renal vascular lesion of LN. It comprises of immune complex deposition in the walls of small arteries and arterioles which usually appear normal by light microscopy. This lesion is usually clinically silent, and does not confer a higher risk of hypertension or progressive renal disease. [49]
3. Lupus vasculopathy: In lupus vasculopathy, there is noninflammatory degeneration of medial myocytes and subendothelial swelling. IF shows variable staining of the vessel wall and lumen for immunoglobulins (e.g., IgG, IgM, IgA), complements (C3 and C1q) and fibrin.
4. Thrombotic microangiopathy: Associated with haemolytic uremic syndrome (HUS)/thrombotic thrombocytopenic purpura (TTP) syndrome. Associated with antiphospholipid antibodies. Associated with scleroderma/mixed connective tissue disease.
5. Necrotizing vasculitis (Polyarteritis nodosa type).

9.2.3. Immunofluorescence

The IF typically shows full-house IF profile i.e., positivity for immunoglobulins (IgA, IgG, and IgM) and complement components (C3 and C1q). The bright deposition of C1q is rare in other glomerulonephritides except C1q nephropathy. The immune deposition is mesangial in class I and II while predominantly peripheral capillary wall with few mesangial deposits in class III, IV and V LN.

The immunoglobulin deposition may be noted in TBMs, interstitium, arteries and arterioles.

9.2.4. Electron Microscopy

The electron-dense deposits in mesangium are universal in all subclasses; apart from that, subendothelial and subepithelial glomerular electron-dense deposits are also seen.

Electron-dense deposits may be seen within the TBMs (mostly on the interstitial side), in the walls of small arteries/arterioles, venules, and peritubular capillaries, and the interstitium. The tubuloreticular inclusions (interferon foot prints) may be seen in the endothelium. The electron-dense deposits in LN may rarely have an organized substructure with curved paracrystalline structures resembling fingerprints (fingerprint deposits).

10. Sickle Cell Disease

The individuals with sickle cell trait are mostly asymptomatic or rarely develop hyposthenuria due to subclinical infarction of renal medulla. On the contrary, patients of sickle cell disease are more prone to vaso-occlusion. Vessel occlusions in the kidney produce glomerular hypertension, FSGS, interstitial nephritis, and renal infarction. Some of the sickle cell disease patients also present with membranoproliferative pattern of injury.

11. Infectious Diseases

A number of infectious diseases lead to nephrotic-range proteinuria, either due to chronic antigenemia or direct podocytopathic effect of infectious agents. Some of these infectious agents are frequent cause of glomerulonephritides worldwide.

11.1. Human Immunodeficiency Virus (HIV)

Renal involvement is an important complication of HIV infection. The most common glomerular pathology in HIV infected patients is HIV-associated nephropathy (HIVAN). HIVAN is a type of FSGS, with prominence of visceral epithelial cells characteristically leading to collapsing glomerulopathy. There is proliferation of podocytes with pseudocrescent formation, microcystic dilatation of renal tubules, and tubuloreticular inclusions. The collapsing glomerulopathy may result from direct podocytopathic effect of virus. The other forms of glomerular injuries like diffuse proliferative glomerulonephritis and membranoproliferative patterns have also been noted especially in patients co-infected with hepatitis B or C. Other renal lesions include IgAN, MCD and TTP.

11.2. Hepatitis B and C

The hepatitis B carrier state leads to chronic antigenemia. On renal biopsy, the commonest lesion in children is MN, while in adults it leads most commonly to MPGN type 1. The lesions are similar to idiopathic MN or type I MPGN. The viral antigens are found in the renal deposits.

The renal manifestations are present in approximately 30% of chronic hepatitis C infected patients. The renal lesions identified in the order of frequency are cryoglobulinemic glomerulonephritis, MN, and MPGN type 1.

11.3. Syphilis

Secondary syphilis may present with the NS. The renal biopsy reveals features of MN, which is indistinguishable from idiopathic MN except that immune deposits often contain treponemal antigens.

11.4. Leprosy

The renal lesions in leprosy include FSGS, mesangioproliferative glomerulonephritis or renal amyloidosis. The other patterns of injuries found less commonly are diffuse proliferative glomerulonephritis and MPGN.

11.5. Malaria

The chronic malaria may lead to MPGN pattern of injury and consequent proteinuria. The mesangioproliferative glomerulonephritis is also reported.

11.6. Schistosomiasis

Schistosoma mansoni is most commonly associated with clinical renal disease, and the glomerular lesions are classified as: Class I- mesangioproliferative glomerulonephritis; cla ss II - extracapillary proliferative glomerulonephritis; class III - MPGN; class IV - FSGS; and class V- amyloidosis.[1]

11.7. Other Parasites

The other parasites causing glomerular injury and nephrotic-range proteinuria include toxoplasma, leishmania and Wuchereria Bancrofti and trichinella. [1]

Conclusion

In summary, the spectrum of diseases underlying NS in adults is highly variable. Secondary causes are more common in adult NS as compared with childhood NS and renal biopsy is imperative for an accurate diagnosis of the underlying cause of the condition.

References

[1] Glassock RJ, Cohen AH. The primary glomerulopathies. *Dis. Mon.* 1996;42:329-83.

[2] Habib R, Kleinknecht C, editors. The primary nephrotic syndrome of childhood: Classification and clinicopathologic study of 406 cases. New York: Appleton-Century-Crofts; 1971.

[3] Waldherr R, Gubler MC, Levy M, Broyer M, Habib R. The significance of pure diffuse mesangial proliferation in idiopathic nephrotic syndrome. *Clin. Nephrol.* 1978;10:171-179.

[4] Hull RP, Goldsmith DJ. Nephrotic syndrome in adults. *BMJ.* 2008;336:1185-9.

[5] D'Agati V. The many masks of focal segmental glomerulosclerosis. *Kidney Int.* 1994;46:1223-1241.

[6] Korbet SM. Primary focal segmental glomerulosclerosis. *J. Am. Soc. Nephrol.* 1998;9: 1333-1340.

[7] Haas M, Spargo BH, Coventry S. Increasing incidence of focal-segmental glomerulosclerosis among adult nephropathies: a 20-year renal biopsy study. *Am. J. kidney Dis.* 1995;26:740-750.

[8] Korbet SM, Genchi RM, Borok RZ, Schwartz MM. The racial prevalence of glomerular lesions in nephrotic adults. *Am. J. kidney Dis.* 1996;27:647-651.

[9] White R, Glasgow EF, Mills RJ. Clinicopathologic study of nephrotic syndrome in childhood. *Lancet.* 1970;1:1353-1359.

[10] Fogo AB, Kashgarian M. Diagnostic Atlas of Renal Pathology: A Companion to Brenner & Rector's the Kidney, 9th ed. Philadelphia: Elsevier/Saunders; 2012.

[11] D'Agati VD, Fogo AB, Bruijn JA, Jennette JC. Pathologic classification of focal segmental glomerulosclerosis: a working proposal. *Am. J. Kidney Dis.* 2004;43:368-382.

[12] Carome MA, Moore J Jr. Nephrotic syndrome in adults. A diagnostic and management challenge. *Postgrad. Med.* 1992;92:209-215.

[13] Buyukbabani N, Droz D. Distribution of the extracellular matrix components in human glomerular lesions. *J. Pathol.* 1994;172:199-207.

[14] Ikeda S, Makino H, Ota Z. Alterations in glomerular extracellular matrix components in glomerulonephritis. *Nippon. Jinzo. Gakkai. Shi.* 1993;35:941-947.

[15] Kanahara K, Yorioka N, Ogawa T, Taniguchi Y, Takemasa A, Hirabayashi A, Yamakido M. An immunohistochemical study of extracellular matrix components and integrins in human glomerular diseases. *Nippon. Jinzo. Gakkai. Shi.* 1994;36:355-364.

[16] Jennette JC, Iskandar SS, Dalldorf FG. Pathologic differentiation between lupus and nonlupus membranous glomerulopathy. *Kidney Int.* 1983;24:377-385.

[17] Bannister KM, Howarth GS, Clarkson AR, Woodroffe AJ. Glomerular IgG subclass distribution in human glomerulonephritis. *Clin. Nephrol.* 1983;19:161-165.
[18] Doi T, Mayumi M, Kanatsu K, Suehiro F, Hamashima Y. Distribution of IgG subclasses in membranous nephropathy. *Clin. Exp. Immunol.* 1984;58:57-62.
[19] Kuroki A, Shibata T, Honda H, Totsuka D, Kobayashi K, Sugisaki T. Glomerular and serum IgG subclasses in diffuse proliferative lupus nephritis, membranous lupus nephritis, and idiopathic membranous nephropathy. *Intern. Med.* 2002;41:936-942.
[20] Haas M. IgG subclass deposits in glomeruli of lupus and nonlupus membranous nephropathies. *Am. J. Kidney Dis.* 1994;23:358-364.
[21] Sethi S, Gamez JD, Vrana JA, Theis JD, Bergen HR 3rd, Zipfel PF, Dogan A, Smith RJ. Glomeruli of Dense Deposit Disease contain components of the alternative and terminal complement pathway. *Kidney Int.* 2009;75:952-960.
[22] Pickering MC, D'Agati VD, Nester CM, Smith RJ, Haas M, Appel GB, Alpers CE, Bajema IM, Bedrosian C, Braun M, Doyle M, Fakhouri F, Fervenza FC, Fogo AB, Frémeaux-Bacchi V, Gale DP, Goicoechea de Jorge E, Griffin G, Harris CL, Holers VM, Johnson S, Lavin PJ, Medjeral-Thomas N, Paul Morgan B, Nast CC, Noel LH, Peters DK, Rodríguez de Córdoba S, Servais A, Sethi S, Song WC, Tamburini P, Thurman JM, Zavros M, Cook HT. C3 glomerulopathy: consensus report. *Kidney Int.* 2013;84:1079-1089.
[23] Walker PD, Ferrario F, Joh K, Bonsib SM. Dense deposit disease is not a membranoproliferative glomerulonephritis. *Mod. Pathol.* 2007;20:605-616.
[24] Fervenza FC, Smith RJ, Sethi S. Association of a novel complement factor H mutation with severe crescentic and necrotizing glomerulonephritis. *Am. J. Kidney Dis.* 2012;60:126-132.
[25] Madaio MP, Harrington JT. The diagnosis of glomerular diseases: acuteglomerulonephritis and the nephrotic syndrome. *Arch. Intern. Med.* 2001;161:25-34.
[26] Estacio RO, Schrier RW. Diabetic nephropathy: pathogenesis, diagnosis, and prevention of progression. *Adv. Intern. Med.* 2001;46:359-408.
[27] Ritz E, Stefanski A. Diabetic nephropathy in type II diabetes. *Am. J. Kidney Dis.* 1996;27:167-194.
[28] Osterby R. Glomerular structural changes in type 1 (insulin-dependent) diabetes mellitus: causes, consequences, and prevention. *Diabetologia.* 1992;35:803-812.
[29] Monga G, Mazzucco G, di Belgiojoso GB, Confalonieri R, Sacchi G, Bertani T. Pattern of double glomerulopathies: a clinicopathologic study of superimposed glomerulonephritis on diabetic glomerulosclerosis. *Mod. Pathol.* 1989;2:407-414.
[30] Iskandar SS, Falk RJ, Jennette JC. Clinical and pathologic features of fibrillary glomerulonephritis. *Kidney Int.* 1992;42:1401-1407.
[31] Pirani CL, Silva FG, Appel GB. Tubulo-interstitial disease in multiple myeloma and other nonrenal diseases. In: Cotran R, Brenner B, Stein J, editors. Tubulo-Interstitial Nephropathies. Volume 10 of Contemporary Issues in Nephrology. New York, NY: Churchill Livingstone; 1983.p.287-334.
[32] Start DA, Silva FG, Davis LD, D'Agati V, Pirani CL. Myeloma cast nephropathy: immunohistochemical and lectin studies. *Mod. Pathol.* 1988;1:336-347.
[33] Nasr SH, Markowitz GS, Stokes MB, Seshan SV, Valderrama E, Appel GB, Aucouturier P, D'Agati VD. Proliferative glomerulonephritis with monoclonal IgG

deposits: a distinct entity mimicking immune-complex glomerulonephritis. *Kidney Int.* 2004;65:85-96.

[34] Lin J, Markowitz GS, Valeri AM, Kambham N, Sherman WH, Appel GB, D'Agati VD. Renal monoclonal immunoglobulin deposition disease: the disease spectrum. *J. Am. Soc. Nephrol.* 2001;12:1482-1492.

[35] Gallo G, Kumar A. Hematopoietic disorders. In: Silva FG, D'Agati VD, Nádasdy T, editors. Renal Biopsy Interpretation. New York, NY: Churchill Livingstone; 1996.p.259-282.

[36] Ronco PM, Alyanakian MA, Mougenot B, Aucouturier P. Light chain deposition disease: a model of glomerulosclerosis defined at the molecular level. *J. Am. Soc. Nephrol.* 2001;12:1558-1565.

[37] Kisilevsky R. Amyloid and amyloidoses: Differences, common themes, and practical considerations. *Mod. Pathol.* 1991;4:514-518.

[38] Ogg CS, Cameron JS, Williams DG, Turner DR. Presentation and course of primary amyloidosis of the kidney. *Clin. Nephrol.* 1981;15:9-13.

[39] Woo P. Amyloidosis in children. *Baillieres Clin. Rheumatol.* 1994;8:691-697.

[40] Isaac J, Herrera GA. Renal biopsy as a primary diagnostic tool in plasma cell dyscrasias. *Pathol. Case Rev.* 1998;3:183-189.

[41] Pronovost PH, Brady HR, Gunning ME, Espinoza O, Rennke HG. Clinical features, predictors of disease progression and results of renal transplantation in fibrillary/immunotactoid glomerulopathy. *Nephrol. Dial. Transplant.* 1996;11:837-842.

[42] Tubbs RR, Gephardt GN, McMahon JT, Hall PM, Valenzuela R, Vidt DG. Light chain nephropathy. *Am. J. Med.* 1981;71:263-9.

[43] Jais JP, Knebelmann B, Giatras I, De Marchi M, Rizzoni G, Renieri A, Weber M, Gross O, Netzer KO, Flinter F, Pirson Y, Dahan K, Wieslander J, Persson U, Tryggvason K, Martin P, Hertz JM, Schröder C, Sanak M, Carvalho MF, Saus J, Antignac C, Smeets H, Gubler MC. X-linked Alport syndrome: natural history and genotype-phenotype correlations in girls and women belonging to 195 families: a "European Community Alport's Syndrome Concerted Action" study. *J. Am. Soc. Nephrol.* 2003;14:2603-10.

[44] van der Loop FT, Monnens LA, Schröder CH, Lemmink HH, Breuning MH, Timmer ED, Smeets HJ. Identification of COL4A5 defects in Alport's syndrome by immunohistochemistry of skin. *Kidney Int.* 1999;55:1217-1224.

[45] Bohle A, Wehrmann M, Greschniok A. Renal morphology in essential hypertension: analysis of 1177 unselected cases. *Kidney Int.* 1998;54:S205-S206.

[46] McCluskey R. Lupus Nephritis. East Norwalk, CT: Appleton-Century-Crofts; 1975.

[47] Churg J, Sobin L. Renal Disease: Classification and Atlas of Glomerular Diseases. Tokyo: Igaku-Shoin; 1982.

[48] Churg J, Bernstein J, Glassock R. Renal Disease: Classification and Atlas of Glomerular Diseases. New York: Igaku-Shoin; 1995.

[49] Banfi G, Bertani T, Boeri V, Faraggiana T, Mazzucco G, Monga G, Sacchi G. Renal vascular lesions as a marker of poor prognosis in patients with lupus nephritis. Gruppo Italiano per lo Studio della Nefrite Lupica (GISNEL). *Am. J. Kidney Dis.* 1991;18:240-248.

In: Nephrotic Syndrome: Etiology, Pathogenesis and Pathology ISBN: 978-1-63482-154-4
Editor: Muhammed Mubarak

Chapter 9

Successful Running of an Electron Microscopy Unit in a Developing Country: Problems and Challenges

Javed I. Kazi and Muhammed Mubarak*
Pathology, Histopathology Department,
Sindh Institute of Urology and Transplantation,
Karachi, Pakistan

Abstract

Electron microscope (EM) is one of the most important ancillary techniques available to the modern day histopathologist for the investigation of human disease. It is, at the same time, the most expensive tool to use with huge costs of the instrument and its maintenance and operation.

As a consequence, its availability and the utility for scientific investigation is not uniform across the world. In the field of diagnostic surgical pathology, EM is most useful in the areas of renal, skin, and tumor pathology. Its role in the latter field has decreased markedly during the past few years with the increasing availability of immunohisto-chemistry (IHC) and other molecular techniques. Its use is, however, still indispensable in the accurate diagnosis of renal glomerular, and some skin diseases. This review is focused on the role of EM in the diagnosis and management of renal diseases in general and glomerular diseases in particular in developing countries and the problems and challenges faced in running such a facility in the low-income countries.

Keywords: Electron microscope, developing countries, histopathology, immunohisto-chemistry, nephropathology, uropathology

---

* Address of Correspondence: Muhammed Mubarak, Histopathology Department, Sindh Institute of Urology and Transplantation (SIUT), Karachi, Pakistan, Email: drmubaraksiut@yahoo.com

1. Introduction

The practice of histopathology is still in the early evolutionary phase in many developing countries including Pakistan, when it has already entered into the modern era of molecular pathology in most developed countries. [1, 2]

As depicted clearly by Zubair et al. [3] a vast majority of lesions which should be biopsied are never biopsied in practice, and even many surgical specimens removed from the patient are not subjected to the histopathological evaluation, especially at many small hospitals.

And worse enough, if the biopsy specimens are sent to the laboratories, their complete pathological evaluation is not done due to non-availability of sophisticated techniques, like immunohistochemistry (IHC), molecular techniques, and electron microscopy (EM) in a vast preponderance of these diagnostic centers.

Only a few centers in Pakistan, mostly in the private sector, are doing quality histopathology practice. [3] In rest of the laboratories, the majority of which are in the public sector institutions, the histopathological diagnosis is still rendered on just hematoxylin and eosin (HE) stained slides.

Even special tinctorial stains, like Masson's trichrome and silver based stains are not available in these laboratories, or if available, the quality of reagents and the tests is suboptimal. [2] There are very few well trained and qualified technologists and the few that are being produced these days by the larger centers are moving out of the country for a better future. [3] In the backdrop of above facts, the concept and the actual practice of subspecialties in histopathology in Pakistan is at its primitive stage, to say the least, as in most other developing countries. Even the few centers of repute claiming to practice quality histopathology seem to be lacking this subspecialty practice in the field of histopathology. [3] It is thus obvious that the conditions are likely to be even worse in the practice of subspecialties. Only occasional centers practice subspecialty histopathology at par with the centers in the developed part of the world.

2. The Success Story

The histopathology department at Sindh Institute of Urology and Transplantation (SIUT) may be considered one prototype par excellence in the subspecialties of nephropathology, uropathology, and renal transplant pathology. SIUT started as an eight-bedded urology ward in the Civil Hospital, Karachi, Pakistan. With the sheer dedication, determination, devotion to cause, untiring efforts and hard work of Professor Rizvi and his team, it has progressed from a small beginning to its present status as a centre of excellence in kidney and urologic diseases in Pakistan.

In 1991 it was granted the status of an institute by an Act of the Provincial Assembly of Sindh and has become one of the leading nephro-urological and transplant centers in the world (www.siut.org). Soon after its inception, the nephrology, urology and kidney transplant activities expanded quite rapidly due to the quality free service and a sharp need was felt of a full-fledged histopathology department to cater for the above specialties and growing numbers of cases of other tissues and organs.

3. Establishment of Histopathology Department at SIUT

This was established in 1995 by the first author (JIK), who brought with him a vast experience and training in the field, both in Pakistan and abroad at the leading centers in the world at that time. His PhD training involved working under Professor Raja Sinniah at National University of Singapore. He then spent four yours at Addenbrooke's Hospital, University of Cambridge, England, which was one of the biggest renal and liver transplant centers in England in those days. Immediately before taking charge of the department, he worked for six months with Professor Peter Furness, at the University of Leicester for gaining further renal and transplant pathology experience. Their joint work on renal transplant pathology resulted in a few landmark publications in some of the best international peer-reviewed journals at that time. [4-8]

4. Establishment of EM Unit at SIUT

With the increasing nephrological and renal transplant activity, an urgent need was also felt for the establishment of the EM unit from the beginning. The same was established in 1998 with the help of generous grant by Rangoonwala family. Professor Peter Furness was very instrumental in realizing this goal. He was generous enough to spare one of his senior EM technologists for two weeks to train our own technologists in the processing and cutting of tissue specimens for ultrastructural examination and to start the EM unit. With the help of the technologist from Leicester University, we were able to train four of our senior technicians to independently process and prepare the TEM samples for ultrastructural examination. There was no trained EM biomedical engineer available in the city at that time, but we were lucky to have one physicist who had experience of working on X-ray diffraction machine. He was already working at SIUT as a consultant and with the help of engineers from Japan; he was able to operate the unit for day to day diagnostic service needs. Indeed, his honesty, dedication, and hard work have been the major factors for continuous functioning of the only EM unit in the country.

5. What We Do?

Although, the department was initially established with a view to cater to the diagnostic needs of nephrology, urology, and the renal transplant departments, but with continued expansion of the institutional activities and establishment of more departments, it has now almost turned into one of the major general histopathology departments in the country. As a result, apart from the above specimens, we see receive many samples from gastroenterology and gastrointestinal and hepatic surgery departments and little bit of everything.

Both the authors of this report are qualified general pathologists with extensive foreign training of the principal author in Singapore and UK (JIK) with subspecialty training in renal and transplant pathology. The other author (MM) is a product of the former and is indigenously trained and qualified. He also spent three months at the Pathology Department of Academic Medical Center, Amsterdam. The extensive training and experience of both authors has contributed to the continued growth and expansion of the departmental diagnostic facilities and research.

Our department is equipped with the state of the art equipment and all the necessary modalities required for optimal evaluation of all biopsy material in general and the nephropathology and renal transplant pathology, in particular. We also enjoy a very close liaison with our clinical colleagues, which is vitally important for the accurate diagnosis of pathological lesions in all above subspecialties, particularly in the practice of renal pathology. [9] With the establishment and successful running of a separate oncology unit, our tumor pathology practice is also expanding very rapidly and it may surpass many other centers because we provide all the treatment free of cost. In this article, our main focus is on the challenges and difficulties encountered in running a transmission EM (TEM) unit in a developing country.

6. Our Experience with the Use of TEM

We have been using the facility of TEM for the diagnosis of medical renal diseases on renal biopsies since the last 15 years. It is the only functional and working EM unit in the field of diagnostic surgical pathology in the whole country. We have also reviewed our experience on the diagnostic utility of EM in the accurate diagnosis of renal glomerular diseases underlying nephrotic syndrome (NS) in an unselected cohort of both adults and children and in childhood NS. These experiences have been published in peer-reviewed international journals of repute and have been cited by many researchers. [10, 11] Using the definitions of diagnostic usefulness of EM employed by Western researchers, we observed that EM study was useful in 94.5 percent of cases. [12-19] There can be some argument on the relevance of these definitions in the context of developing nations, but we believe that these definitions are equally applicable to developing countries as they are to developed countries, as the practice of science should be similar everywhere. [2] In view of these considerations, in two of our previous studies, we have clearly shown that the role of ultrastructural investigation in the diagnostic evaluation of renal biopsies in overall NS and in childhood NS is no less important in developing countries than in industrialized countries. [10, 11] Indeed, its use in the above clinical conditions is as pertinent in developing countries like Pakistan as in any developed country of the world. Very few reports from other developing countries are available on the usefulness of ultrastructural study of renal biopsies. [20-22] We also receive some samples from other institutes from around the country for an ultrastructural study, mostly the renal biopsies, but sometimes other samples, such as nasal mucosa for ciliary abnormalities, tumors, and skin specimens. If EM is so helpful in the diagnostic pathology, then the question arises as to why EM instruments or electron microscopists are not widely available or used in the developing countries? The answer to this question is complex and is partly related to the cost of the instrument and its maintenance. However, there are many other factors contributing to this state of affairs in these countries. As the users of the only functional TEM facility in the country for the last 15 years, we have the first hand experience of the problems encountered and the challenges faced in the installation, maintenance and continued functioning of such a facility in a developing country. We will elaborate on these issues one by one, as under:

7. The Procurement of the Instrument

The exorbitant cost of the instrument is one major, but not the sole factor, accounting for the small number of TEM units in the developing countries. In fact, an informal survey by the authors of this chapter has shown that the main problem is not the availability of the sophisticated EM device in Pakistan. There is no dearth of TEM devices in the country. According to the best of our knowledge, there are around ten TEM instruments in the whole country, but all of them are in a non-operational state, and nearly all of these are in public sector institutions. It is easy to get the device ordered and installed, but extremely difficult to maintain it and keep it in working order.

8. Maintenance and Continued Functioning

The continued functioning of the unit requires, besides many other requirements, the dedication, hard work, honesty and sincerity on the part of the operator, which are rare commodities in the developing countries. A dedicated, air conditioned and dust proof laboratory building, separate from the main laboratory, is the ideal place for setting up the EM unit. We have installed the machine in the basement of the new premises of SIUT, i.e., Dewan Farooq Medical Complex (DFMC). This place was found to be ideal for the installation of the EM instrument. The problem of electricity failures and voltage changes jeopardize smooth functioning of the instrument. Sudden power failures lead to abrupt closure of the instrument and cause a fault in the machine. To circumvent this problem, we have our own electricity generator in the new premises to cater to the continuous demands of electric supply in the hospital.

9. The Trained Manpower

There is a severe shortage of trained manpower in EM at all levels including pathologists, scientists, engineers, and EM technologists in developing countries. As mentioned above, we had to hire temporarily (for two weeks) an EM technologist from University of Leicester, UK to train our technologists about the processing, cutting and staining of the EM tissue. Similarly, histopathologists trained in the use and interpretation of TEM are also scarce in developing countries. One of the principal authors of this article (JIK) had extensive training and experience in the use of TEM for the pathologic study of renal and renal allograft biopsies. Another major problem is the lack of trained bio-medical engineers who can provide continued technical support. Lately, our EM instrument has developed some defect, and we had to request Japanese company to send an engineer to fix the problem.

10. Consumables and Reagents

The continued and uninterrupted supply of chemicals and reagents is necessary for continued functioning of any laboratory equipment. The chemicals and reagents required for tissue processing for fine structural study are expensive, difficult to procure and handle and need extreme care in their use.

Majority of them are also toxic and potentially carcinogenic. Almost all of these are manufactured in developed countries and many of these are tightly regulated by the controlling agencies of developed countries.

Because, we do not have any local vendor in Pakistan, we have to order these directly from the foreign companies. Once, we encountered a problem in the staining of the ultra thin sections for EM study.

A lot of search on the internet and communication with some experts in developed countries led us to redress the problem. Extreme care has to be exercised in the use of water and stains in order to prevent contamination of the slides with dust and bacteria, etc. The safe disposal of toxic wastes is also a challenge, as are the toxic fumes of the reagents used in the preparation of EM samples. A fume hood cabinet has to be used to process and prepare the tissues and reagents.

11. Photography

The TEM photomicrographs are necessary for the accurate interpretation of fine structural alterations in tissues observed under the TEM. Although, it seems a simple and straightforward job, in a developing country, even photography for EM is fraught with problems.

Lately, the glassy paper is not available in the market, forcing us to use low quality paper for photography. Very few photographers are skilled in developing and printing the TEM photographs, which are black and white, and not colored. Nowadays, new models of EM incorporate personal computers and digital imaging software as an option with the instrument.

12. Ultrastructural Research- Lowest Priority

The last but not the least factor, is that the research is the least priority in many developing countries.

This is mainly because of very low allocation of funds for this activity by the governments in these countries. The above, coupled with the overall pessimistic attitude of people towards research in developing nations, result in little interest by the pathologists and physicians in ultrastructural research.

Conclusion

In conclusion, there are numerous hurdles and challenges in smoothly running a diagnostic EM facility in a developing country like Pakistan. With sheer hard work, commitment, dedication, and will, these can be tackled, and fruitful service can be provided, as in our case.

References

[1] Kazi JI, Mubarak M. Histopathology in present era. *J. Pak. Med. Assoc.* 2009;59:1-2.

[2] Furness PN, Kazi JI. Laboratory investigation of renal biopsy specimen. *J. Nephrol. Urol. Transplant.* 1998; 1:19-26.

[3] Ahmed Z, Qureshi A, Khurshid A. The practice of histopathology in a developing country: difficulties and challenges; plus a discussion on terrible disease burden we carry. *J. Clin. Pathol.* 2009;62:97-101.

[4] Kazi JI, Furness PN, Nicholson M. Diagnosis of early acute renal allograft rejection by evaluation of multiple histological features using a Bayesian Belief Network. *J. Clin. Path.* 1998;51:108-113.

[5] Kazi JI, Furness PN, Nicholson M, Ahmed E, Akhtar E, Naqvi A, Rizvi A. Interinstitutional variation in the performances of Bayseian Belief Network for the diagnosis of acute renal graft rejection. *Transplant. Proc.* 1999;31:3152.

[6] Furness PN, Kazi JI, Levesley J, Taub N, Nicholson M. A neural network approach to the diagnosis of early acute allograft rejection. *Transplant. Proc.* 1999;31:3151.

[7] Furness PN, Levesley J, Luo Z, Taub N, Kazi JI, Bates WD, Nicholson ML. A neural network approach to the diagnosis of early acute renal transplant rejection. *Histopathology.* 1999;35:461-467.

[8] Jain S, Curwood V, Kazi JI, White SA, Furness PN, Nicholson M. Acute rejection in protocol renal transplant biopsies-institutional variations. *Transplant. Proc.* 2000;32: 616.

[9] Abbas K, Mubarak M, Kazi JI, Muzaffar R. Pattern of morphology in renal biopsies of nephrotic syndrome patients. Correlation with immunoglobulin and complement deposition and serology. *J. Pak. Med. Assoc.* 2009;59:540-543.

[10] Mubarak M, Kazi JI. Role of immunoflourescence and electron microscopy in the evaluation of renal biopsies in nephrotic syndrome in a developing country. *Ultrastruct. Pathol.* 2009;33:260-264.

[11] Mubarak M, Kazi J. Study of nephrotic syndrome in children: importance of light, immunoflourescence and electron microscopic observations to a correct classification of glomerulopathies. *Nefrologia.* 2013;33:237-242.

[12] Dische FE, Parsons V. Experience in the diagnosis of glomerulonephritis using combined light microscopical, ultrastructural and immunofluorescence techniques-an analysis of 134 cases. *Histopathology.* 1977;1:331-362.

[13] Turner DR. Advances in understanding the morphology of glomerular disease. *J. Clin. Path.* 1981;34:1207-1213.

[14] Spargo BH. Practical use of electron microscopy for the diagnosis of glomerular disease. *Hum. Pathol.* 1975;6:405-420.
[15] Haas MA. Reevaluation of routine electron microscopy in the examination of native renal biopsies. *J. Am. Soc. Nephrol.* 1997;8:70-76.
[16] Pearson JM, McWilliam LJ, Coyne JD, Curry A. Value of electron microscopy in diagnosis of renal disease. *J. Clin. Path.* 1994;10:209-215.
[17] Rivera A, Magliato S, Meleg-Smith S. Value of electron microscopy in the diagnosis of childhood nephrotic syndrome. *Ultrastruct. Pathol.* 2001;25:313-320.
[18] Collan Y, Hirsimäki P, Aho H, Wuorela M, Sundström J, Tertti R, Metsärinne K. Value of electron microscopy in kidney biopsy diagnosis. *Ultrastruct. Pathol.* 2005;29:461-468.
[19] Wagrowska-Danilewicz M, Danilewicz M. Current position of electron microscopy in the diagnosis of glomerular diseases. *Pol. J. Pathol.* 2007;58:87-92.
[20] Tighe JR, Jones NF. The diagnostic value of routine electron microscopy of renal biopsies. *Proc. Roy. Soc. Med.* 1970;47:126-128.
[21] Sementilli A, Moura LA, Franco MF. The role of electron microscopy for the diagnosis of glomerulopathies. *Sao Paulo Med. J.* 2004;122:104-109.
[22] Elhefnawy NG. Contribution of electron microscopy to the final diagnosis of renal biopsies in Egyptian patients. *Pathol. Oncol. Res.* 2011;17:121-125.

In: Nephrotic Syndrome: Etiology, Pathogenesis and Pathology ISBN: 978-1-63482-154-4
Editor: Muhammed Mubarak

Chapter 10

Focal Segmental Glomerulosclerosis

A. V. Vanikar**, *K. V. Kanodia, R. D. Patel and L. K. Nigam
Department of Pathology, Laboratory Medicine, Transfusion Services
and Immunohematology, IKDRC-ITS, Ahmedabad, India

Abstract

Focal and segmental glomerulosclerosis (FSGS) is a pattern of glomerular injury characterized by segmental sclerosis and/or hyalinosis involving some but not all the glomeruli. It is primarily a morphological diagnosis, and the term, FSGS, describes the characteristic distribution of the lesions in the affected glomeruli. It is emerging as the leading cause of nephrotic syndrome, not only in adults but, also in children, in many parts of the world. The lesion can occur in a wide variety of clinical settings and can occur in primary or secondary form. The subclassication of FSGS into primary and secondary forms is of utmost importance in determining optimal treatment and prognostication of the disorder. Primary FSGS, also known as idiopathic FSGS, is a clinicopathological syndrome characterized by heavy proteinuria and biopsy findings of FSGS, and there must be no evidence of an antecedent glomerulonephritis, a systemic disease with glomerular involvement or evidence of glomerular immune complex deposition. Secondary FSGS may result from diverse pathogenic mechanisms including heritable mutation of podocyte proteins, viral infections, toxins and medications. FSGS may also be mediated by adaptive structural/functional responses to diverse insults in the setting of reduced or normal nephron numbers. In this chapter, we will describe the nomenclature, classification, etiopathogenesis, morphology, clinical presentation and prognosis of the lesion. The discussion of treatment is beyond the scope of this chapter.

---

* Address for correspondence: Dr. Aruna V Vanikar, MD, Professor and Head, Department of Pathology, Laboratory Medicine, Transfusion Services and Immunohematology, and Professor, Department of Stem Cell Biology and Regenerative Medicine, G.R. Doshi and K.M. Mehta Institute of Kidney Diseases & Research Centre and Dr. H.L. Trivedi Institute of Transplantation Sciences, Civil Hospital Campus, Asarwa, Ahmedabad, India.E-mail: vanikararuna@yahoo.com; ikdrcad1@sancharnet.in.

Keywords: FSGS, pathologic variants, nephrotic syndrome, pathogenesis, proteinuria, renal biopsy

1. Introduction

Focal and segmental glomerulosclerosis (FSGS) is a pattern of glomerular injury characterized by segmental sclerosis and/or hyalinosis involving some but not all the glomeruli. It can occur in primary or secondary form. Primary FSGS, also called as idiopathic FSGS, is a clinicopathological syndrome characterized by heavy proteinuria and biopsy findings of FSGS, and there must be no evidence of an antecedent glomerulonephritis, a systemic disease with glomerular involvement or evidence of glomerular immune complex deposition. Secondary FSGS may result from diverse pathogenic mechanisms including heritable mutations of podocyte proteins, viral infections, toxins and medications. [1] FSGS may also be mediated by adaptive structural/functional responses to diverse insults in the setting of reduced or normal nephron numbers.

Since the first description by Fahr and Rich, several different histological variants of FSGS have been described. [2, 3] Recently, a group of nephropathologists proposed a standardized pathological classification system for FSGS based entirely on light microscopic examination known as Columbia classification. [4] Five histological variants of FSGS are described in this classification which is now universally followed; "not otherwise specified" (NOS) also called as classical, perihilar, cellular, tip lesion and collapsing variant. The prognostic significance of this classification is in a stage of evolution.

There are two aspects of differentiation of primary form from secondary form of FSGS, morphological and clinical. For the pathological diagnosis, the morphologic lesion must fall within the spectrum of FSGS with absence of antecedent glomerular injury/ involvement including systemic disease and absence of immune complex deposition. Clinically, the patient should have absence of any underlying cause or systemic disease or family history leading to segmental glomerular scarring.

The causes of secondary FSGS include drugs, viruses, immunological diseases, physical agents and hereditary diseases. [1] Morphologic variants can be divided into two forms, those associated with podocyte injury and those due to other mechanisms.

2. Terminology and Synonyms

The segmental sclerosis is imperative for FSGS. It should be distinguished from segmental scarring in which glomerular architecture is disrupted by deposition of mainly collagen type III. Hyalinosis, defined by deposition of eosinophilic, acellular material within the sclerotic areas and capillaries was formerly considered as mandatory for diagnosis of FSGS; however, it was found that not all types of FSGS have hyalinosis, not all the time is hyalinosis observed, and that other glomerular pathologies also show hyalinosis despite not having features of FSGS.

FSGS is a progressive lesion, in which increasing number of glomeruli get segmentally sclerosed, and the lesion of segmental sclerosis in an individual glomerulus eventually progresses to global sclerosis.

3. History

The first description of FSGS was given by Fahr in 1925 in a patient with lipoid nephrosis. [2] It took 25 years to describe the pathogenesis of FSGS when Rich described the cases of FSGS in autopsy findings of children who died of nephrosis or uremia and intercurrent infections. [3] In 1970, Churg, Habib and White described the histological classification of minimal change disease (MCD) and FSGS in children with nephrotic syndrome (NS) for the International Study of Kidney Diseases in Children (ISKDC). [5] Schwartz and Lewis had postulated that segmental scar of FSGS may begin with epithelial cell damage. [6] Subsequent studies have confirmed the central role of podocyte injury in primary/ secondary forms of FSGS.

4. Clinical Presentation

The incidence of FSGS varies from 10% to 78% in different countries/regions. [7-16] There is no reliable information about the incidence of FSGS in adults. In children, FSGS patients tend to be older than children with MCD and it is more common amongst males than females. They have higher incidence of hematuria, hypertension, renal insufficiency and have less selective proteinuria.

Laboratory tests like tumor necrosis factor (TNF)-α in supernatant fluid from cultured peripheral blood mononuclear cells [17], blood mRNA and protein levels of vascular endothelial growth factor (VEGF) and tumor growth factor (TGF)- β1[18], plasma and urinary endothelin-1 levels [19], insertion/ deletion alleles in ACE gene [20-22] urinary podocyte excretion rates [23] and genome wide m-RNA expression profiling [24] are some of the advanced tests believed to help in diagnosis of primary FSGS. In addition, Ki-67 (MIB-1), a proliferation marker is positive in podocytes in collapsing glomerulopathy (CG). [25]

5. Pathologic Findings

5.1. Gross/Macroscopic Findings

Recent information is scarce, however autopsy findings of Fahr showed enlarged, pale, swollen kidneys on autopsy. In chronic renal failure (CRF), these kidneys were symmetrically contracted and scarred.

The first image of FSGS was published in 1925 in a remarkably accurate drawing by Fahr in an Atlas of Human Pathology. [2] Fahr described patients with the glomerular pathology of FSGS in his autopsy series of "definitely characterized nephrosis" and these kidneys were enlarged and swollen with pale yellow fat filled cortices. The kidneys showed symmetric contraction in patients with CRF or after prolonged dialysis. [2]

5.2. Histopathology

FSGS is a common and nonspecific pattern of glomerular injury encountered in human renal biopsies. However it can be missed since it is a focal lesion. Primary FSGS need to be differentiated from the nonspecific pattern of focal and segmental glomerular scarring (secondary FSGS) that can follow a variety of inflammatory, proliferative, thrombotic and hereditary conditions affecting the glomeruli.

Certain general features described below help in establishing the diagnosis of FSGS on renal biopsies.

1. Number of glomeruli involved: The diagnosis is established even when only one glomerulus is involved.
2. Site: FSGS has zonal distribution, beginning in the juxtamedullary junctional area. So it is important to note whether this junctional area has been included.
3. Size: Glomerular hypertrophy often accompanies FSGS.
4. Glomerular lesion is focal: Some, not all glomeruli are involved in FSGS.

   It is also segmental: A segment of glomerular capillary tuft [lobule(s)] is involved.
5. Synechiae: Adhesion of glomerular tuft to Bowman's capsule, called synechiae is often seen early in the process of sclerosis.
6. Sclerosis: There is an increased collagenous extracellular matrix expanding the mesangium with resultant obliteration of capillary lumina.
7. Hyalinosis: Accumulation of glassy, accelullar, Periodic acid-Schiff (PAS) positive, and silver negative [stained by Jone's methaneamine silver stain (JMS)]. It contains glycoproteins, proteins and lipids.
8. Intraglomerular location of sclerosis: This helps to determine the type of FSGS. It is often possible if looked for diligently to determine whether the segmental sclerosis is located at hilar pole, tubular pole or neither or both sites or peripheral areas. So it is imperative to precisely identify the location of a segmental lesion. Columbia classification is based on the site of location of glomerular sclerosis. It is necessary to identify the location of segmental lesion in relationship to well defined glomerular landmarks.
9. Hypercellularity: The hypercellularity of segmental lesion is caused by proliferation of mesangial cells, epithelial cells and sometimes is accompanied with leucocytic infiltration. Schwartz et al. found glomerular hypercellularity, primarily owing to podocyte proliferation in 54% of the renal biopsy specimens. [26] The proliferating cells in Bowman's space appear to originate from podocytes which are the visceral epithelial cells. It is very difficult to identify the cells, but morphologically these cells have abundant chromophilic cytoplasm with vesicular nuclei and these cells are attached to the glomerular basement membrane (GBM). Mature podocytes do not proliferate and the proliferating cells do not generally express mature podocyte markers. By electron microscopy, the normal podocytes appear as polarized cells

with small basal membrane domain facing the GBM and large apicolateral domain facing the urinary space. They contain main cell body which divides into large extensions, the primary processes, from which originate numerous small extensions, known as foot processes. In FSGS, these cells undergo marked changes in the cell shape and form, with changes in immunohistochemical markers. So these cells are phenotypically altered podocytes. A monolayer of these cells overlays the sclerotic segment in the Bowman's space, loosely cohesive and unattached to the Bowman's capsule. This is in contrast to epithelial cell crescents, where the parietal epithelial cells are firmly adherent to the Bowman's capsule.

The podocyte alterations play an important role in the development of segmental glomerulosclerosis. The accumulation of leucocytes, foam cells and cellular debris also causes hypercellularity of the sclerotic segment. Foam cells are monocytes/ macrophages present in solidified areas and in glomerular capillary lumina. Foam cells are a frequent constituent of "tip" lesion.

Mesangial cell proliferation is also a cause of glomerular hypercellularity in FSGS; this is usually a diffuse change throughout the glomerulus and is seen in all the glomeruli.

5.3. Classification

FSGS can be classified in a variety of ways. The two more commonly used classifications are: (1) Etiological: primary and secondary FSGS (Table 1); and (2) Morphological classification (Table 2). During the past 20 years, a number of publications have addressed the morphological heterogeneity of primary and secondary FSGS. The early descriptions of Rich depicted discrete segmental scars with hyalinosis predominantly affecting juxtamedullary glomeruli. [27] The lesions of FSGS differed in both their topographic location within the glomerular tuft and the quality of endocapillary and extracapillary alterations. To achieve uniformity in approach to the pathological classification of FSGS, an international group of renal pathologists with mutual interest in FSGS convened at Columbia University, New York in November 2000. They reached a consensus and the classification evolved thereof is based entirely on an assessment of glomerular light microscopy features such as the location and the quality of the segmental lesion. The only shortcoming of Columbia classification is that it does not include immunofluorescence and electron microscopy examination which may be required to exclude other causes of sclerosis.

Table 1. Etiologic Classification of FSGS

Primary (idiopathic) FSGS
Secondary FSGS
1. Familial/genetic
A. Mutations in α-actinin 4
B. Mutations in podocin
C. Mutations in WT-1

Table 1. (Continued)

D. Mutations in β integrin
2. Virus-associated
A. HIV-1 (HIV-associated nephropathy)
B. Parvovirus B19
3. Drug-induced
A. Heroin (heroin nephropathy)
B. Interferon-α
C. Lithium
D. Pamidronate
4. Mediated by adaptive structural-functional responses
A. Reduced renal mass
Oligomeganephronia
Unilateral renal agenesis
Renal dysplasia
Reflux nephropathy
Sequelae to cortical necrosis
Surgical renal ablation
Chronic allograft nephropathy
Any advanced renal disease with reduction in functioning nephrons
B. Initially normal renal mass
Hypertension
Atheroemboli or other acute vaso-occlusive processes
Obesity
Cyanotic congenital heart disease
Sickle cell anemia

5.4. FSGS Variants

5.4.1. Glomerular lesions

5.4.1.1. FSGS, Not Otherwise Specified (NOS) or Classic FSGS

The most common morphological pattern of FSGS, which is the classic FSGS, constitutes the generic lesion of FSGS. This category requires that the other morphologic categories (perihilar, cellular, tip, and collapsing variants) be excluded. It is defined by focal and segmental consolidation of capillary tufts by increased extracellular matrix, obliterating the glomerular capillary lumina with or without podocyte hyperplasia. Mesangial hypercellularity and glomerulomegaly may be present [Figure 1(a, b)].Mesangial hypercellularity is more prevalent in pediatric FSGS in early disease course. The segmental lesions may affect more than one lobule. The number of glomeruli affected by the segmental lesions depends on the severity of the disease and also depends on the number of serial sections of renal biopsy examined.

Table 2. Morphologic Classification Algorithm of FSGS

Variant	Location of Defining Lesions	Distribution of Defining Lesions	Defining Features	Hyaline	Adhesion	Podocyte Hypertrophy/ Hyperplasia	Glomeru-lomegaly	Mesangial Hypercellularity	Arteriolar Hyalinosis
1.FSGS (NOS)	Anywhere	Segmental	Segmental increase in matrix obliterating capillary lumina (also segmental collapse without overlying podocyte hyperplasia) Exclude 2,3,4, and 5	+/–	++/–	–/+	+/–	–/+	+/–
2.FSGS perihilar variant	Perihilar	Segmental	At least 1 glomerulus with perihilarhyalinosis +/– sclerosis >50% of glomeruli with segmental lesions must have perihilar sclerosis and/or hyalinosis Exclude 3,4, and 5	++/–	+++/–	–/+	+++/–	–/+	++/–
3.FSGS cellular variant	Anywhere	Segmental	At least 1 glomerulus with segmental endocapillaryhypercellularity occluding lumina, +/– foam cells, +/– karyorrhexis Exclude 4 and 5	–/+	–/+	++/–	–/+	–/+	–/+
4. FSGS tip variant	At tip domain	Segmental	At least 1 segmental lesion involving tip domain (outer 25% of tuft next to origin of proximal tubule). The tubular pole must be identified. Lesion must have either an adhesion or confluence of podocytes with parietal or tubular cells at the tubular lumen or neck Lesions can be sclerosing (in <25% of tuft) or cellular (in <50% of tuft). No perihilar sclerosis Exclude 5	+/–	+++/–	++/–	–/+	–/+	–/+
5. FSGS collapsing variant	Anywhere	Segmental or global	At least 1 glomerulus with collapse and overlying podocyte hypertrophy and hyperplasia	–/+	–/+	+++/– Often with droplets/ vacuoles	–/+	–/+	–/+

NOTE : Plus (+) and minus (–) indicate the range of possible findings in all the involved glomeruli of a given biopsy specimen with the most frequent finding to the left and the least frequent finding to the right.

NOS variant

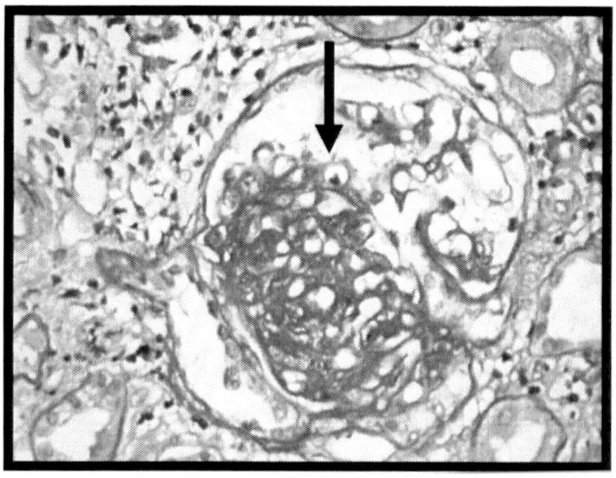

Figure 1a (PAS, ×200)

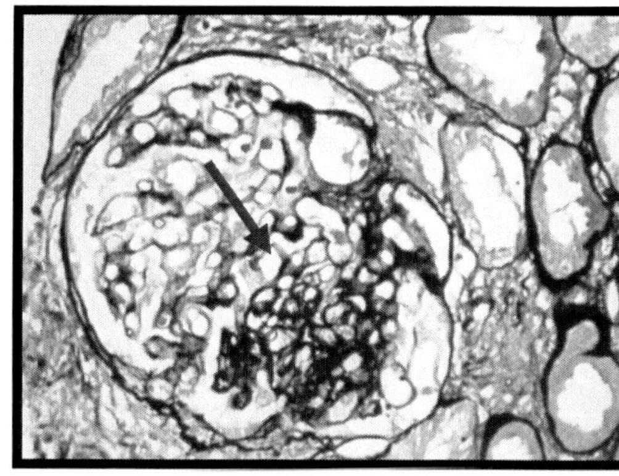

Figure 1b (JSM, ×200)

Figure 1(a, b): Consolidation of the capillary tuft with loss of capillary architecture (shown by arrow)

5.4.1.2. Tip Lesion

Howie and Brewer first described the tip lesion in an adult patient with various segmental glomerular lesions. [28] Its location is adjacent to the origin of the proximal convoluted tubule, i.e., the peripheral 25% of the glomerular tuft next to origin of the proximal tubule. [29] The tip lesion involves only a small portion of the glomerular tuft comprising one or two lobules. The diagnosis of the tip lesion requires that the collapsing variant be excluded. The lesion is characterized by swollen, hypertrophied visceral epithelial cells with parietal or tubular epithelial cells at the tubular pole. The affected lobules may display endocapillary hypercellularity with foam cells and hyalinosis (Figure 2). Sometimes, the affected segment may herniate in to the tubular lumen. There is frequent association of the tip lesion with other forms of FSGS and global glomerulosclerosis. Patients with tip lesion usually present with NS and have excellent response to steroids, resembling that of MCD.

Tip Lesion

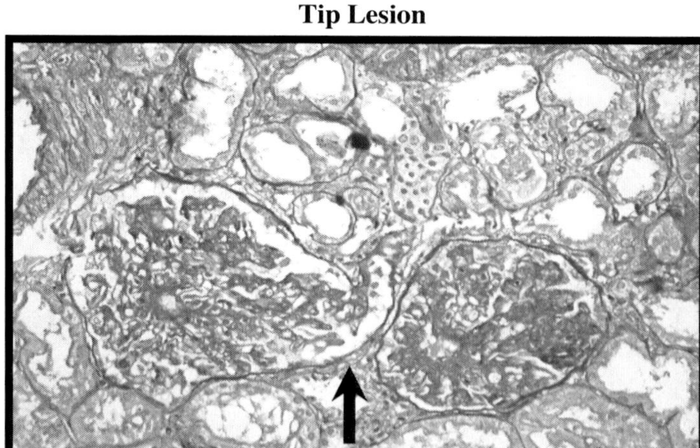

Figure 2. On the left side glomerulus, herniation of tuft into the proximal tubule (arrow), on right glomerulus showing classical variant of FSGS progressing to global sclerosis, (PAS, ×100)

5.4.1.3. Perihilar Variant

There must be at least one glomerulus with perihilar hyalinosis, with or without sclerosis and more than 50% of glomeruli with segmental lesions must have perihilar sclerosis or hyalinosis. Glomerulomegaly and adhesions are common. There is often arteriolar hyalinosis, sometimes in continuity with hyalinosis in the perihilar segment. Podocyte hyperplasia and hypertrophy may be present, as in NOS, but typically are less frequent than in other variants. There is absence of mesangial hypercellularity in perihilar variant (Figure 3). Other glomeruli may show lesions of segmental and/or global sclerosis. These lesions have been reported to be more frequent in adults in secondary forms mediated by glomerular hyperfiltration, as in obesity, cyanotic congenital heart disease, reflux nephropathy, renal agenesis, dysplasia, oligomeganephronia, or any advanced renal disease with reduced number of functioning nephrons.

Perihilar

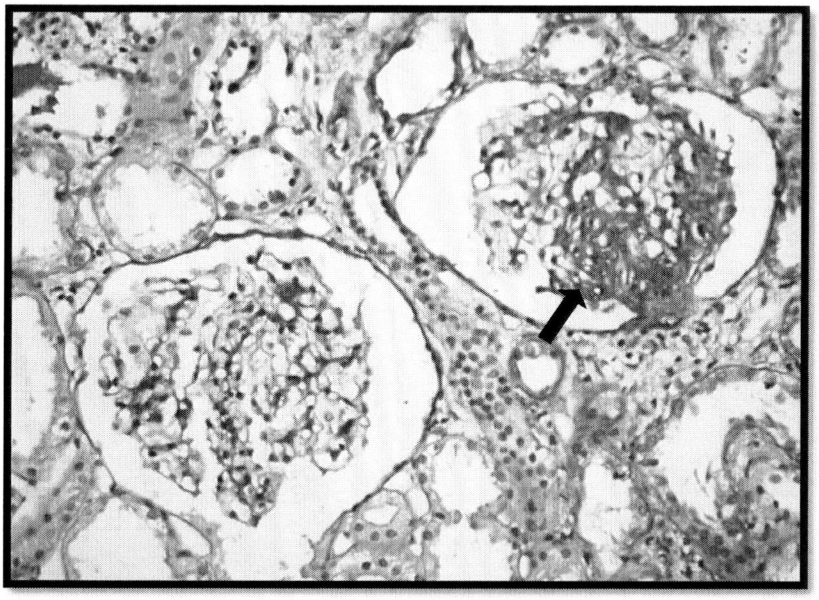

Figure 3. Glomerulus with perihilar sclerosis (arrow) and hyalinosis (PAS, ×200).

5.4.1.4. Cellular Variant

The cellular variant of FSGS was first described by Schwartz and Lewis in 1985, but the two terms collapsing and cellular lesion have been used interchangeably or synonymously leading to diagnostic confusion. [6, 26] After Columbia classification and studies by Thomas et al. and Stokes et al., cellular lesion has been introduced as a distinct entity. [30, 31]

The more restrictive definition of cellular variant was proposed as "only forms of FSGS with predominantly endocapillary hypercellularity". The initial pathogenic event in FSGS is podocyte injury. As a result, there can be extracapillary hypercellularity caused by proliferation of podocytes. However, this proliferation is less marked as compared to that seen in CG. These cells tend to be plump, rounded and poorly cohesive. (Figure 4) The diagnosis of cellular variant mandates exclusion of collapsing and tip variants. The cellular variant may be responsive to immunosuppressive therapy. [31]

Cellular FSGS

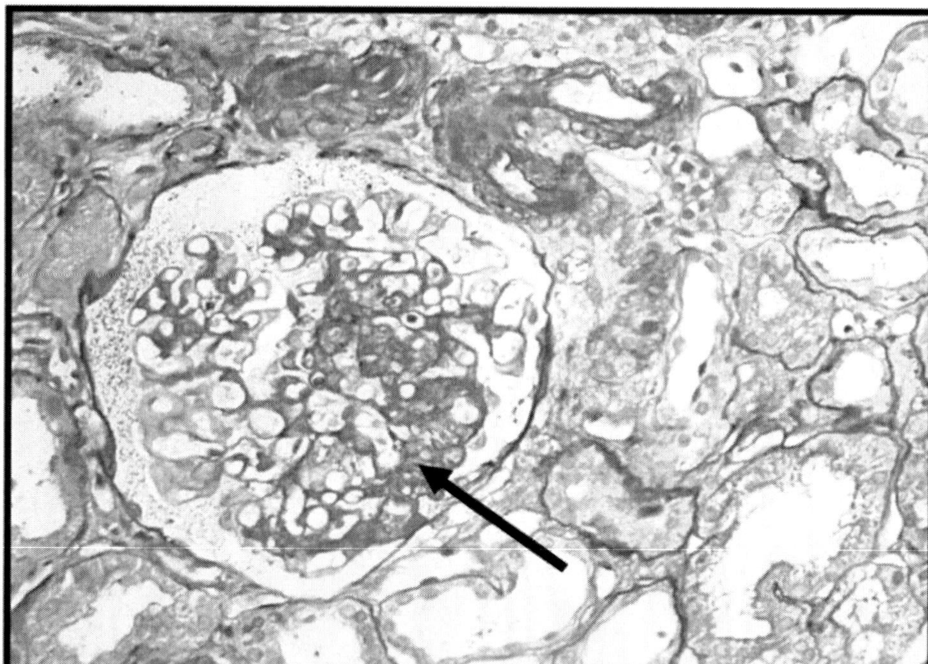

Figure 4. Glomerulus with segmental endocapillary hypercellularity (arrow) (PAS, ×400).

5.4.1.5. Collapsing Variant

The collapsing variant is also known as CG. The term glomerular collapse was first introduced by Weiss et al. in 1986 to describe an unusual clinicopathologic complex of severe NS, rapidly progressive renal failure and glomerular collapse occurring in six human immunodeficiency virus (HIV) negative black patients. [32]

Initially, CG was described as malignant FSGS in 1978 due to the clinical presentation of rapidly progressive NS leading to end-stage renal disease (ESRD). In the era of HIV pandemic, this form of glomerular injury came to be identified as "HIV associated nephropathy" (HIVAN). [33-38]

The characteristic features of CG are segmental and global collapse of glomerular capillaries, wrinkling and retraction of the GBM and marked hypertrophy and hyperplasia of podocytes. The podocytes have enlarged, open, vesicular nuclei with prominent nucleoli and rare mitotic figures. The podocytes may be crowded but are loosely cohesive and fill the urinary space forming pseudo-crescents (Figures 5 and 6). The podocytes display a dysregulated phenotype with increased rate of proliferation and apoptosis. [39-44] The injured podocytes exhibit reduced expression of cyclin kinase inhibitors p27 and p17, promoting permissive cellular proliferation. These cells lose their mature podocyte markers such as synaptopodin, WT-1, GLEPP-1, and C3b receptor, and CALLA. [25] Podocytes become less cohesive and shed in to the urinary space. The trans-differentiation of podocyte to macrophage/monocyte phenotype also has been described. CG is distinguished from the cellular form by the absence of endocapillary hypercellularity, and the usual lack of hyalinosis, foam cells and adhesions to the Bowman's capsule.

Collapsing FSGS

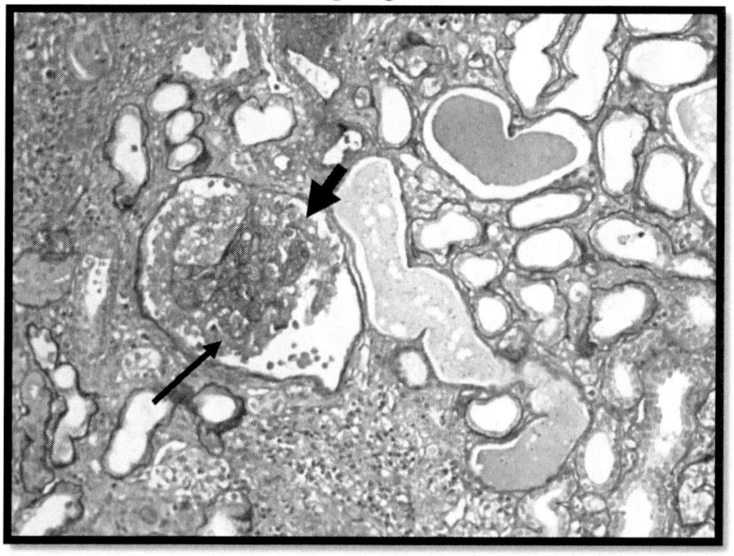

Figure 5. Global collapse of capillary tuft (thick arrow) with podocytic proliferation (thin arrow) forming pseudocrescent. (PAS, ×200).

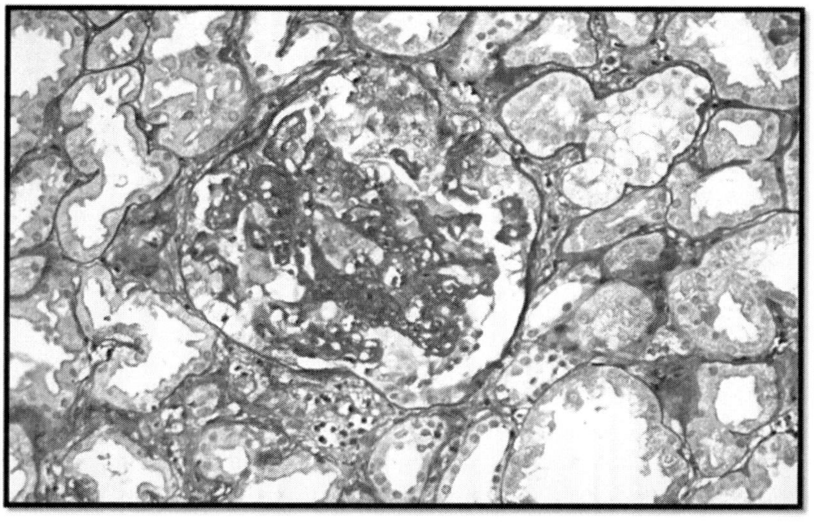

Figure 6. Global collapse of capillary tuft secondary to CNI toxicity in renal allograft biopsy. (PAS, ×200).

The clinical manifestations of CG are generally more severe with massive proteinuria, hypoalbuminemia and hypercholesterolemia with high serum creatinine level despite a shorter time course from clinical onset to biopsy examination. Patients with CG are at high risk of progressing to ESRD and are unresponsive to steroid therapy. [45-49] A collapsing pattern of FSGS may also occur *de novo* or as a recurrent disease in an allograft post renal transplant due to calcineurin inhibitor/mTOR toxicity and renal ischemia injury associated with moderate to severe arteriosclerosis. [50-53]

5.4.2. Tubulointerstitial Lesions

Long standing proteinuria leads to progressive tubulointerstitial damage. The amount of tubular damage is proportional to the degree and extent of glomerular involvement. [54-63] Tubules may show degenerative and regenerative changes including epithelial simplification, enlarged hyperchromatic nuclei and nucleoli. Proximal tubules frequently contain intracellular lipid and protein resorption droplets. As the glomerular lesion progresses to chronic renal insufficiency, the extent of tubular atrophy also increases. Even with the normal glomerular morphology, the presence of atrophic tubules in a biopsy from a patient with NS should raise suspicion of FSGS. [64]

In CG, 40% cases show dilated proximal tubules with protein casts (microcyst formation). Tubular epithelial simplification and flattening with rare tubulitis has also been noted. [25, 64] Interstitial fibrosis accompanies tubular loss and atrophy. Interstitial cellular infiltration is minimal with chronic inflammatory cells and rarely with foam cells.

5.4.3. Vascular Lesions

The vascular lesions of arteriolar hyalinosis and arterial intimal fibrosis are both related to hypertension and progressive course of FSGS. [55-57] Lee and Spargo noted more severe epithelial cell injury, higher serum creatinine and more urinary albumin excretion in patients with arteriolar hyalinosis as compared to patients without hyalinosis. [65]

5.5. Immunofluorescence Studies

There is typically focal and segmental deposition of IgM and C3 in the sclerosed and hyaline areas. [55-58, 66, 67] Sometimes, less intense staining of IgA, IgG and albumin is also noted. [56, 68, 69] A renal biopsy showing diffuse mesangial or granular IgG or IgA, especially when associated with electron dense deposits, should not be diagnosed as primary FSGS.

5.6. Electron Microscopy

The lesion of segmental sclerosis shows wrinkling and retraction of the GBMs and accumulation of intramembranous hyaline with resulting narrowing or occlusion of the capillary lumina. The sclerotic segment may contain foamy macrophages, cellular debris, lipid droplets, granular matrix, fibrils and electron dense deposits. The major ultrastructural finding of FSGS is the complete effacement of foot processes, accompanied by podocyte alterations that include hyperplasia, hypertrophy, increased organelle content and focal microvillous transformation. [56, 57, 66, 70-72] The hypertrophied podocytes display rounded cell bodies that adhere to GBM with frequent loss of primary processes. There may be detachment of podocytes. The degree of foot process fusion varies from being mild to severe, and depends on the severity of the proteinuria. In the areas of foot process effacement, there is loss of recognizable slit diaphragms (SDs) and matrix like condensation of cytoskeletal filaments oriented parallel to the direction of GBM itself. Although the lesions of FSGS are focal at the light microscopic level, the podocyte alterations are relatively diffuse at the electron microscopy level.

The basal lamina and mesangium may show changes in FSGS but they are less diagnostically specific than podocyte pathology. The lamina densa is often irregular in thickness and may contain electron lucent areas with cytoplasmic inclusions and invaginations or membrane fragments. The mesangium shows increased matrix with active mesangial cells with prominent rough endoplasmic reticulum, Golgi apparatus and cytoplasmic processes undergo necrosis, which contributes to hypocellular appearance of the sclerotic areas.

6. Prognostic Indicators

The clinical presentation of FSGS patients is different from other NS patients, both in children and adults. These patients have more frequent hematuria, hypertension, renal insufficiency and are unresponsive to steroids. In addition, they frequently progress to uremia as well as renal failure leading to death. [73-76] The presence of nephrotic-range proteinuria (>3 gm/day in adults), elevated serum creatinine at presentation and steroid resistant proteinuria are adverse clinical prognostic factors for FSGS; and the collapsing variant, interstitial fibrosis and tubular atrophy are the adverse histological predictors of FSGS. [77]

It has been observed that patients with non-nephrotic proteinuria have excellent long-term outcome in spite of not receiving treatment compared to nephrotic-range proteinuria. In contrast, patients with massive proteinuria (>10 gm/day) have worse prognosis. [75-78] Ten year patient survival with non-nephrotic proteinuria was 90% *vs.* 30% with nephrotic-range proteinuria. [55, 73, 74, 78, 79] Patients with serum creatinine >1.3 mg/dL have poor renal survival than patients with serum creatinine <1.3 mg/dL. [73, 74, 80] Serum creatinine is more important predictor than proteinuria which is again more significant than other factors.

While comparing FSGS of children and adults, the age is not a significant predictor for survival or disease progression. However, hypertension is more progressive in adults *vs.* children. [56] Racial predilection is more for Africans followed by Asians and then Americans. If the patients respond to steroid therapy, they have better outcome than others. [80]

In a study by Stokes et al. cellular, collapsing and tip variants showed greater frequency and severity of NS, and shorter time to biopsy compared to NOS variant. [29, 31, 81]

Predictors of ESRD for all FSGS patients included initial serum creatinine, percentage of glomeruli showing global sclerosis, percentage of glomeruli showing CG lesions, chronic tubulo-interstitial injury score, and lack of remission response. [4, 5, 26, 31, 45, 54, 61, 66, 73, 80] CG had the highest rate of renal insufficiency at presentation, most extensive glomerular involvement and chronic tubulo-interstitial disease, fewest remissions and highest rate of ESRD. Patients with tip lesions were older and showed the highest remission rate and lowest rate of ESRD. Cellular variant showed intermediate rates of remission and ESRD compared to CG and tip lesions. [4, 31]

In tip lesion, poor prognosticators were severity of proteinuria at presentation and percentage of associated peripheral lesions. Tip lesions were found to closely resemble minimal change disease with respect to high incidence of NS, severity of proteinuria, short duration from onset to biopsy, and absence of chronic tubulointerstitial disease. Thus within the MCD/FSGS spectrum, tip lesion is a distinctive and prognostically favourable clinicopathologic entity. [4]

In a study in adult Dutch population, the histology, proteinuria at renal biopsy and immunosuppressive therapy did not predict a remission. [16] In the same study, prognosis of patients with perihilar FSGS was comparable to NOS variant with stable renal function at 10 years follow-up in both groups. Many patients with tip lesion were found to undergo spontaneous remission in their study.

7. FSGS in Renal Allografts

The pathogenetic mechanisms for recurrence include role of genetic diseases, humoral factors, baro-trauma, glomerular hypertrophy, podocyte dysfunction and hyperlipidemia.

Studies of familial FSGS have demonstrated mutations in SD and podocyte proteins that are critical in forming and maintaining the glomerular filtration barrier (GFB). [82-91] The SD complex comprises of several proteins like nephrin, P-cadherin, CD2AP, ZO-1, FAT, podocin and possibly Neph 1. This complex interacts via cytoplasmic F-actin/ α-actinin-4complex with the apical (podocalyxin) and basal ($\alpha_3\beta_1$ integrin) domains of the podocyte. Mutations in *NPHS1* (nephrin), *NPHS2* (podocin), *CD2AP* and *ACTN4* (α-actinin-4) have been implicated in glomerular pathology and dysfunction in human beings. FSGS is also seen in inherited syndromes like nail-patella syndrome, Galloway-Mowat syndrome and Charcot-Marie-Tooth disease. [92, 93]

De novo FSGS can occur in following settings: (i) adult recipients of pediatric kidneys or small size donors with large body mass index (BMI) of recipients resulting into hyperfiltration injury; (ii) in long standing grafts with nephron loss and fibrosis resulting into hyperfiltration injury; (iii) in grafts with severe vascular disease resulting into presumed glomerular hypoperfusion and subsequent CG; (iv) secondary injury like calcineurin inhibitor or sirolimus toxicity; and (v) new onset primary FSGS. [94]

Secondary FSGS usually occurs months to years after transplantation. Perihilar and classic variants are most common forms of secondary FSGS. However based on the morphology alone, primary FSGS cannot always be distinguished from secondary FSGS. In a study by Bhathena et al. in renal allografts of 2 years or older, they found that the mean glomerular diameter of 148 μm before transplant increased to 203 ± 10 μm in kidneys with FSGS vs.158 ± 8.32 μm without FSGS. [95] These findings support the hypothesis that FSGS develops in conjunction with glomerular hypertrophy. Collapsing FSGS presents with modest proteinuria or NS. The affected grafts often show severe small vessel disease or arteriolar hyalinosis associated with calcineurin inhibitor toxicity and even thrombotic microangiopathy, transplant endarteritis/arteriopathy or transplant glomerulitis. In this situation, ischemia results into glomerular hypoperfusion and tuft collapse. The outcome of these cases is poor resulting into graft failure within one year. [96-98] Whenever a large size recipient receives kidney from small size donor, these biopsies disclose FSGS with crescents or mesangial prominence and clinical presentation is severe hypertension, heavy proteinuria and eventually renal failure. [99]

7.1 Recurrent FSGS

FSGS recurs in 30 to 37% of the grafts and is associated with increased graft failure rate. [100-108] The second graft has high chances of recurrence up to 80%. [103, 107, 109] Recurrence can occur at about 7.5 months post-transplant in adults and in about 2 weeks in children. [105, 106] In an Indian study, the recurrence was noted any time between 8 days to 2 years. [108] The risk factors for recurrence are younger age at onset, rapid progression of the original disease, dialysis duration, immunosuppressive therapy and histological type of FSGS in native kidney. [101, 102, 106, 107, 110, 111] Collapsing FSGS and diffuse mesangial hypercellularity, [102, 107, 112-114] and pre-adolescent age [107, 113] have higher chances of recurrence. The chances of recurrence are 5 times higher in children as compared to adults and the chances are higher with living donors than deceased donors. [113, 114, 115]

8. Pathogenesis of FSGS

The study of renal transplants has given new insights in understanding the pathogenesis of FSGS. The pathologic changes begin as wide spread effacement of foot processes, villous transformation of cytoplasm (in 1-2 weeks) followed by podocyte detachment or dropout and segmental tuft sclerosis with accumulation of intracapillary foam cells (within 2 months). [116] Displaced SDs similar to those seen in aminonucleoside treated rats have been observed. [117] Podocytes show profound changes in adhesion molecules and signs of trans-differentiation into macrophage like cells. [118, 119] Podocyte foot processes are restored after treatment with plasmapheresis. [106] This finding suggests that post-transplant FSGS is associated with circulating factors. In a mouse model of FSGS, bone marrow transplant from a healthy mouse into mouse with FSGS ameliorated the disease and when bone marrow of FSGS mouse was administered into the healthy mouse, it resulted into occurrence of FSGS. This suggested that FSGS is a stem cell disorder. [120] In a study of living donor renal allograft recipients by Vanikar et al., [108] 12 patients in whom stem cells were infused in thymus, no recurrence was noted in any kind of FSGS over a follow-up of 8 years, whereas in groups where stem cells were not infused in thymus, but were infused into portal circulation alone, recurrence was noted in 28.6% out of 7 patients over a follow up of 2.6 years. Patients who were administered proteosome inhibitor, Bortezomib, had higher incidence of recurrence of FSGS in 1 out of 3 patients within 1 year of transplantation. This indicated that there was role of central thymic tolerance to prevent FSGS.

8.1 Humoral Factors

Immunoglobulins, Cytokines and Growth Factors, Circulating Factors

IgM deposits with complement and sometimes other immunoglobulins have been found in scarred portions of glomeruli; however, their direct role in the pathogenesis of FSGS has still not been established. Some cytokines and growth factors have been implicated in the pathogenesis of FSGS, since peripheral blood of patients with FSGS was found to have elevated cytokines.

Albumin permeability (P_{alb})was found to be elevated in patients with recurrent FSGS. In one study, it was found that plasma from patients with primary FSGS when injected in to rats led to occurrence of FSGS. [121] However, substantial evidence of circulating factors in recurrence of FSGS has not been well established.

8.2 Hemodynamic Injury and Glomerular Hypertrophy

Glomerular Hypertension

Glomerular hypertension has been implicated in the progression of renal disease in the remnant kidney model and the same mechanism may apply to FSGS in human beings. Glomerular hypertrophy appears to be independently associated with development of FSGS. Fogo et al. demonstrated that the patients with the first biopsy showing MCD and large glomeruli were more likely to develop FSGS on a second biopsy. [122] It is believed that in remnant kidney model, the expression of large T antigen may alter production of collagen, and proteoglycans; and platelet-derived growth factor (PDGF) in vitro played a role in inducing glomerular hypertrophy. Growth factors and cytokines like PDGF, TGF β, TGF-α, insulin like growth factor 1, growth hormone, epidermal growth factor, IL-1 and IL-6, TNF-α, basic fibroblast growth factor (FGF), endothelin and plasminogen activator inhibitor-1 (PAI-1) are involved in glomerular scarring.

Hyperlipidemia and Obesity

Epidemiologic studies have shown that low high density lipoproteins (HDL) cholesterol and high triglycerides increased the relative risks of developing renal dysfunction associated with obesity initiated metabolic syndromes (OIMS) associated with FSGS. [123-125] The excess excretory load seen in obesity is associated with adaptive changes in glomerular filtration rate (GFR) like hyperfiltration, afferent arteriolar dilatation and glomerular capillary hypertension typically noted in reduced nephron number noted in chronic kidney disease (CKD). Adverse adaptation to excess renal sodium retention in obesity (mediated by angiotensin-2 and sympathetic activation) induce hyperfiltration and afferent vasodilatation leading to proteinuria and glomerular injury. The excess intracellular lipids in OIMS may also have toxic effects on renal cells.

Cellular Injury

Barisoni et al. demonstrated loss of mature podocyte differentiation markers WT-1, CALLA, C3b receptor, GLEPP-1, podocalyxin and synaptopodin, and increased proliferation in the involved podocytes in CG and HIVAN. [39-41] These phenotypic alterations are not seen in any other proteinuric disease. Apoptosis may be associated with gradual podocyte death in FSGS. Apoptosis, detachment of podocytes with urinary excretion and lack of proliferation of podocytes are the main causes of podocytopenia which eventually leads to scarring in classic FSGS. Kriz et al. described the stereotyped response to injury beginning with foot process effacement, progression through cell body attenuation and pseudocyst formation to detachment of podocytes from the GBM and loss into urinary space. [126] When the denuded area of GBM created by podocyte loss meets the parietal epithelium, these cells attach to the capillary basement membrane. This begins the sequence of events leading to formation of adhesion, which is posited as the earliest "committed" lesion in the development of FSGS. Filtration continues through the podocyte-deprived capillaries into the expanding paraglomerular space leading to invasion of the lesion by interstitial fibroblasts, organization and enlargement of the lesion, and progression to global glomerulosclerosis. Once the capillary is denuded, hydraulic forces will favour the paraglomerular accumulation of filtrate and will accelerate the progression of glomerular lesion. [127] These observations demonstrate that podocyte injury is the most likely common element linking diverse diseases associated with FSGS and glomerular scarring.

IgM Nephropathy

IgM nephropathy (IgMN) is an understudied and therefore ill-understood clinicopathological condition characterized by dominant IgM deposits in the glomerular mesangium. Clinically, patients usually present with steroid dependent or steroid-resistant NS or subnephrotic proteinuria. It is more prevalent in Asian countries affecting patients of all ages with slightly more male predilection. Incidence has been reported to be 4.8 to 7.8% of all biopsies. [128-130] FSGS constitutes about 16% of IgMN in adults and about 10% in children and these cases are accompanied by hypertension, marked proteinuria and biopsies have more interstitial fibrosis and tubular atrophy than other FSGS lesions. These patients tend to develop ESRD within 1 year and are not amenable to steroids. [128-132]

8.3 Secondary Forms of FSGS

Several diseases or disorders are known to cause FSGS. Study of mechanisms of the lesion formation in these cases can improve our understanding of the evolution and management of primary FSGS.

8.3.1 Secondary to Structural Functional Adaptations

FSGS with Reduced Renal Mass (Reduced Nephrons) and Glomerulomegaly

Rennke and Klein postulated that nephron loss causes compensatory hypertrophy of remnant glomeruli with increased volume, which in combination with increased glomerular pressure due to systemic hypertension or other poorly understood factors, leads to injury and loss of podocytes. The end result is capillary collapse and mesangial sclerosis. [133]

Chronic Pyelonephritis and Reflux Nephropathy

Kincaid-Smith demonstrated FSGS in 88 out of 195 patients with atrophic pyelonephritis. [134] Morphometric studies have shown an increase in diameter and surface area of glomeruli in pediatric and adult patients of reflux nephropathy. These eventually lead to focal podocyte detachment and tuft adhesion to Bowman's capsule. These findings support the hypothesis that adaptive changes following nephron loss due to atrophic pyelonephritis and reflux nephropathy place stress on the podocytes and lead to progressive loss of renal function.

Oligomeganephronia

This is a rare congenital anomaly in which renal hypoplasia occurs without dysplasia or other urinary tract abnormalities. [135] It was first described in infants with polydypsia, polyuria, vomiting, fever and growth retardation. These infants grew up to adolescence with proteinuria, slow loss of renal functions to lead to galloping deterioration and eventually death around 15 years of age. Renal biopsies in the initial stages showed marked enlargement in the size of glomeruli, tubules and juxtaglomerular apparatus without any other morphological changes. The enlargement can vary from 2 to 12 times the normal size. Later on, these progressed to FSGS.

Postulated mechanisms for decreased nephrogenesis include deficient metanephric blastema or a defect in growth and branching of the ureteric bud. [135] Oligomeganephronia is usually sporadic malformation; however, genetic basis also can be responsible. Familial occurrence has been reported with chromosomal abnormalities like branchio-oto-renal, acro-renal and renal coloboma syndromes. PAX-2, a nuclear transcription factor, is critical for the development of kidney, ear and eye. Mutations in PAX-2 have been observed in above mentioned syndromes.

Unilateral Renal Agenesis

The incidence of unilateral renal agenesis is reported to be about 1:1000 in autopsies of children. About 50% of these children also have associated abnormalities in the lower urinary tract. Morphometry has shown about 1.75 times glomerular diameter enlargement and 5 times increased volume of glomeruli in these cases. [136] The frequency with which FSGS occurs in unilateral renal agenesis is not known, but one study has shown that FSGS was present in 2 out of 7 autopsies of unilateral renal agenesis. [137]

Nephrectomy and More Extensive Surgical Ablation

There are some reports of occurrence of FSGS in remnant kidneys following elective donor nephrectomy for kidney transplantation; however, several reports state that FSGS is not seen even after a long follow-up of 8 to 46 years. [137-139]

Cholestrol Atheroembolization

Renal atheroembolization or atheroembolic renal disease (AERD) is a common complication of atherosclerosis, peripheral vascular disease, male gender, recent invasive vascular procedures, hypercholesterolemia and hypertension. The clinical syndrome associated with AERD includes acute on chronic renal failure, but Greenberg et al. reported the association of AERD, FSGS and nephrotic-range proteinuria. [140]

Morbid Obesity

Kasiske and Crosson described 17 patients with morbid obesity (BMI of 41) and found that 9 of these had FSGS. [141] Kambham et al. analysed 71 obese patients (BMI $\geq$ 40) and found that 57 patients had FSGS and 14 had only glomerulomegaly. [142] Compared with non-obesity-related FSGS, these patients had higher proportion of global glomerulosclerosis, glomerulomegaly and mild increase in arteriolar disease but lower proportion of segmental scarring and less widely distributed foot process effacement. These patients rarely develop edema and full NS like the non-obese patients with primary FSGS. In addition, predictors of poor outcome in these patients were serum creatinine and proteinuria at the time of presentation. Progression of FSGS and ESRD in morbid obesity has the same etiopathogenesis as that of obesity and hyperlipidemia described in primary FSGS.

Cyanotic Congenital Heart Disease

The glomerular pathology seen in young patients dying of congenital cyanotic heart disease (CCHD) include glomerular enlargement, mesangial expansion and dilatation and congestion of glomerular capillaries. [143] CCHD *per se* do not cause FSGS; however, glomerulomegaly can result from prolonged hypoxia, polycythemia, hyperviscosity and increased pressure in right ventricle. In a study by Flanagan et al. it was observed that patients who were more than 21 years old and cyanotic in spite of surgical manipulation, were at increased risk of proteinuria and renal insufficiency. [144] However, FSGS was still not an established association in their studies as well as in other studies. [144-146]

Type-I Glycogen Storage Disease

This is an autosomal recessive disease with decreased glucose-6-phosphatase activity and accumulation of glycogen in liver and kidney. These patients have elevated GFR due to mechanisms still not understood and this is believed to lead to glomerular lesions. [147-149]

8.3.2 Genetic Causes

The following schema describes inherited FSGS due to mutations in various genes.

- Autosomal recessive FSGS
- Nephrin (NPHS-1 mutations)
- Podocin (NPHS-2 mutations)
- Autosomal dominant FSGS
    - Localized to 11q21-22
    - Localized to 19q/13 (*ACTN4* mutations) α-actinin-4
    - Others
- *CD2AP* mutations
- Syndromic FSGS
    - WT1 mutations
        - Diffuse mesangial sclerosis
        - Denys-Drash syndrome
    - Frasier syndrome
    - Nail-Patella syndrome
    - Alport's syndrome

Galloway Mowat syndrome

Autosomal dominant progressive nephropathy with FSGS and sensori-neural deafness

Autosomal recessive FSGS with neurologic findings

Mitochondrial DNA mutations (mtMTTL1)

MELAS syndrome

Neuro-sensory deafness, maternally inherited diabetes mellitus, and progressive renal disease

Congenital Nephrotic Syndrome [CNS] (Finnish-Type NPHS1 Mutation)

Congenital nephrotic syndrome (CNS) is a distinct entity with autosomal recessive inheritance, most common in Finland with gene frequency of 1:200, incidence of 10-12.5 per 100,000 live births, and presenting at birth. The newborn has a typical face with profound motor and mental retardation, and NS. Proteinuria begins during gestation. Microhematuria is often present with mild aminoaciduria and glycosuria. There is elevated alpha-feto protein (AFP) between 15th to 20^{th}weeks of gestation. The responsible gene, *NPHS-1*, was identified by genome-wide screening of the affected Finnish families and was localized to the long arm of chromosome 19 (19q13). In Finland, two mutations of NPHS-1 gene are found to be responsible for most of the cases of CNS. Finn-major is a deletion of nucleotides 121-122, and Finn-minor encodes a premature termination. [149] Non-Finnish populations rarely have these mutations. The mutations are distributed throughout the gene, and defective nephrin synthesis and podocyte dysfunction leads to uncontrollable proteinuria.

Grossly, the kidneys are enlarged and may have cortical cysts usually in the deeper cortex. The glomerular pathology is not diagnostic of CNS. Tubular dilatation is the most common finding. Few glomerular abnormalities may be present at birth but fetal glomeruli, mesangial sclerosis and global sclerosis can be seen in variable proportions. The GBM is ultrastructurally and biochemically normal. The proximal convoluted tubules are dilated with low lipid-containing epithelium. This has been described as microcystic disease or 'a string of sausages'. In some affected nephrons, the urinary space of glomerulus is dilated. Electron microscopy shows widespread effacement of podocyte foot processes. SDs are not seen between the adjacent pedicles and nephrin is usually not expressed. Tubular protein resorption droplets may be seen. Immunoglobulins and complement components can be seen in glomeruli from scarred areas.

Death usually occurs in first year of life due to sepsis. Usually, they do not die of renal failure. If untreated, survival beyond 4 years has been unheard of. Recurrent disease after transplantation is not expected, but Patrakka et al. reported NS in 13 out of 51 grafts of children with *NPHS1*mutations. [150] Recurrent FSGS post-transplant in CNS appears to have different pathogenesis from original disease since all the children had Finn-major/ minor genotype associated with absence of nephrin in native kidneys, however, anti-nephrin antibodies developed in 4 out of 9 patients supporting immune pathogenesis.

Autosomal Recessive FSGS and Steroid-Resistant Nephrotic Syndrome

Fuchshuber et al. described a familial form of steroid resistant NS with recessive transmission, early onset, rapid progression to ESRD and lack of recurrence after transplantation. [151] The gene was mapped on a locus on chromosome 1q25-1q31. The gene, *NPHS2,* encodes podocin, an integral membrane protein that is exclusively expressed in the podocytes of fetal and mature kidney. [152] Podocin is a member of stomatin protein family of lipid raft-associated proteins which are critical for arrangement of SD. [153] Podocin is proposed to act as a scaffold protein to maintain or regulate the integrity of the SD. [154] Subsequently the study of non-familial steroid resistant NS in children and adults has shown homozygous or compound heterozygous *NPHS2* mutations in up to 30% of the affected individuals. [82, 83, 85,155,157] All these individuals present with steroid resistant NS or heavy proteinuria rapidly progressing to ESRD. Although it was described between 3 months to 5 years of age, it may present before the age of 3 months. Strong association between R229q allele and FSGS, high BMI, microalbuminuria and diabetes, has been described by Tsukaguchi, Periera, et al. and others. [83, 85, 90, 92, 155, 156, 158] Most of the patients were reported as MCD in the early course and FSGS later on. Later studies have shown variable response of FSGS to transplantation like absence of recurrence, recurrence with steroid response and recurrence of steroid responsive proteinuria.

Autosomal Dominant FSGS

A relatively less common condition of familial FSGS compared to CNS and steroid resistant NS is known to affect individuals in successive generations of few families. The disease was mapped to chromosome 19q13 and demonstrated missense mutations in *ACTN4,* the gene encoding alpha-actinin-4. This actin-cross-linking protein is localized to the foot processes of podocytes. Morphological injury described is MCD, mesangial proliferative glomerulonephritis and FSGS.

CD2-associated Protein (CD2AP) Mutations

CD2-associated protein (CD2AP) is expressed in lymphoid cells and epithelium. CD2AP knockout mice were found to develop glomerulosclerosis, massive proteinuria and eventually died shortly after birth. Heterozygous state in humans is believed to confer susceptibility to FSGS like mice. [160, 161]

Syndromic FSGS

FSGS occurs in several inherited systemic syndromes listed previously.

Diffuse Mesangial Sclerosis

Habib and Bois reported 6 cases of diffuse mesangial sclerosis (DMS) in nephrotic infants and later analyzed 40 patients with DMS. [161] When NS develops early in patients with DMS, it may often be confused with Finnish type of CNS. However, its rapid course to ESRD and glomerular pathology helps establish its diagnosis. All the glomeruli show mesangial sclerosis, and the matrix initially has a fibrillar appearance with deeper glomeruli least affected. With the disease progression, mesangial matrix accumulates to obliterate glomerular capillaries. Epithelial cells become prominent to persist in spite of tuft retraction, but crescents are unusual. [162] Tubules are dilated and atrophic and may contain hyaline casts. Nonspecific mesangial IgM and C3 deposits are seen in the periphery of sclerotic glomeruli. Electron microscopy shows mesangial collagen fibrils, and the GBM is split and wavy because of zones of subepithelial lucent widening. In Habib's series, patients progressed to ESRD usually by the age of 4 years. Ten patients underwent transplantation and none had recurrence.

The Denys-Drash Syndrome

The glomerular pathology of Denys-Drash syndrome (DDS) is similar to DMS and progresses rapidly to ESRD. [163, 165] In addition, the triad includes male sex with pseudohermaphroditism and predisposition to development of Wilms' tumor; however, all the components may not manifest in every individual.Habib reported six such children, none of whom had recurrence posttransplantation. [162] This syndrome is caused by germ-line mutation in exons 8 or 9 of *WT1* that produce a premature stop codon and a truncated protein with increased affinity for the wild type *WT1*.

Frasier Syndrome

It comprises male pseudohermaphroditism (XY chromosome, female external genitalia with streak ovaries), progressive nephropathy and ovarian tumors (gonadoblastoma). [166] It is caused by *WT1* donor splice site of intron 9 leading to defective alternative splicing of *WT1* and an altered ratio of WT1 positive/negative KTS isoforms. [167, 168] In contrast to the characteristic pathology of DMS and DDS, FSGS is the characteristic pathology. Patients with Frasier syndrome have a more progressive form of FSGS, low incidence of Wilms' tumor and a higher risk of gonadal tumors. [169-171]

Mutant Mitochondrial DNA

The MELAS syndrome (mitochondrial myopathy, encephalopathy, lactic acidosis, and stroke) is caused by A3243G mutation in the mitochondrial gene *MTTL1,* which encodes $tRNA^{Leu}$ and the same mutation may be associated with neurosensory deafness, diabetes mellitus and progressive renal disease. [172-179] Analysis of *MTTL1* in MELAS patients reveals that 80% haveA3243G mutation, 7.5% have T3271C, and 7.5% to 10%A3253G. The renal disease mainly manifests as tubular dysfunction and usually presents with FSGS, proteinuria or NS. Extrarenal manifestations of deafness and diabetes follow renal manifestations. These patients may progress to renal failure; however, the disease does not recur after transplantation. The sclerosis begins at hilum to envelop the entire tufts subsequently; however, unlike the other secondary forms, the glomerular volume does not increase. The mutations in mitochondrial DNA owing to age and oxidative stress, accumulate in the long-lived cells of muscles and neurons, and podocytes, thus manifesting with the syndromic constellation.

8.3.3 Miscellaneous Secondary Forms of FSGS

FSGS has been identified in nephrotic patients treated with interferon-α for hepatitis C virus infection/hematologic malignancies, and in patients with HIV infection. CG has also been found to be associated with thrombotic microangiopathy and autoimmune diseases.

Conclusion

In conclusion, FSGS is one of the most common glomerular pattern of injury observed in a wide variety of primary and secondary renal glomerular diseases. It is highly heterogeneous disorder with varied etiology, pathogenesis, pathology, clinical presentation and prognosis. Its accurate diagnosis and classification is of paramount importance in the optimal management and prognostication of the disorder.

References

[1] D'Agati V. The many masks of focal segmental glomerulosclerosis. *Kidney Int.* 1994;46:1223-1241.

[2] Fahr T. Pathologische anatomie des morbus brightii. In: Henke F, Lubarsch O, editors. Handbuch der Speziellen Pathologischen Anatomie und Histologie (Vol 6). Berlin: Springer; 1925. p. 156.

[3] Cameron JS. The enigma of focal segmental glomerulosclerosis. *Kidney Int. Suppl.* 1996;S57:119-131.

[4] D'Agati V, Fogo A, Bruijn J, Jennette J. Pathologic classification of focal segmental glomerulosclerosis: a working proposal. *Am. J. Kidney Dis.* 2004;43:368-382.

[5] Churg J, Habib R, White R. Pathology of the nephrotic syndrome in children: A report for the International Study of Kidney Disease in Children. *Lancet.* 1970;160:1299-1302.

[6] Schwartz MM, Lewis EJ. Focal segmental glomerular sclerosis: The cellular lesion. *Kidney Int.* 1985;28:968-974.

[7] Kitiyakara DC, Kopp JB, Eggers DP. Trends in the epidemiology of focal segmental glomerulosclerosis. *Semin. Nephrol.* 2003;23:172-182.

[8] Barisoni L, Valeri A, Radhakrishnan J. Focal segmental glomerulosclerosis: A 20-year epidemiological perspective. *J. Am. Soc. Nephrol.* 1994;5:347.

[9] Haas M, Meehan SM, Karrison TG, Spargo BH. Changing etiologies of unexplained adult nephrotic syndrome: A comparison of renal biopsy findings from 1976-1979 and 1995-1997. *Am. J. Kidney Dis.*1997;30:621-631.

[10] Haas M, Spargo BH, Coventry S. Increasing incidence of focal-segmental glomerulosclerosis among adult nephropathies: A 20-year renal biopsy study. *Am. J. Kidney Dis.* 1995;26:740-750.

[11] Korbet SM, Genchi RM, Borok RZ, Schwartz MM. The racial prevalence of glomerular lesions in nephrotic adults. *Am. J. Kidney Dis.* 1996; 27:647-651.

[12] Carbone L, D'Agati V, Cheng JT, Appel GB. Course and prognosis of human immunodeficiency virus-associated nephropathy. *Am. J. Med.* 1989; 87:389-395.

[13] Pakasa M, Mangani N, Dikassa L. Focal and segmental glomerulosclerosis in nephrotic syndrome: A new profile of adult nephrotic syndrome in Zaire. *Mod. Pathol.* 1993;6: 125-128.

[14] Pontier PJ, Patel TG. Racial differences in the prevalence and presentation of glomerular disease in adults. *Clin. Nephrol.* 1994;42:79-84.

[15] Gulati S, Sharma AP, Sharma RK, Gupta A. Changing trends of histopathology in childhood nephrotic syndrome. *Am. J. Kidney Dis.* 1999;34:646-650.

[16] Deegens JKJ, Steenbergen EJ, Borm GF, Wetzel JFMS. Pathological variants of focal segmental glomerulosclerosis in an adult Dutch population- epidemiology and outcome. *Nephrol. Dial. Transplant.* 2008;23:186-192.

[17] Bakr A, Shokeir M, El Chenawi F. Tumor necrosis factor-alpha production from mononuclear cells in nephrotic syndrome. *Pediatr. Nephrol.* 2003;18:516-520.

[18] Cheong HI, Lee JH, Hahn H, Park HW, Ha IS, Choi Y. Circulating VEGF and TGF-beta1 in children with idiopathic nephrotic syndrome. *J. Nephrol.* 2001;14:263-269.

[19] Chen HC, Guh JY, Chang JM, Tsai JC, Hwang SJ, Lai YH. Plasma and urinary endothelin-1 in focal segmental glomerulosclerosis. *J. Clin. Lab. Anal.* 2001;15:59-63.

[20] Hori C, Hiraoka M, Yoshikawa N, Tsuzuki K, Yoshida Y, Yoshioka K, Fujisawa K, Tsukahara H, Ohshima Y, Mayumi M. Significance of ACE genotypes and medical treatments in childhood focal glomerulosclerosis. *Nephron.* 2001;88:313-319.

[21] Lee DY, Kim W, Kang SK, Koh GY, Park SK. Angiotensin-converting enzyme gene polymorphism in patients with minimal-change nephrotic syndrome and focal segmental glomerulosclerosis. *Nephron.* 1997;77:471-473.

[22] Lowik MM, Levtchenko EN, Monnens LA, van den Heuvel LP. WT-1 and NPHS2 mutation analysis in patients with non-familial steroid-resistant focal-segmental glomerulosclerosis. *Clin. Nephrol.* 2003;59:143-146.

[23] Hara M, Yanagihara T, Kihara I. Urinary podocytes in primary focal segmental glomerulosclerosis. *Nephron.* 2001;89:342- 347.

[24] Alcorta D, Preston G, Munger W,Sullivan P, Yang JJ, Waga I, Jennette JC, Falk R. Microarray studies of gene expression in circulating leukocytes in kidney diseases. *Exp. Nephrol.* 2002;10:139-149.

[25] Farris B. Focal Segmental Glomerulosclerosis. In: Colvin RB, Chang, Farris AB, Kambham N, Cornell LD, Meehan SM, Liapis H, Seshan SV, Bonsib SM, Jain S, Vasilyev A, editors. Diagnostic Pathology: Kidney Diseases. Canada: Amirsys Publishing Inc; 2011. p. 2-34.

[26] Schwartz MM, Evans J, Bain R, Korbet SM. Focal segmental glomerulosclerosis: Prognostic implications of the cellular lesion. *J. Am. Soc. Nephrol.* 1990;10:1900-1907.

[27] Rich AR. A hitherto undescribed vulnerability of the juxtamedullary glomeruli in lipoid nephrosis. *Bull. Johns Hopkins Hosp.* 1957;100:173-186.

[28] Howie AJ, Brewer DB. The glomerular tip lesion: A previously undescribed type of segmental glomerular abnormality. *J. Pathol.* 1984;142:205-220.

[29] Stokes MB, Markowitz GS, Lin J, Valeri AM, D'Agati VD. Glomerular tip lesion: A distinct entity within the minimal change disease/focal segmental glomerulosclerosis spectrum. *Kidney Int.*2004;65:1690-1702.

[30] Thomas DB, Franceschini N, Hogan SL, Ten Holder S, Jennette CE, Falk RJ, Jennette JC. Clinical and pathological characteristics of focal segmental glomerulosclerosis pathologic variants. *Kidney Int.* 2006;69:920-926.

[31] Stokes MB, Valeri AM, Markowitz GS, D'Agati VD. Cellular focal segmental glomerulosclerosis: Clinical and pathologic features. *Kidney Int.* 2006;70:1783-1792.

[32] Weiss MA, Daquioag E, Margolin EG, Pollak VE. Nephrotic syndrome, progressive irreversible renal failure and glomerular "collapse": A new clinicopathologic entity? *Am. J. Kidney Dis.* 1986;7:20-28.

[33] Gardenswartz MN, Lerner CW, Seligson GR, Zabetakis PM, Rotterdam H, Tapper ML, Michelis MF, Bruno MS. Renal disease in patients with AIDS: A clinicopathologic study. *Clin. Nephrol.* 1984;21:197- 204.

[34] Pardo V, Aldana M, Colton RM,Fischl MA, Jaffe D, Moskowitz L, Hensley GT, Bourgoignie JJ. Glomerular lesions in the acquired immunodeficiency syndrome. *Ann. Intern. Med.* 1984;101:429-434.

[35] Rao TK, Filippone EJ, Nicastri AD, Landesman SH, Frank E, Chen CK, Friedman EA. Associated focal and segmental glomerulosclerosis in the acquired immunodeficiency syndrome. *N. Engl. J. Med.* 1984;310:669-673.

[36] Bourgoignie JJ, Meneses R, Ortiz C, Jaffe D, Pardo V. The clinical spectrum of renal disease associated with human immunodeficiency virus. *Am. J. Kidney Dis.* 1988;12: 131-137.

[37] Bourgoignie JJ, Meneses R, Pardo V. The nephropathy related to acquired immune deficiency syndrome. *Adv. Nephrol. Necker. Hosp.* 1988;17:113-126.

[38] Casanova S, Mazzucco G, Barbiano di Belgiojoso G, Motta M, Boldorini R, Genderini A, Monga G. Pattern of glomerular involvement in human immunodeficiency virus-infected patients: An Italian study. *Am. J. Kidney Dis.* 1995;26:446-453.

[39] Barisoni L, Kriz W, Mundel P, D'Agati V. The dysregulated podocyte phenotype: A novel concept in the pathogenesis of collapsing idiopathic focal segmental glomerulosclerosis and HIV-associated nephropathy. *J. Am. Soc. Nephrol.* 1999;10: 51-61.

[40] Yang Y, Gubler MC, Beaufils H. Dysregulation of podocyte phenotype in idiopathic collapsing glomerulopathy and HIV-associated nephropathy. *Nephron.* 2002;91:416-423.

[41] Bariety J, Nochy D, Mandet C, Jacquot C, Glotz D, Meyrier A. Podocytes undergo phenotypic changes and express macrophagic-associated markers in idiopathic collapsing glomerulopathy. *Kidney Int.* 1998;53:918-925.

[42] Barisoni L, Mokrzycki M, Sablay L,Nagata M, Yamase H, Mundel P. Podocyte cell cycle regulation and proliferation in collapsing glomerulopathies. *Kidney Int.* 2000;58: 137-143.

[43] Mundel P, Shankland SJ. Podocyte biology and response to injury. *J. Am. Soc. Nephrol.* 2002;13:3005-3015.

[44] Barisoni L, Mundel P. Podocyte biology and the emerging understanding of podocyte diseases. *Am. J. Nephrol.* 2003;23:353-360.

[45] Haas M, Spargo BH, Coventry S. Increasing incidence of focal-segmental glomerulosclerosis among adult nephropathies: A 20-year renal biopsy study. *Am. J. Kidney Dis.* 1995;26:740-750.

[46] Laurinavicius A, Hurwitz S, Rennke HG. Collapsing glomerulopathy in HIV and non-HIV patients: A clinicopathological and follow-up study. *Kidney Int.* 1999;56:2203-2213.

[47] Valeri A, Barisoni L, Appel GB, Seigle R, D'Agati V. Idiopathic collapsing focal segmental glomerulosclerosis: A clinicopathologic study. *Kidney Int.* 1996;50:1734-1746.

[48] Detwiler RK, Falk RJ, Hogan SL, Jennette JC. Collapsing gloemerulopathy: A clinically and pathologically distinct variant of focal segmental glomerulosclerosis. *Kidney Int.* 1994;45:1416-1424.

[49] Grcevska L, Polenakovik M. Collapsing glomerulopathy: Clinical characteristics and follow-up. *Am. J. Kidney Dis.* 1999;33:652-657.

[50] Chun MJ, Korbet SM, Schwartz MM, Lewis EJ. Focal segmental glomerulosclerosis in nephrotic adults: Presentation, prognosis, and response to therapy of the histologic variants. *J. Am. Soc. Nephrol.* 2004;15:2169-2177.

[51] Gupta R, Sharma A, Mahanta PJ, Agarwal SK, Dinda AK. Focal and segmental glomerulosclerosis in renal allograft recipients: A clinic-pathologic study of 37 cases. *Saudi J. Kidney Dis. Transpl.*2013;24:8-14.

[52] Letavernier E, Bruneval P, Mandet C,Duong Van Huyen JP,Péraldi MN, Helal I, Noël LH, Legendre C. High Sirolimus Levels May Induce Focal Segmental Glomerulosclerosis De Novo. *J. Am. Soc. Nephrol.* 2007;2:326-333.

[53] Gupta R, Sharma A, Agarwal S K, Dinda A K. Collapsing glomerulopathy in renal allograft biopsies: A study of nine cases. *Indian J. Nephrol.* 2011;21:10-13.

[54] Churg J, Habib R, White R. Pathology of the nephrotic syndrome in children: A report for the International Study of Kidney Disease in Children. *Lancet.* 1970;760:*1299*-1302.

[55] Beaufils H, Alphonse JC, Guedon J, Legrain M. Focal glomerulosclerosis: Natural history and treatment. *Nephron.* 1978;21:75-85.

[56] Newman WJ, Tisher CC, McCoy RC, Gunnels JC, Krueger RP, Robinson RR. Focal glomerular sclerosis: Contrasting clinical patterns in children and adults. *Medicine.* 1976;55:67-87.

[57] Velosa JA, Donadio JV, Holley KE. Focal sclerosing glomerulonephropathy: A clinicopathologic study. *Mayo Clin. Proc.* 1975;50:121-133.

[58] Hyman LR, Burkholder PM. Focal sclerosing glomerulonephropathy with hylanosis. *J. Pediatr.* 1974;84:217-225.

[59] Yoshikawa N, Ito H, Akamatsu R, Matsuyama S, Hasegawa O, Nakahara C, Matsuo T. Focal segmental glomerulosclerosis with and without nephrotic syndrome in children. *J. Pediatr.* 1986;109:65-70.

[60] Bonsib SM. Focal-segmental glomerulosclerosis. The relationship between tubular atrophy and segmental sclerosis. *Am. J. Clin. Pathol.* 1999;111:343-348.

[61] Gubler MC, Waldherr R, Levy M. Idiopathic nephrotic syndrome with focal and segmental sclerosis and/or hyalinosis: Clinical course response to therapy, and long-term outcome. In: Strauss J, editor. Nephrotic Syndrome: Current Concepts in Diagnosis and Management. New York: Garland; 1979. p. 193.

[62] Hyman LR, Burkholder PM. Focal sclerosing glomerulonephropathy with segmental hyalinosis. A clinicopathologic analysis. *Lab. Invest.* 1973;28:533-544.

[63] Eddy AA. Experimental insights into the tubulointerstitial disease accompanying primary glomerular lesions. *J. Am. Soc. Nephrol.* 1994;5:1273-1287.

[64] Schwartz MM. Focal Segmental Glomerulosclerosis. In: Heptinstall's Pathology of the Kidney. 6th ed. Philadelphia: Wolters Kluwer/ Lippincott Wiliams & Wilkins; 2007. p. 155-204.

[65] Lee HS, Spargo BH. Significance of renal hyaline arteriolosclerosis in focal segmental glomerulosclerosis. *Nephron.* 1985;4:86-93.

[66] Habib R, Kleinknecht C. The primary nephrotic syndrome of childhood: Classification and clinicopathologic study of 406 cases. In: Sommers SC, editor. Pathology Annual. New York: Appleton-Century Crofts; 1971. p. 427.

[67] Jenis EH, Teichman S, Briggs WA,Sandler P, Hollerman CE, Calcagno PL, KnieserMR, Jensen GE, Valeski JE. Focal segmental glomerulosclerosis. *Am. J. Med.* 1974;57:695-705.
[68] Schoeneman MJ, Bennett B, Greifer I. The natural history of focal segmental glomerulosclerosis with and without mesangial hypercellularity in children. *Clin. Nephrol.* 1978;9:45-54.
[69] Hyman LR, Burkholder PM. Focal sclerosing glomerulonephropathy with segmental hyalinosis. A clinicopathologic analysis. *Lab. Invest.* 1973;28:533-544.
[70] A report of the Southwest Pediatric Nephrology Study Group. Focal segmental glomerulosclerosis in children with idiopathic nephrotic syndrome. *Kidney Int.*1985;27: 442-449.
[71] Yoshikawa N, Ito H, Akamatsu R,Matsuyama S, Hasegawa O, Nakahara C, Matsuo T. Focal segmental glomerulosclerosis with and without nephrotic syndrome in children. *J. Pediatr.* 1986;109:65-70.
[72] Rumpelt HJ, Thoenes W. Intraglomerular (immune) deposits in focal and segmental sclerosing glomerulopathy (-nephritis) (focal sclerotic lesion, hyalinose segmentaire et focale). *Clin. Nephrol.* 1973;1:367-371.
[73] Rydel JJ, Korbet SM, Borok RZ, Schwartz MM. Focal segmental glomerular sclerosis in adults: Presentation, course and response to treatment. *Am. J. Kidney Dis.* 1995;25: 534-542.
[74] Korbet SM, Schwartz MM, Lewis EJ. Primary focal segmental glomerulosclerosis: Clinical course and response to therapy. *Am. J. Kidney Dis.* 1994;23:773-783.
[75] Cameron JS. The natural history of glomerulonephritis. In: Black D, Jones NF, editors. Renal Disease. Oxford: Blackwell; 1979. p.329.
[76] Cameron JS. The problem of focal segmental glomerulosclerosis. In: Kincaid-Smith P, d'Apice AJF, Atkins RC, editors. Progress in Glomerulonephritis. New York: Wiley; 1979. p. 209.
[77] Wehrmann M, Bohle A, Held H, Schumm G, Kendziorra H, Pressler H. Long-term prognosis of focal sclerosing glomerulonephritis: An analysis of 250 cases with particular regard to tubulointerstitial changes. *Clin. Nephrol.* 1990;33:115-122.
[78] Cameron JS, Turner DR, Ogg CS, Chantler C, Williams DG. The long-term prognosis of patients with focal segmental glomerulosclerosis. *Clin. Nephrol.* 1978;10:213-218.
[79] Mongeau JG, Robitaille PO, Clermont MJ, Merouani A, Russo P. Focal segmental glomerulosclerosis (FSGS) 20 years later. From toddler to grown up. *Clin. Nephrol.* 1993;40:1-6.
[80] Ingulli E, Tejani A. Racial differences in the incidence and renal outcome of idiopathic focal segmental glomerulosclerosis in children. *Pediatr. Nephrol.* 1991;5:393-397.
[81] Alexopoulos E, Stangou M, Papagianni A, Pantzaki A, Papadimitrou M. Factors influencing the course and the response to treatment in primary focal segmental glomerulosclerosis. *Nephrol. Dial. Transplant.* 2000;15:1348-1356.
[82] Caridi G, Bertelli R, Carrea A, Di Duca M, Catarsi P, Artero M, Carraro M, Zennaro C, Candiano G, Musante L, Seri M, Ginevri F, Perfumo F, Ghiggeri GM. Prevalence, genetics, and clinical features of patients carrying podocin mutations in steroid-resistant nonfamilial focal segmental glomerulosclerosis. *J. Am. Soc. Nephrol.* 2001;12: 2742-2746.

[83] Caridi G, Bertelli R, Scolari F, Sanna-Cherchi S, Di Duca M, Ghiggeri GM. Podocin mutations in sporadic focal-segmental glomerulosclerosis occurring in adulthood. *Kidney Int.* 2003;64:365.

[84] Bertelli R, Ginevri F, Caridi G, Dagnino M, Sandrini S, Di Duca M, Emma F, Sanna-Cherchi S, Scolari F, Neri TM, Murer L, Massella L, Basile G, Rizzoni G,Perfumo F, Ghiggeri GM. Recurrence of focal segmental glomerulosclerosis after renal transplantation in patients with mutations of podocin. *Am. J. Kidney Dis.* 2003;41: 1314-1321.

[85] Ruf RG, Lichtenberger A, Karle SM, Haas JP, Anacleto FE, Schultheiss M, Zalewski I, Imm A, Ruf EM, Mucha B, Bagga A, Neuhaus T, Fuchshuber A,Bakkaloglu A, Hildebrandt F; Arbeitsgemeinschaft Für Pädiatrische Nephrologie Study Group. Patients with mutations in NPHS2 (podocin) do not respond to standard steroid treatment of nephrotic syndrome. *J. Am. Soc. Nephrol.* 2004;15:722-732.

[86] Weber S, Gribouval O, Esquivel EL, Morinière V, Tête MJ, Legendre C, Niaudet P, Antignac C. NPHS2 mutation analysis shows genetic heterogeneity of steroid-resistant nephrotic syndrome and low post-transplant recurrence. *Kidney Int.* 2004;66: 571-579.

[87] Salzer U, Prohaska R. Stomatin. Flotillin-1, and flotillin-2 are major integral proteins of erythrocyte lipid rafts. *Blood.* 2001;97:1141-1143.

[88] Simons M, Schwarz K, Kriz W, Holzman LB. Involvement of lipid rafts in nephrin phosphorylation and organization of the glomerular slit diaphragm. *Am. J. Pathol.* 2001;159:1069-1077.

[89] Schwarz K, Simons M, Reiser J, Moin AS, Christian F. Podocin, a raft-associated component of the glomerular slit diaphragm, interacts with CD2AP and nephrin. *J. Clin. Invest.* 2001;108:1621-1629.

[90] Caridi G, Bertelli R, Di Duca M, Dagnino M, Emma F, Onetti Muda A, Scolari F, Miglietti N, Mazzucco G, Murer L, Carrea A, Massella L, Rizzoni G, Perfumo F, Ghiggeri GM. Broadening the spectrum of diseases related to podocin mutations. *J. Am. Soc. Nephrol.* 2003;14:1278-86.

[91] Mathis BJ, Kim SH, Calabrese K, Seidman JC, Seidman CE, Pollack MR. A locus for inherited focal segmental glomerulosclerosis maps to chromosome 19q13. *Kidney Int.* 1998;53:282-286.

[92] Pereira AC, Pereira AB, Mota GF, Cunha RS, Herkenhoff FL, Pollak MR, Mill JG, Krieger JE. NPHS2 R229Q functional variant is associated with microalbuminuria in the general population. *Kidney Int.* 2004;65:1026-1030.

[93] Kaplan JM, Kim SH, North KN,*Kim SH*, *North KN*, Rennke H, Correia LA, Tong HQ, Mathis BJ, Rodríguez-Pérez JC. Mutations in ACTN4, encoding alpha-actinin-4, cause familial focal segmental glomerulosclerosis. *Nat. Genet.* 2000;24:251-256.

[94] Colvin R B, Nickeleit V. Renal Transplant Pathology. In: Heptinstall's Pathology of the Kidney. 6th ed. Philadelphia: Wolters Kluwer/ Lippincott Wiliams & Wilkins; 2007. p. 1347-1490.

[95] Bhathena DB. Glomerular size and the association of focal glomerulosclerosis in long-surviving human renal allografts. *J. Am. Soc. Nephrol.* 1993;4:1316-1326.

[96] Meehan SM, Pascual M, Williams WW, Tolkoff-Rubin N,Delmonico FL, Cosimi AB, Colvin RB. De novo collapsing glomerulopathy in renal allografts. *Transplantation.* 1998;65:1192-1197.

[97] Stokes MB, Davis CL, Alpers CE. Collapsing glomerulopathy in renal allografts: A morphological pattern with diverse clinicopathologic associations. *Am. J. Kidney Dis.* 1999;33:658-666.

[98] Nadasdy T, Allen C, Zand MS. Zonal distribution of glomerular collapse in renal allografts: Possible role of vascular changes. *Hum. Pathol.* 2002;33:437-441.

[99] Neumayer HH, Huls S, Schreiber M, Riess R, Luft FC. Kidneys from pediatric donors: Risk versus benefit. *Clin. Nephrol.* 1994;4:94-100.

[100] Schwarz A, Krause PH, Offermann G, Keller F. Recurrent and de novo renal disease after kidney transplantation with or without cyclosporine A. *Am. J. Kidney Dis.* 1991;17:524-531.

[101] Leumann EP, Tisher CC. Recurrence of focal segmental glomerulosclerosis in the transplanted kidney. *Acta. Pathol. Microbiol. Immunol. Scand.* 1980;94:69-76.

[102] Striegel JE, Sibley RK, Fryd DS, Mauer SM. Recurrence of focal segmental sclerosis in children following renal transplantation. *Kidney Int.* 1986;19:S44-50.

[103] Zimmerman CE. Renal transplantation for focal segmental glomerulosclerosis. *Transplantation.* 1980;29:172.

[104] O'Meara Y, Green A, Carmody M, Donohoe J, Campbell E, Browne O, Walshe J. Recurrent glomerulonephritis in renal transplants; Fourteen years' experience. *Nephrol. Dial. Transplant.* 1989;4:730-734.

[105] Tejani A, Stablein DH. Recurrence of focal segmental glomerulosclerosis post transplantation: A special report of the North American Pediatric Renal Transplant Cooperative Study. *J. Am. Soc. Nephrol.* 1992;2:S258-S263.

[106] Artero M, Biava C, Amend W, Tomlanovich S, Vincenti F. Recurrent focal glomerulosclerosis: Natural history and response to therapy. *Am. J. Med.* 1992;92:375-383.

[107] Weber S, Tonshoff B. Recurrence of focal segmental glomerulosclerosis in children after transplantation: Clinical and genetic aspects. *Transplantation.* 2005;80:S128-S134.

[108] Vanikar AV, Trivedi HL, Shah PR, Kanodia KV, Patel RD, Modi PR, Dave SD, Singhai AM, Shah VR, Trivedi VB, Shankar V. Single-center experience on renal transplantation in primary focal and segmental glomerulosclerosis using hematopoietic stem cell transplantation in thymus, bone marrow, portal and peripheral circulation. *Saudi J. Kidney Dis. Transpl.* 2013;24:15-21.

[109] Hosenpud J, Piering WF, Garancis JC, Kauffman HM. Successful second kidney transplantation in a patient with focal glomerulosclerosis: A case report. *Am. J. Nephrol.* 1985;5:299-304.

[110] Pinto J, Lacerda G, Cameron JS, Turner DR, Bewick M, Ogg CS. Recurrence of focal segmental glomerulosclerosis in renal allografts. *Transplantation.* 1981;32:83-89.

[111] Broyer M, Gagnadoux MF, Guest G. Kidney transplantation in children: Results of 383 grafts performed at Infants Malades Hospital from 1973 to 1984. *Adv. Nephrol. Necker. Hosp.* 1987;16:307-333.

[112] Maizel SE, Sibley RK, Horstman JP, Kjellstrand CM, Simmons RL. Incidence and significance of recurrent focal segmental glomerulosclerosis in renal allograft recipients. *Transplantation.* 1981;32:512-516.

[113] Senggutuvan P, Cameron JS, Hartley RB. Recurrence of focal segmental glomerulosclerosis in transplanted kidneys: Analysis of incidence and risk factors in 59 allografts. *Pediatr. Nephrol.* 1990;4:21-28.

[114] Detwiler RK, Falk RJ, Hogan SL, Jennette JC. Collapsing glomerulopathy: A clinically and pathologically distinct variant of focal segmental glomerulosclerosis. *Kidney Int.* 1994;45:1416-1426.

[115] Schwarz A, Krause PH, Offermann G, Keller F. Recurrent diseases in the renal allograft. *Am. J. Kidney Dis.* 1991;17:524-531.

[116] Verani RR, Hawkins EP. Recurrent focal segmental glomerulosclerosis: A pathological study of the early lesion. *Am. J. Nephrol.* 1986;6:263-270.

[117] Harrison DJ, Jenkins D, Dick J. An unusual inter podocyte cell junction and its appearance in a transplant graft kidney. *J. Cli. Pathol.* 1988;41:155-157.

[118] Bariety J, Bruneval P, Hill G,Irinopoulou T, Mandet C, Meyrier A. Posttransplantation relapse of FSGS is characterized by glomerular epithelial cell transdifferentiation. *J. Am. Soc. Nephrol.* 2001;12:261-274.

[119] Kemeny E, Mihatsch MJ, Durmuller U, Gudat F. Podocytes loose their adhesive phenotype in focal segmental glomerulosclerosis. *Clin. Nephrol.* 1995;43:71-83.

[120] Nishimura M, Toki J, Sugiura K. Focal segmental glomerular sclerosis, a type of intractable chronic glomerulonephritis, is a stem cell disorder. *J. Exp. Med.* 1994;179: 1053-1058.

[121] Savin VJ, McCarthy ET, Sharma M. Permeability factors in focal segmental glomerulosclerosis. *Semin. Nephrol* 2003;23:147-160.

[122] Fogo AB. Animal models of FSGS: Lessons for pathogenesis and treatment. *Semin. Nephrol.* 2003;23:161-171.

[123] National Cholesterol Education Program (NCEP) Expert Panel on Detection, Evaluation, and Treatment of High Blood Cholesterol in Adults (Adult Treatment Panel III). Third Report of the National Cholesterol Education Program (NCEP) Expert Panel on Detection, Evaluation, and Treatment of High Blood Cholesterol in Adults (Adult Treatment Panel III) final report. *Circulation.* 2002;106:3143-421.

[124] Bagby SP. Obesity-initiated metabolic syndrome and the kidney: A recipe for chronic kidney disease? *J. Am. Soc. Nephrol.* 2004;15:2775-2791.

[125] Chen J, Muntner P, Hamm LL, Jones DW, Batuman V, Fonseca V, Whelton PK, He J. The metabolic syndrome and chronic kidney disease in U.S. adults. *Ann. Intern. Med.* 2004;140:167-174.

[126] Kriz W, Gretz N, Lemley KV. Progression of glomerular diseases: Is the podocyte the culprit? *Kidney Int.* 1998;54:687-697.

[127] Rennke HG. How does glomerular epithelial cell injury contribute to progressive glomerular damage? *Kidney Int.* 1994;45:S58-S63.

[128] Myllymäki J, Saha H, Mustonen J. IgM nephropathy: clinical picture and long-term prognosis. *Am. J. Kidney Dis.* 2003;41:43-50.

[129] Singhai AM, Vanikar AV, Goplani KR. Immunoglobulin M nephropathy in adults and adolescents in India: a single center study of natural history. *Indian J. Pathol. Microbiol.* 2011;54:3-6.

[130] Tejani A, Nicastri AD. Mesangial IgM nephropathy. *Nephron.* 1983;35:1-5.

[131] Vanikar AV. IgM nephropathy; can we still ignore it. *J. Nephropathol.* 2013;2:98-103.

[132] Vanikar AV, Kanodia KV, PatelRD, Suthar KS,PatelHV, Gumber, Trivedi HL. IgM nephropathy in India: a single centre experience. *Indian J. Pediatr.* 2012;79:1025-1027.

[133] Rennke HG, Klein PS. Pathogenesis and significance of nonprimary focal and segmental glomerulosclerosis. *Am. J. Kidney Dis.* 1989;13:443-456.

[134] Kincaid-Smith P. Glomerular lesions in atrophic pyelonephritis and reflux nephropathy. *Kidney Int. Suppl.* 1975;4:S81-S83.

[135] Salomon R, Tellier AL, Attie-Bitach T, Amiel J, Vekemans M, Lyonnet S, Dureau P, Niaudet P, Gubler MC, Broyer M. PAX2 mutations in oligomeganephronia. *Kidney Int.* 2001;59:457-462.

[136] Bhathena DB, Julian BA, McMorrow RG, Baehler RW. Focal sclerosis of hypertrophied glomeruli in solitary functioning kidneys of humans. *Am. J. Kidney Dis.* 1985;5:226-232.

[137] Kiprov DD, Colvin RB, McCluskey RT. Focal and segmental glomerulosclerosis and porteinuria associated with unilateral renal agenesis. *Lab. Invest.* 1982;46:275-281.

[138] Gutierrez-Millet V, Nieto J, Praga M, Usera G, Martinez MA, Morales JM. Focal glomerulosclerosis and proteinuria in patients with solitary kidneys. *Arch. Intern. Med.* 1986;146:705-709.

[139] Zucchelli P, Cagnoli L, Casanova S, Donini U, Pasquali S. Focal glomerulosclerosis in patients with unilateral nephrectomy. *Kidney Int.* 1983;24:649-655.

[140] Greenberg A, Bastacky SI, Iqbal A, Borochovitz D, Johnson JP. Focal segmental glomerulosclerosis associated with nephrotic syndrome in cholesterol atheroembolism: Clinicopathological correlations. *Am. J. Kidney Dis.* 1997;29:334-344.

[141] Kasiske BL, Crosson JT. Renal disease in patients with massive obesity. *Arch. Intern. Med.* 1986;146:1105-1109.

[142] Kambham N, Markowitz GS, Valeri AM, Lin J, D'Agati VD. Obesity-related glomerulopathy: An emerging epidemic. *Kidney Int.* 2001;59:1498-1509.

[143] Spear GS. The glomerulus in cyanotic congenital heart disease and primary pulmonary hypertension: A review. *Nephron.* 1964;29:238-248.

[144] Flanagan MF, Hourihan M, Keane JF. Incidence of renal dysfunction in adults with cyanotic congenital heart disease. *Am. J. Cardiol.* 1991;68:403-406.

[145] Hida K, Wada J, Yamasaki H,Nagake Y, Zhang H, Sugiyama H, Shikata K, Makino H. Cyanotic congenital heart disease associated with glomerulomegaly and focal segmental glomerulosclerosis: Remission of nephrotic syndrome with angiotensin converting enzyme inhibitor. *Nephrol. Dial Transplant.* 2002;17:144-147.

[146] Dittrich S, Haas NA, Buhrer C, Müller C, Dähnert I, Lange PE. Renal impairment in patients with long-standing cyanotic congenital heart disease. *Acta. Paediatr.*1998;87: 949-954.

[147] Baker L, Dahlem S, Goldfarb S, Kern EF, Stanley CA, Egler J, Olshan JS, Heyman S. Hyperfiltration and renal disease in glycogen storage disease, type I. *Kidney Int.* 1989;35:1345-1350.

[148] Wolfsdorf JI, Crigler JF Jr. Effect of continuous glucose therapy begun in infancy on the long-term clinical course of patients with type I glycogen storage disease. *J. Pediatr. Gastroenterol. Nutr.* 1999;29:136-143.

[149] Kestila M, Lenkkeri U, Mannikko M, Lamerdin J, McCready P, Putaala H, Ruotsalainen V, Morita T, Nissinen M, Herva R, Kashtan CE, Peltonen L, Holmberg

C,Olsen A, Tryggvason K. Positionally cloned gene for a novel glomerular protein "nephrin" is mutated in congenital nephrotic syndrome. *Mol. Cell.* 1998;1:575-582.

[150] Patrakka J, Ruotsalainen V, Reponen P,Qvist E, Laine *J*, Holmberg C. Recurrence of nephrotic syndrome in kidney grafts of patients with congenital nephrotic syndrome of the Finnish type: Role of nephrin. *Transplantation.* 2002;73:394-403.

[151] Fuchshuber A, Jean G, Gribouval O,Gubler MC, Broyer M, Beckmann JS, Niaudet P, Antignac C. Mapping a gene (SRN1) to chromosome 1q25-q31 in idiopathic nephrotic syndrome confirms a distinct entity of autosomal recessive nephrosis. *Hum. Mol. Genet.* 1995;4:2155-2158.

[152] Boute N, Gribouval O, Roselli S,Benessy F, Lee H, Fuchshuber A, Dahan K. NPHS2, encoding the glomerular protein podocin, is mutated in autosomal recessive steroid-resistant nephrotic syndrome. *Nat. Genet.* 2002;24:349-354.

[153] Simons M, Schwarz K, Kriz W, Miettinen A, Reiser J, Mundel P, Holthöfer H. Involvement of lipid rafts in nephrin phosphorylation and organization of the glomerular slit diaphragm. *Am. J. Pathol.* 2001;159:1069-1077.

[154] Schwarz K, Simons M, Reiser J, Saleem MA, Faul C, Kriz W, Shaw AS, Holzman LB, Mundel P. Podocin, a raft-associated component of the glomerular slit diaphragm, interacts with CD2AP and nephrin. *J. Clin. Invest.* 2001;108:1621-1629.

[155] Karle SM, Uetz B, Ronner V, Glaeser L, Hildebrandt F, Fuchshuber A. Novel mutations in NPHS2 detected in both familial and sporadic steroid-resistant nephrotic syndrome. *J. Am. Soc. Nephrol.* 2002;13:388-393.

[156] Frishberg Y, Rinat C, Megged O,Shapira E, Feinstein S, Raas-Rothschild A. Mutations in NPHS2 encoding podocin are a prevalent cause of steroid-resistant nephrotic syndrome among Israeli-Arab children. *J. Am. Soc. Nephrol.* 2002;13:400-405.

[157] Winn MP. Not all in the family: Mutations of podocin in sporadic steroid-resistant nephrotic syndrome. *J. Am. Soc. Nephrol.* 2002;13:577-579.

[158] Tsukaguchi H, Sudhakar A, Le TC, Nguyen T, Yao J, Schwimmer JA, Schachter AD, Poch E, Abreu PF, Appel GB, Pereira AB, Kalluri R, Pollak MR. NPHS2 mutations in late-onset focal segmental glomerulosclerosis: R229Q is a common disease-associated allele. *J. Clin. Invest.* 2002;110:1659-1666.

[159] Shih NY, Li J, Karpitskii V, Nguyen A, Dustin ML. Congenital nephrotic syndrome in mice lacking CD2-associated protein. *Science.* 1999;*286:312*-315.

[160] Kim JM, Wu H, Green G. CD2-associated protein haplo insufficiency is linked to glomerular disease susceptibility. *Science.* 2003;*300:1298-1300.*

[161] Habib R, Bois E. Heterogeneity of early onset nephrotic syndromes in infants (nephrotic syndrome "in infants"). Anatomical, clinical and genetic study of 37 cases [in French]. *Helv. Paediatr. Acta.* 1973;*28:91*-107.

[162] Habib R, Gubler MC, Niaudet P, Gagnadoux MF. Congenital/infantile nephrotic syndrome with diffuse mesangial sclerosis: Relationship with Drash Syndrome. In: Bartsocas CS, editor. Genetics of Kidney Disorders: Progress in Clinical and Biological Research. New York: Liss; 1989. p. 193.

[163] Denys P, Malvaux P, Van Den Berghe H. Association of an anatomo-pathological syndrome of male pseudohermaphroditism, Wilms' tumor, parenchymatous nephropathy and XX/XY mosaicism [in French]. *Arch. Fr. Pediatr.* 1967;24:719-729.

[164] Drash A, Sherman F, Hartmann WH, Blizzard RM. A syndrome of pseudohermaphroditism, Wilms' tumor, hypertension, and degenerative renal disease. *J. Pediatr.* 1970;76:585-593.

[165] Eddy AA, Mauer SM. Pseudohermaphroditism, glomerulopathy, and Wilms tumor (Drash syndrome): Frequency in end-stage renal failure. *J. Pediatr.* 1985;106:584-587.

[166] Frasier SD, Bashore RD, Mosier HD. Gonadoblastoma associated with pure gonadal dysgenesis in monzygous twins. *J. Pediatr.* 1964;64:*740*-745.

[167] Klamt B, Koziell A, Poulat F,Poulat F, Wieacker P, Scambler P, Berta P. Frasier syndrome is caused by defective alternative splicing of WT1 leading to an altered ratio of WT1 +/- KTS splice isoforms. *Hum. Mol. Genet.* 1998;7:709-714.

[168] Barbaux S, Niaudet P, Gubler MC,Grünfeld JP, Jaubert F, Kuttenn F, Fékété CN, Souleyreau-Therville N, Thibaud E, Fellous M, McElreavey K. Donor splice-site mutations in WT1 are responsible for Frasier syndrome. *Nat. Genet.* 1997;17:467-470.

[169] McTaggart SJ, Algar E, Chow CW, Powell HR, Jones CL. Clinical spectrum of Denys-Drash and Frasier syndrome. *Pediatr. Nephrol.* 2001;16:335-339.

[170] Moorthy AV, Chesney RW, Lubinsky M. Chronic renal failure and XY gonadal dysgenesis: "Frasier syndrome" a commentary on reported cases. *Am. J. Med. Genet.* 1987;3:297-302.

[171] Auber F, Lortat-Jacob S, Sarnacki S,Jaubert *F*, Salomon R, Thibaud E. Surgical management and genotype/phenotype correlations in WT1 gene-related diseases (Drash, Frasier syndromes). *J. Pediatr. Surg.* 2003;38:124-129.

[172] Goto Y, Nonaka I, Horai S. A mutation in the Trna (Leu)(UUR) gene associated with the MELAS subgroup of mitochondrial encephalomyopathies. *Nature.* 1990;*348*:651-653.

[173] DiMauro S, Schon EA. Mitochondrial respiratory-chain diseases. *N. Engl. J. Med.* 2003;348:2656-2668.

[174] Guery B, Choukroun G, Noel LH, Clavel P, Rötig A, Lebon S, Rustin P. The spectrum of systemic involvement in adults presenting with renal lesion and mitochondrial tRNA (Leu) gene mutation. *J. Am. Soc. Nephrol.* 2003;14:2099-2108.

[175] Doleris LM, Hill GS, Chedin P, Nochy D, Bellanne-Chantelot C. Focal segmental glomerulosclerosis associated with mitochondrial cytopathy. *Kidney Int.* 2000;58:1851-1858.

[176] Hameed R, Raafat F, Ramani P,Gray G, Roper HP, Milford DV. Mitochondrial cytopathy presenting with focal segmental glomerulosclerosis, hypoparathyroidism, sensorineural deafness, and progressive neurological disease. *Postgrad. Med. J.* 2001;77:523-526.

[177] Hotta O, Inoue CN, Miyabayashi S,Furuta T, Takeuchi A, Taguma Y. Clinical and pathologic features of focal segmental glomerulosclerosis with mitochondrial tRNALeu (UUR) gene mutation. *Kidney Int.* 2001;59:1236-1243.

[178] Jansen JJ, Maassen JA, van der Woude FJ. Mutation in mitochondrial tRNA(Leu(UUR)) gene associated with progressive kidney disease. *J. Am. Soc. Nephrol.* 1997;8:1118-1124.

[179] Mochizuki H, Joh K, Kawame H,Imadachi A, Nozaki *H*, Ohashi T, Usui N, Eto Y, Kanetsuna Y, Aizawa S. Mitochondrial encephalomyopathies preceded by de-Toni-Debre-Fanconi syndrome or focal segmental glomerulosclerosis. *Clin. Nephrol.* 1996;46: 347-352.

Index

#

10q23, 62
10q24, 62, 66

A

accounting, 30, 110, 115, 143, 165
acid, 20, 68, 89, 172
acidosis, 51
acquired immunodeficiency syndrome (AIDS), 193
acute glomerulonephritis, 8
acute nephritic syndrome, 87
acute rejection, 167
acute renal failure, 6, 7, 23, 87, 131
adaptation(s), 133, 184
ADH, 130
adhesion(s), 15, 17, 20, 24, 25, 26, 60, 61, 65, 109, 112, 175, 177, 179, 183, 185, 186
adolescents, 9, 103, 118, 198
adulthood, 4, 64, 67, 68, 119, 196
adults, v, 103, 129, 198
advancement, 112, 115
aetiology, 73
African Americans, 72, 80, 132
age, 2, 3, 6, 46, 49, 58, 59, 61, 64, 68, 69, 70, 71, 82, 84, 101, 102, 103, 113, 125, 132, 136, 143, 181, 183, 186, 189, 190
agonist, 20
albumin, 2, 4, 13, 14, 21, 22, 130, 131, 145, 180
albuminuria, 21, 28, 71, 129
aldehydes, 35
aldosterone, 11, 12, 17, 18, 19, 20, 27, 28
allele, 64, 72, 76, 80, 189, 200
allergy, 35
Alpha enolase, 35
alters, 60
amiloride, v, vii, 11, 12, 13, 15, 16, 17, 18, 19, 20, 21, 22, 23, 26
amino acid(s), 38, 63, 69, 72
amyloidosis, 3, 4, 83, 85, 86, 96, 100, 102, 130, 146, 148, 149, 150, 157, 160
ANCA, 48, 50, 53, 55, 136
anchoring, 13, 24, 62, 70
anemia, 174
angiogenesis, 19
angiotensin, 192
angiotensin converting enzyme (ACE), 63, 171, 192, 199
aniridia, 69
antibody(s), 31, 32, 34, 35, 36, 38, 39, 42, 43, 47, 50, 51, 55, 110, 150, 152
antidiuretic hormone, 130
Anti-GBM disease, 111
antigen, 24, 31, 32, 33, 35, 37, 38, 42, 43, 47, 48, 110, 184
anti-inflammatory agents, 130, 136
anti-inflammatory drugs, 91, 111
antiphospholipid antibodies, 155
Anti-PLA2R, 53
APL, 48
apoptosis, 70, 178
Argentina, 11
arteries, 27, 153, 155, 156
arterioles, 88, 144, 145, 153, 155, 156
arteriosclerosis, 180
arthritis, 91, 95
Asian countries, 185
assessment, 82, 84, 97, 173
asymmetry, 21
asymptomatic, 61, 65, 69, 81, 107, 151, 156
atherosclerosis, 20, 28, 99, 186
atopy, 5, 130, 131
atrophy, 71, 85, 89, 92, 105, 106, 113, 115, 151, 153, 180, 181, 185, 194

autoantibodies, 31, 32, 33, 34, 35, 39, 44, 48, 49
autoimmune disease(s), 54, 153, 190
autoimmunity, 44, 53
autosomal dominant, 60, 62, 67, 68, 69, 71, 151
autosomal recessive, 60, 62, 63, 66, 70, 71, 75, 151, 152, 187, 188, 200

B

bacteria, 166
Bangladesh, 122
basal lamina, 115, 135, 181
base pair, 72
basement membrane, 4, 11, 12, 29, 30, 33, 36, 47, 49, 54, 58, 62, 65, 66, 85, 86, 90, 91, 94, 98, 104, 112, 114, 115, 117, 125, 131, 137, 140, 142, 143, 144, 145, 146, 147, 151, 152, 172, 185
basophils, 120
benign, 46, 110, 153
biomarkers, 73, 80
biosynthesis, 62, 66, 70, 71, 79
birefringence, 96, 149
birth weight, 61
births, 188
blindness, 66
blood, 11, 12, 19, 23, 24, 28, 33, 49, 51, 52, 58, 86, 129, 145, 154, 171
blood flow, 19
blood pressure, 11, 12, 19, 26, 28
blood vessels, 86, 129, 145, 154
body mass index (BMI), 182, 187, 189
bone marrow, 183, 197
bone marrow transplant, 183
brain, 51
branching, 96, 150, 186
Brazil, 64, 122
breakdown, 35, 54
BSR, 55

C

C3 glomerulopathies, 48, 49, 53, 54, 141
C3 nephritic factor, 49, 141
Ca^{2+}, 27, 62
calcium, 17, 18, 19, 27, 65, 67
cancer, 24, 25
capsule, 49, 60, 65, 88, 109, 115, 142, 145, 146, 151, 152, 172, 173, 179, 186
carcinoma, 91, 102, 111
cardiovascular morbidity, 20
cascades, 15, 52
catabolism, 130
cataract, 66
catecholamines, 14
categorization, 109
category a, 95
cathepsin G, 25
cation, 61, 77
causation, 57
C-C, 122
cell body, 4, 172, 185
cell cycle, 193
cell division, 17, 72
cell line(s), 16
cell signaling, 71
cell surface, 13, 15, 16, 63
cellular, 24, 38, 71, 108, 109, 134, 135, 177, 178, 181, 184, 192
cellular immunity, 71
cellulitis, 7, 10
challenges, viii, 9, 73, 161, 164, 167
Charcot-Marie-Tooth disease (CMT), 67
chemicals, 166
chemokines, 16
chemotaxis, 17
childhood, 46, 63, 64, 67, 69, 71, 74, 75, 79, 117, 118, 119, 121, 123, 124, 127, 130, 158, 164, 168, 192, 194
childhood cancer, 69
children, v, 101, 103, 117, 118, 119, 154, 171, 191, 194
China, 36
cholangitis, 111
cholesterol, 63, 95, 184, 199
chromosomal abnormalities, 186
chromosome, 61, 63, 65, 67, 68, 69, 70, 71, 72, 75, 77, 78, 108, 151, 188, 189, 190, 196, 200
chromosome 10, 65
chronic inflammatory cells, 180
chronic kidney disease (CKD), 67, 73, 108, 184, 198
chronic renal failure, 7, 78, 87, 143, 171, 186, 201
chymotrypsin, 16
cilium, 62
circulation, 14, 16, 32, 43, 44, 45, 50, 59, 73, 183, 197
classification, 47, 55, 60, 89, 92, 99, 100, 103, 108, 109, 112, 114, 124, 125, 126, 139, 143, 154, 158, 167, 169, 170, 171, 172, 173, 177, 191
cleavage, 25, 43, 45
climates, 83
clinical diagnosis, 138
clinical presentation, 2, 13, 86, 87, 95, 96, 101, 103, 104, 107, 114, 115, 146, 169, 178, 181, 183, 191
clinical syndrome, 1, 7, 57, 186
cloning, 57, 61, 68, 76, 78

closure, 165
CNS, 4, 58, 61, 62, 63, 64, 65, 69, 74, 104, 120, 188, 189
cochlea, 151
coding, 63, 72, 73
codon, 190
coenzyme, 70, 78, 79
cognitive development, 66
collagen, 17, 47, 107, 118, 138, 150, 151, 152, 170, 184, 189
collapsing glomerulopathy, 193, 194, 197, 198
colon, 23, 136
colon cancer, 23
communication, 166
complement, vii, 29, 30, 32, 33, 38, 41, 42, 43, 44, 45, 46, 47, 48, 49, 50, 51, 52, 53, 54, 55, 95, 104, 105, 113, 115, 123, 126, 138, 139, 141, 142, 155, 159, 167, 184, 188
complications, 1, 5, 6, 7, 10, 16, 21, 39, 51, 63, 69, 96, 118
condensation, 135, 181
conductivity, 21
configuration, 114
congenital heart disease, 108, 133, 174, 177, 199
congenital NS
  diffuse mesangial sclerosis, 133, 187
  Finnish type, 3, 61, 104, 189, 200
Congo red staining, 96, 149, 150
connective tissue, 42, 91, 110, 118, 155
consensus, 36, 45, 54, 82, 84, 154, 159, 173
consolidation, 174
constituents, 16
consumption, 50
contamination, 166
controversial, 15, 113, 109, 116, 134
coronary heart disease, 6
correlation(s), 17, 19, 32, 34, 59, 63, 75, 78, 87, 95, 97, 106, 107, 118, 126, 127, 128, 144, 160, 199, 201
correlation analysis, 126
cortex, 19, 28, 83, 84, 89, 188
corticosteroids, 82
creatinine, 2, 58, 101, 102, 153, 179, 180, 181, 187
crescentic glomerulonephritis, 105, 122
crescents, 115
  cellular, 24, 38, 71, 108, 109, 134, 135, 177, 178, 181, 184, 192
CRF, 171
Croatia, 119, 120
CRP, 48
cure, 83
cyanotic, 177, 187, 199
cyanotic congenital heart disease, 108, 133, 174, 199
cyclophosphamide, 107, 123
cyclosporine, 16, 24, 65, 122, 197
cytokines, 11, 13, 14, 16, 32, 39, 42, 47, 52, 59, 184
cytokinesis, 62, 72
cytoplasm, 15, 35, 62, 68, 70, 71, 132, 172, 183
cytoplasmic tail, 15
cytoskeleton, 4, 19, 20, 28, 58, 59, 60, 62, 63, 68, 70, 71, 135

D

decay, 45
defects, 4, 20, 52, 66, 151, 160
deficiency(s), 5, 42, 44, 48, 49, 54, 66, 70, 74, 78, 79, 95, 126, 193
deficit, 151
deformability, 19
degradation, 16, 25
dense deposit disease, 54, 83, 115, 159
Denys-Drash syndrome (DDS), 61, 190
depolymerization, 67
derivatives, 15
destruction, 58
detachment, 12, 13, 109, 114, 180, 183, 185, 186
detectable, 33, 35, 146
detection, 34, 48, 149
developed countries, 81, 82, 84, 162, 164, 166
developed nations, 149
developing countries, vii, viii, 82, 84, 96, 161, 162, 164, 165, 166
developing nations, 164, 166
diabetes, 4, 59, 70, 105, 159, 188, 189, 190
diabetes mellitus, 3, 143
diabetic glomerulosclerosis, 93, 143, 144, 145, 159
diabetic kidney disease, 145
diabetic nephropathy, 21, 80, 96, 130, 133, 143, 159
diabetic retinopathy, 144
diacylglycerol, 65
diagnostic criteria, 105, 109
dialysis, 51, 80, 171, 183
diaphragm, 4, 57, 62, 109, 114, 118, 130, 196, 200
diastolic blood pressure, 153
differential diagnosis, 138
diffuse LN, 154
diffuse mesangial sclerosis, 133, 187
dilation, 20
dimerization, 63
direct measure, 53
disease activity, 5, 51, 106
disease gene, 73, 146
disease progression, 73, 89, 141, 146, 160, 181, 189
disequilibrium, 72

disorder, 4, 57, 59, 66, 71, 72, 74, 84, 100, 111, 148, 153, 169, 183, 191, 198
displacement, 34
dissociation, 28, 32
distribution, 87, 134, 159, 169, 172, 197
diuretic, 11, 13, 18
diversity, 5
DNA, 68, 69, 133, 188, 190
donors, 24, 182, 183, 197
drug therapy, 63
drugs, 3, 4, 6, 21, 30, 59, 102, 104, 107, 170
drusen, 49
dyscrasia, 146
dysplasia, 66, 71, 133, 174, 177, 186

E

edema, 1, 2, 4, 5, 6, 7, 8, 9, 11, 12, 13, 14, 16, 17, 18, 20, 21, 22, 23, 28, 42, 58, 101, 102, 117, 130, 131, 155, 187
effusion, 6
electricity, 165
electron, viii, 49, 60, 68, 69, 70, 82, 86, 90, 91, 94, 96, 97, 104, 106, 112, 114, 116, 125, 128, 131, 132, 138, 139, 141, 143, 146, 147, 154, 155, 156, 162, 164, 167, 168, 172, 173, 180, 181
electron microscopy, viii, 60, 68, 69, 70, 71, 82, 96, 97, 104, 125, 132, 138, 139, 147, 150, 154, 155, 162, 167, 168, 172, 173, 181, 188, 189
electron-dense deposits, 156
ELISA, 24, 34
emancipator, 122
embolism, 7
emission, 199
encephalopathy, 70, 190
encoding, 60, 77, 189, 196, 200
end stage renal disease (ESRD), 6, 57, 58, 61, 63, 64, 67, 68, 71, 72, 80, 90, 109, 112, 114, 116, 141, 153, 178, 180, 181, 185, 187, 188, 189, 190
endothelial cells, 4, 16, 19, 20, 27, 28, 51, 53, 60, 92
endothelial NO synthase, 19
endothelium, 14, 17, 20, 28, 58, 145, 156
endotoxemia, 25
endotoxins, 14, 45
England, 163
enlargement, 92, 116, 185, 186, 187
entrapment, 108
environmental factors, 44, 57, 65
enzyme(s), 19, 25, 34, 35, 70, 71, 74, 130, 192
enzyme inhibitors, 74
epidemic, 199
epidemiology, 123, 124, 125, 191, 192
epilepsy, 70
epithelia, 27, 151
epithelial cells, 34, 35, 38, 42, 89, 92, 104, 109, 112, 131, 134, 135, 136, 145, 155, 156, 172, 176, 189
epithelium, 185, 188, 189
epitopes, 33, 38
equipment, 82, 164, 166
erythrocyte sedimentation rate, 48
esophagus, 136, 151
ESR, 48
ester, 23
etiology, 4, 29, 53, 83, 87, 95, 103, 105, 110, 148, 191
Europe, 8
European Community, 160
evidence, 5, 9, 15, 27, 29, 31, 32, 46, 50, 52, 60, 64, 75, 91, 97, 107, 113, 121, 169, 170, 184
evolution, 99, 100, 125, 170, 185
examinations, 73
exclusion, 104, 178
excretion, 17, 18, 22, 25, 26, 27, 101, 102, 129, 130, 171, 180, 185
exons, 61, 63, 65, 69, 190
exposure, 6, 51, 125
extracellular matrix, 15, 16, 49, 107, 108, 112, 134, 138, 150, 158, 172, 174
extracts, 31

F

familial nephrotic syndrome, 27
families, 63, 68, 70, 71, 72, 160, 188, 189
family history, 170
family members, 68
fat, 155, 171
FDA, 34
female rat, 136
fever, 186
Fibrillary GN, 102
fibrin, 144, 145, 147, 155
fibrinogen, 14, 17, 145
fibrinolytic, 16, 25
fibroblast growth factor, 184
fibroblasts, 16, 185
fibrosis, 18, 27, 87, 89, 106, 113, 115, 131, 151, 153, 180, 181, 182, 185
filament, 19, 62
filtration, 1, 4, 11, 12, 13, 16, 21, 27, 29, 58, 61, 67, 71, 74, 75, 102, 117, 130, 153, 182, 184, 185
fine tuning, 17
fingerprints, 156
Finland, 61, 188
Finnish type, 3, 61, 104, 189, 200
fluid, 11, 12, 13, 14, 23, 45, 46, 49, 141, 171

fluorescence, 140, 147, 149, 150
Focal LN, 154
focal segmental glomerulosclerosis, vii, viii, 2, 24, 57, 74, 75, 76, 77, 78, 79, 80, 83, 85, 86, 88, 98, 99, 103, 105, 118, 119, 123, 124, 125, 126, 130, 132, 133, 134, 135, 136, 158, 191, 192, 193, 194, 195, 196, 197, 198, 199, 200, 201
cellular, 24, 38, 71, 108, 109, 134, 135, 177, 178, 181, 184, 192
collapsing, 108, 109, 134, 178, 179, 182, 183, 193, 194, 197, 198
NOS, 60, 108, 109, 110, 134, 170, 174, 175, 176, 177, 181, 182
perihilar, 108, 109, 134, 175, 177, 182
tip variant, 134
food, 130
foot processes, 60
foreign companies, 166
formaldehyde, 136
formation, 4, 8, 12, 13, 14, 21, 23, 29, 31, 33, 38, 43, 45, 46, 47, 48, 51, 53, 58, 59, 68, 94, 114, 117, 146, 156, 180, 185
founder effect, 71
fragments, 49, 146, 181
France, 34
Frasier syndrome, 61, 62, 66, 133, 187, 190, 201
functional changes, 21
fusion, 106, 107, 180

G

Galloway-Mowat syndrome, 182
gastrointestinal tract, 51
GBM, 4, 11, 12, 13, 20, 30, 31, 32, 36, 46, 47, 49, 50, 52, 53, 58, 59, 60, 65, 71, 85, 88, 90, 91, 92, 94, 109, 110, 111, 112, 114, 115, 116, 136, 137, 138, 142, 143, 144, 145, 146, 147, 150, 151, 152, 153, 172, 178, 180, 185, 188, 189
gelation, 19, 20
gene expression, 23, 65, 192
gene promoter, 16
gene regulation, 60
genes, 4, 36, 54, 57, 58, 59, 60, 61, 64, 65, 67, 68, 70, 71, 72, 73, 74, 75, 76, 120, 187
genetic alteration, 36
genetic defect, 57, 133, 151
genetic disease, 182
genetic disorders, 74
genetic factors, vii, 36, 57, 60, 68
genetic mutations, 108
genetic predisposition, 104
genetic testing, 9
genetics, 74, 80, 120, 195
genetics, v, 36, 57, 60, 78, 120, 200
genitals, 6
genitourinary tract, 69
genome, 36, 68, 72, 171, 188
genotype, 59, 75, 78, 160, 188, 201
genotyping, 41
geography, 102
Germany, 34
germline mutations, 69
gestation, 188
GFB, 4, 5, 58, 59, 64, 65, 66, 71, 102, 182
GFR, 11, 12, 153, 184, 187
glaucoma, 71
glomerular injury, 46
glomeruli, 153, 159
glomerulomegaly, 177, 185
glomerulopathy, 122, 141, 150
glomerulus, 12, 13, 58, 62, 76, 82, 87, 88, 89, 93, 131, 134, 140, 142, 146, 147, 170, 172, 173, 175, 176, 177, 188, 199
glucocorticoid, 58, 71
glucose, 187, 199
glycogen, 187, 199
glycogen storage disease, 108, 133
glycolysis, 35
glycoproteins, 65, 172
glycosaminoglycans, 58
glycosylation, 52, 145
gonadal dysgenesis, 68, 69, 78, 201
gonadoblastoma, 201
gonads, 69
Goodpasture antigen, 47
governments, 166
grading, 100
growth, 14, 25, 52, 62, 65, 71, 72, 106, 122, 164, 184, 186
growth factor, 14, 52, 106, 122, 184
growth hormone, 184
GTPases, 17
guidelines, 82, 84, 97, 142

H

haplotypes, 104
haptoglobin, 51
HE, 28, 80, 122, 162
heart disease, 7, 187
hematuria, 42, 46, 47, 49, 58, 93, 107, 113, 116, 131, 132, 150, 151, 154, 155, 171, 181
hemolytic anemia, 51
hemolytic uremic syndrome, 41, 48, 54
hemorrhage, 47
hepatitis, 30, 95, 118, 130, 136, 156, 157, 190

Hepatitis B, 3, 91, 94, 110, 111, 133, 136, 157
Hepatitis C, 91, 94, 118, 136
hepatocytes, 42
heritability, 69
herniate, 176
heroin, 133, 174
heterogeneity, 33, 59, 63, 69, 73, 76, 100, 114, 124, 126, 173, 196
high blood pressure, 71, 113
high density lipoprotein, 184
highly active antiretroviral therapy, 25
histamine, 14
histochemistry, 49
histology, 6, 61, 64, 65, 67, 68, 102, 105, 182
histopathology, viii, 1, 60, 81, 101, 122, 127, 161, 163, 167, 172
HIV, 3, 25, 59, 80, 88, 94, 108, 113, 130, 133, 156, 173, 178, 190, 193
HIV-1, 173
HIVAN, 59, 72, 73, 156, 178, 184
HLA, 33, 36, 37, 40, 104
homeostasis, 6, 19, 67
hormone(s), 18, 26, 27, 68, 78, 130
human development, 151
human immunodeficiency virus, 130, 178, 191, 193
human leukocyte antigen, 104
Hunter, 37
hyaline, 88, 96, 109, 148, 149, 153, 155, 180, 189, 194
hyalinosis, 145, 170, 172, 175
hydatid, 136
hydrocarbons, 125
hydrogen peroxide, 34
hydrolysis, 65
hypercalciuria, 27
hypercellularity, 172, 175
hypercholesterolemia, 6, 58, 179, 186
hyperfiltration, 12, 59, 153, 177, 182, 184
hyperkalemia, 12, 51
hyperlipidemia, 1, 2, 7, 101, 102, 117, 130, 182, 184, 187
hyperplasia, 95, 174, 175, 177, 178, 180
hypersensitivity, 44, 46, 47, 48, 130
hypertension, 6, 11, 12, 14, 21, 27, 28, 42, 46, 49, 58, 59, 72, 73, 80, 87, 88, 114, 115, 117, 130, 132, 133, 134, 150, 153, 155, 156, 160, 171, 174, 180, 181, 183, 184, 185, 186, 201
hypertrophy, 107, 114, 172, 175, 177, 178, 180, 182, 184, 185
hypoalbuminemia, 1
hypocomplementemia, 114, 115
hyponatremia, 51
hypoparathyroidism, 201
hypoplasia, 133, 186
hypovolemia, 11, 12, 13
hypoxia, 39, 187

I

identification, 27, 39, 41, 65, 73, 118
idiopathic, vii, 7, 8, 9, 10, 23, 29, 30, 36, 37, 39, 40, 53, 58, 73, 75, 89, 90, 95, 100, 101, 102, 103, 107, 108, 110, 113, 117, 118, 119, 121, 125, 126, 136, 138, 153, 155, 157, 158, 159, 169, 170, 173, 192, 193, 195, 200
IFN-β, 59
IgA nephropathy, 48, 55, 85, 86, 87, 88, 93, 98, 107, 145
IgM nephropathy, 85, 86, 93, 103, 104, 121, 122, 131, 185, 198, 199
image, 171
IMF, 113
immune response, 5, 17, 33, 42, 130
immune system, 5, 9, 42
immunity, 5
immunization, 31, 35
immunocompromised, 7
immunofluorescence, 34, 39, 49, 60, 104, 127, 138, 140, 142, 146, 147, 148, 167, 173
immunoglobulin(s), 29, 49, 53, 83, 91, 95, 104, 114, 123, 126, 135, 138, 139, 142, 145, 146, 155, 156, 160, 167, 184, 188
immunohistochemistry, 96, 160, 161, 162
immunosuppression, 24, 73
immunosuppressive agent, 5
impregnation, 112, 125
imprinting, 69
in utero, 61, 64
in vitro, 11, 13, 16, 17, 63, 67, 184
in vivo, 25, 26, 54
incidence, 2, 8, 58, 64, 84, 99, 103, 108, 118, 125, 132, 136, 158, 171, 182, 183, 186, 188, 190, 191, 193, 195, 198
income, 161
India, 29, 36, 37, 119, 121, 123, 125, 129, 169, 198, 199
individuals, 8, 12, 13, 35, 62, 65, 84, 116, 156, 189
induction, 15
industrialized countries, 164
infants, 61, 65, 186, 189, 199, 200
infarction, 156
infection, 6, 7, 46, 53, 59, 63, 91, 94, 136, 156, 190
infectious agents, 130, 156
inflammation, 17, 18, 27, 41, 42, 45, 47, 48, 49, 50, 52, 85, 89, 90, 155
inflammatory cells, 47, 53, 92, 140

inflammatory disease, 146, 148
inflammatory mediators, 47
inheritance, 61, 62, 64, 68, 72, 151, 188
inherited disorder, 67
inhibition, 19, 23, 27
inhibitor, 19, 25, 45, 153, 180, 182, 183, 184, 199
innate immunity, 5
inositol, 65
INS, 101, 102, 103, 105, 106, 107, 108, 110, 113, 117
insertion, 63, 171
institutions, 162, 165
insulin, 14, 159, 184
integrin(s), 12, 13, 15, 16, 17, 21, 24, 25, 26, 158, 173, 182
integrity, 65, 189
interferon(s), 23, 42, 59, 133, 156, 174, 190
interstitial nephritis, 133, 156
intracellular calcium, 67
intraocular, 65
intron, 69, 190
ion channels, 67
ion transport, 22
ions, 19, 20, 34
Iran, 121, 124
ischemia, 34, 152, 153, 180, 182
Islam, 122

J

Japan, 163

K

K^+, 17, 26
karyotype, 69
keratinocytes, 16, 25
ketones, 35
kidney transplantation, 59, 73, 197
Korea, 36

L

labeling, 107
lactate dehydrogenase, 51
lactic acid, 70, 190
lamination, 153
Laminin, 65, 76, 77
laminin-5, 65
L-arginine, 19
LDL, 31
lead, 7, 41, 48, 50, 51, 59, 61, 63, 64, 67, 82, 89, 92, 132, 134, 139, 146, 151, 152, 156, 157, 165, 186, 187
leakage, 1, 2, 18, 19, 110
lecithin, 95
lens, 65, 66, 84
leprosy, 130, 136, 149, 157
leukocytes, 192
liberation, 47
ligand, 31, 38
light, 41, 49, 52, 60, 82, 85, 86, 88, 96, 104, 127, 128, 130, 131, 134, 137, 140, 141, 144, 146, 147, 148, 149, 154, 155, 167, 170, 173, 181
light microscopy, 140
lipids, 32, 172, 184
lipodystrophy, 141
lipoid nephrosis, 171, 192
lipoproteins, 14
lithium, 133
liver, 4, 95, 142, 149, 163, 187
liver disease, 95
liver transplant, 163
localization, 35, 38, 139
loci, 36
locus, 65, 67, 72, 77, 78, 188, 196
low risk, 64
lumen, 143, 155, 175, 176
Luo, 167
lupus, 3, 4, 30, 37, 46, 48, 54, 73, 80, 83, 91, 95, 107, 136, 139, 153, 154, 155, 158, 159, 160
lupus nephritis, 47, 85, 86, 93, 133
lymphocytes, 22
lymphoid, 189
lymphoma, 3, 102, 130
lysine, 69

M

MAC, 30, 32, 33, 36, 43, 46, 47, 51, 53, 110
macromolecules, 59
macrophages, 12, 16, 42, 173, 180
malaria, 3, 94, 111,130, 136, 157
malignancy, 30, 33, 136
management, 7, 8, 10, 13, 21, 31, 34, 37, 55, 82, 83, 98, 101, 102, 117, 125, 129, 158, 161, 185, 191, 201
manipulation, 187
Mannose binding lectin, 33
mapping, 31, 65, 70, 71, 72, 78
marrow, 183
mass, 19, 59, 88, 174, 182

matrix, 16, 51, 52, 58, 65, 85, 88, 90, 93, 107, 109, 114, 137, 140, 144, 145, 147, 149, 175, 180, 181, 189
matrix metalloproteinase, 16
maturation process, 58
MCP, 50, 51
mechanical properties, 19, 28
mechanical stress, 59
medical, vii, 1, 7, 73, 81, 82, 83, 164, 165, 192
medulla, 84
Megalin, 31
mellitus, 4, 105, 143, 190
membranes, 46, 65, 142
membranoproliferative glomerulonephritis (MPGN), 14, 37, 41, 49, 54, 83, 100, 113, 114, 115, 116, 117, 126, 127, 128, 130, 139, 140, 141, 142, 150, 157, 159
membranous glomerulonephritis, 37, 38, 39, 84, 99, 100, 125, 126, 136
membranous nephropathy, 2, 3, 8, 14, 29, 30, 36, 37, 38, 39, 40, 52, 55, 98, 99, 100, 111, 125, 126, 130, 137, 138, 139, 159
mental retardation, 69, 151, 188
mercury, 91, 111, 136
mesangial cell proliferation, 173
mesangial cells, 48, 52, 88, 90, 92, 93, 94, 104, 106, 110, 172, 181
mesangial proliferative glomerulonephritis (MesPGN), 90, 93, 106, 107, 121, 122, 123, 189
mesangiocapillary glomerulonephritis, 94, 126, 127
mesenteric vessels, 20
messengers, 65
meta-analysis, 22
metabolic pathways, 32
metabolic syndrome, 18, 184, 198
metabolism, 6, 146
metastatic cancer, 59
methylprednisolone, 16, 24
Mg^{2+}, 27
MHC, 39
mice, 11, 13, 17, 31, 64, 66, 69, 76, 78, 189, 200
microalbuminuria, 143
microorganisms, 42
MicroRNAs (miRNAs), 73, 80
microscope, 161
microscopy, 35, 52, 68, 71, 82, 85, 86, 88, 96, 97, 104, 131, 134, 137, 138, 140, 141, 147, 149, 150, 154, 155, 173, 188, 189
migration, 15, 16, 25, 65, 68, 71
minimal change disease, 13, 84, 85, 86, 89, 102, 103, 119, 120, 122, 124, 130, 131, 132, 171, 182, 192
minimal change nephrotic syndrome, 27, 58, 117, 119, 120, 121, 123, 124
miscarriage, 35
mitochondria, 60, 70
mitochondrial DNA, 190
mitogen, 24
models, 11, 12, 18, 33, 41, 42, 64, 117, 166, 198
modifications, 63
modifier gene, 65
molecular mimicry, 33
molecular pathology, 162
molecular weight, 16, 31
molecules, 5, 13, 14, 15, 16, 20, 41, 43, 44, 45, 46, 58, 61, 73, 106, 183
monoclonal antibody, 38
monolayer, 65, 173
monomers, 20
monozygotic twins, 69, 78
Moon, 77, 124, 125
morbidity, 12, 153
morphology, 85, 87, 97, 104, 123, 160, 167, 169, 180, 182
morphometric, 125
mortality, 12, 20, 22, 153
MPO, 50
MR, 28, 54, 76, 77, 79, 80, 121, 196, 200
mRNA(s), 15, 17, 22, 107, 171
mucosa, 164
multiple myeloma, 159
muscle mass, 133
muscles, 66, 190
mutant, 64, 67, 68, 71, 72, 79
mutation(s), 4, 9, 40, 41, 44, 50, 51, 57, 58, 59, 60, 61, 63, 64, 65, 66, 67, 68, 69, 70, 71, 73, 75, 76, 77, 78, 79, 104, 120, 124, 133, 141, 151, 159, 169, 170, 182, 187, 188, 189, 190, 192, 195, 196, 199, 200, 201
mutational analysis, 71
myofibroblasts, 20
myopathy, 70, 190

N

Na^+, 13, 17, 22, 26, 27
NAD, 47
NADPH oxidoreductase, 32
Nail-patella syndrome, 3, 133
natural killer cell, 15, 24
necrosis, 131, 133, 174, 181, 192
necrotizing glomerulonephritis, 88, 159
nephrectomy, 69, 186, 199
Nephrin, 61, 75, 108, 120, 133, 187
nephritic syndrome, 52, 93, 95, 123, 139, 141
nephritis, 4, 29, 30, 31, 35, 37, 38, 47, 54, 73, 80, 83, 85, 86, 93, 107, 133, 138, 139, 154, 159, 160, 195

nephrocalcinosis, 18, 27
nephrologist, 54, 81, 83, 97
nephron, 12, 13, 14, 17, 18, 26, 169, 170, 182, 184, 185, 186
nephrosclerosis, 153
nephrosis, 11, 12, 17, 22, 26, 63, 75, 76, 77, 171, 200
Netherlands, 34
neural network, 167
neuroblastoma, 136
neurological disease, 201
neurons, 67, 190
neutrophils, 12, 50
New Zealand, 8, 113
Nigeria, 118
nitric oxide, 19, 27, 28, 113
nitric oxide synthase (NOS), 27, 28, 60, 108, 109, 110, 134, 170, 174, 175, 176, 177, 181, 182
nitrite, 28
nodular glomerulosclerosis, 144
nodules, 144, 146
North Africa, 71
North America, 197
NPHS1, 60, 61, 62, 63, 64, 65, 73, 75, 76, 108, 120, 133, 182, 188
NPHS2, 60, 61, 62, 63, 64, 65, 73, 75, 76, 109, 120, 124, 133, 182, 189, 192, 196, 200
NSAIDs, 130
nuclear receptors, 68
nuclei, 172, 178, 180
nucleotides, 188

O

obesity, 59, 88, 108, 133, 134, 145, 174, 177, 184, 187, 198, 199
occlusion, 87, 92, 94, 180
oedema, 8, 117
oligomeganephronia, 133, 174, 186
organ(s), 32, 142, 151, 153, 162
organelle, 180
osmotic pressure, 14, 23
ovarian tumor, 190
ovaries, 190
oxidative stress, 27, 190
oxygen, 34, 106

P

pain, 6
Pakistan, viii, 1, 41, 57, 76, 81, 98, 101, 118, 121, 123, 161, 162, 163, 164, 165, 166, 167
PAN, 17, 22, 26
paradigm shift, 31
parallel, 14, 90, 112, 135, 181
parasites, 157
parathyroid hormone, 18
parenchyma, 6, 7, 82, 84, 85
PAS, 84, 87, 88, 89, 93, 94, 144, 172, 176, 177, 178, 179
patella, 3, 66, 71, 133, 151, 182
pathogenesis, vii, 1, 2, 4, 5, 7, 8, 9, 16, 17, 29, 31, 33, 34, 35, 36, 37, 38, 41, 42, 50, 53, 55, 59, 60, 65, 68, 73, 74, 79, 87, 95, 97, 101, 103, 105, 106, 108, 117, 118, 120, 122, 123, 130, 159, 170, 171, 183, 184, 188, 191, 193, 198
pathologist, 83, 84, 92
pathology, vii, 3, 70, 81, 82, 84, 95, 96, 97, 98, 101, 103, 117, 122, 125, 126, 127, 131, 156, 161, 162, 163, 164, 171, 181, 182, 187, 188, 189, 190, 191
pathophysiological, 12, 19
pathophysiology, 1, 4, 8, 10, 14, 23, 29, 99, 106, 117, 118, 125
pathways, 17, 41, 42, 43, 44, 47, 50, 53, 61, 70, 99, 106, 113
PDGF, 106, 184
penetrance, 60, 67, 68, 69, 72
peptidase, 31
peptide, 32, 130
perihilar, 108, 109, 134, 175, 177, 182
perinatal, 66
peripheral blood, 171, 184
peripheral blood mononuclear cell, 171
peripheral vascular disease, 186
peritonitis, 6, 7
permeability, 4, 5, 12, 14, 15, 16, 20, 28, 59, 60, 63, 71, 75, 102, 184
permeation, 27
PGN, 14, 126, 127, 130
pH, 72, 146
phagocytosis, 44
pharynx, 149
PHB, 63
phenotype(s), 22, 59, 60, 63, 64, 66, 68, 69, 73, 75, 77, 78, 160, 178, 193, 198, 201
Philadelphia, 97, 158, 194, 196
phosphate, 22
phosphoinositides, 65, 72
phospholipids, 18, 26
phosphorylation, 18, 27, 71, 196, 200
photomicrographs, 166
Pierson syndrome, 61, 62, 66, 77
placenta, 61
plasma membrane, 15, 19, 27, 63, 64, 71
plasma proteins, 1, 2, 4, 6, 14, 88, 102, 108, 109, 134, 145, 153

plasmapheresis, 73, 183
plasmin, v, 8, 11, 14, 19, 22, 25, 27
plasminogen, v, 9, 11, 12, 13, 14, 15, 16, 18, 19, 23, 24, 25, 39, 59, 184
platelet aggregation, 51, 130
platelets, 51, 151
pneumonia, 7
podocin, 109, 133, 187, 189, 196, 200
podocytes, 178, 183, 193, 198
polyarteritis nodosa, 92, 155
polycystic kidney disease, 92
polycythemia, 187
polymerization, 19, 20, 67
polymorphism(s), 31, 40, 64, 113, 120, 192
polypeptide, 78
polyuria, 186
population, 6, 16, 22, 61, 102, 109, 123, 124, 126, 145, 182, 192, 196
post-transplant, 76, 183, 188, 196
potassium, 13, 19, 20, 28
prednisone, 107, 119
preservation, 14
pressure gradient, 14
prevention, 1, 159
primary amyloidosis, 146, 149, 160
primary biliary cirrhosis, 110, 136
primary pulmonary hypertension, 199
private sector, 162
procurement, 82
progesterone, 14
prognosis, 2, 57, 73, 87, 101, 103, 104, 106, 107, 110, 113, 114, 116, 117, 119, 122, 123, 124, 125, 126, 136, 147, 160, 169, 181, 182, 191, 194, 195, 198
pro-inflammatory, 52
proliferation, 15, 24, 42, 52, 62, 69, 88, 90, 92, 93, 105, 106, 107, 113, 121, 123, 131, 140, 156, 158, 171, 172, 173, 177, 178, 179, 184, 193
protection, 19, 42, 51
protective role, 18
protein family, 189
protein kinases, 32
proteinase, 50
proteins, 4, 11, 13, 14, 15, 18, 25, 32, 35, 42, 43, 44, 45, 50, 51, 54, 57, 58, 59, 60, 61, 62, 63, 64, 65, 67, 70, 71, 72, 77, 130, 131, 135, 138, 141, 148, 169, 170, 172, 182, 189, 196
proteoglycans, 138, 150, 184
proteolysis, 15, 16
prototype, 162
proximal convoluted tubules, 188
proximal tubules, 22, 39, 61, 70, 180
pseudocyst, 185
pseudohermaphroditism, 201
public sector, 162, 165
pulmonary embolism, 6, 10
pyelonephritis, 87, 88, 133, 145, 186, 199

R

reactant(s), 138
reactive oxygen, 28, 32, 47
reactive oxygen species (ROS), 106
reagents, 162, 166
receptors, 15, 16, 24, 26, 42, 52, 55, 59, 68, 78, 107, 141
recombination, 72
recovery, 18, 23, 27, 32, 33
recurrence, 5, 32, 59, 64, 69, 71, 76, 109, 139, 141, 182, 183, 184, 188, 190, 196
recycling, 16
red blood cells, 51
reflux nephropathy, 177, 186, 199
Reflux nephropathy, 88, 108, 133, 174
Registry, 98, 120
rejection, 167
relapses, 5, 123
relaxation, 19
remission, 5, 27, 32, 33, 34, 36, 63, 65, 73, 107, 116, 181, 182
remodelling, 62, 70, 71, 140
renal biopsy, 46, 68, 81, 97, 98, 102, 120, 129, 160
renal dysfunction, 17, 42, 47, 54, 109, 110, 129, 184, 199
renal failure, 2, 6, 7, 8, 23, 41, 50, 70, 78, 143, 146, 147, 154, 178, 181, 183, 188, 190, 192, 201
renal medulla, 15, 156
renal replacement therapy, 119, 143
renin, 11, 12, 27, 28, 113, 130
residues, 46
resistance, 21, 51, 58, 64, 72, 107, 132
resolution, 107
response, 2, 15, 22, 32, 36, 38, 42, 57, 58, 59, 60, 82, 103, 104, 105, 106, 109, 119, 121, 176, 181, 185, 189, 193, 194, 195, 197
retardation, 69, 71, 186
reticulum, 63, 64, 77, 181
retina, 65
retinopathy, 144, 151
RH, 24, 26, 96, 121, 123
rheumatoid arthritis, 91, 95, 136
rheumatoid factor, 48
right ventricle, 187
rings, 115
risk(s), 6, 36, 59, 69, 72, 73, 80, 119, 153, 155, 179, 183, 184, 187, 190, 198

risk factors, 6, 183, 198
rituximab, 119
RNA, 73, 171

S

salmon, 149
Saudi Arabia, 118
schema, 145, 187
Schimke immune-osseous dysplasia, 66, 71
schistosomiasis, 130, 136
scleroderma, 111, 155
scope, 29, 81, 82, 129, 169
secrete, 5
secretion, 12, 16, 20
sediments, 130
segmental glomerulosclerosis, 2, 9, 14, 23, 57, 74, 83, 84, 87, 99, 103, 126, 132, 135, 136, 151, 158, 169, 170, 173, 191, 192, 193, 194, 195, 196, 197, 199, 201
selectivity, 18
senescence, 32
sensitivity, 19, 28, 33, 34
sensorineural hearing loss, 70
sensors, 27
sepsis, 188
sequencing, 4, 57, 71, 72, 74
Serbia, 98, 119, 120
serine, 15, 18, 43, 45, 46, 69
serology, 85, 87, 93, 96, 105, 107, 123, 167
serum, 4, 5, 8, 14, 16, 18, 19, 27, 31, 32, 33, 35, 37, 38, 47, 48, 50, 51, 52, 53, 58, 59, 72, 114, 130, 131, 135, 146, 148, 153, 159, 179, 180, 181, 187
serum albumin, 4, 8, 27, 31, 131
sex, 6, 190
shape, 19, 66, 173
shear, 19
shortage, 165
showing, 30, 43, 44, 51, 85, 86, 88, 89, 90, 94, 143, 147, 152, 155, 176, 180, 181, 184
siblings, 63
sickle cell, 156
side chain, 20
side effects, 58
signal transduction, 65
signalling, 58, 60, 61, 64, 67
signs, 5, 6, 66, 183
silver, 82, 84, 87, 91, 94, 112, 114, 116, 137, 138, 140, 150, 162, 172
Singapore, 163
skin, 151, 152, 160, 161, 164
skin diseases, 161
SLE, 4, 46, 47, 48, 54, 105, 110, 130, 136, 138, 153, 154, 155
sleeping sickness, 72
slit diaphragm, 118
smooth muscle, 16, 20, 151
smooth muscle cells, 16
SNP, 31, 33, 64
socioeconomic status, 102
sodium, 8, 11, 12, 13, 16, 17, 18, 19, 20, 21, 22, 26, 27, 28, 118, 130, 184
solid tumors, 69, 136
solidification, 87, 88, 153
South Korea, 34
Spain, 98
species, 28, 32, 47, 106
specific adsorption, 135
spleen, 142, 149
sprue, 95
standardization, 100
state(s), 13, 19, 20, 64, 72, 104, 118, 130, 157, 164, 165, 186, 189
stem cells, 183
steroids, 4, 6, 18, 65, 103, 104, 106, 107, 134, 176, 181, 185
stimulation, 15, 21, 42, 65, 107, 130
stomach, 136
storage, 65, 108, 133, 199
streptococci, 46
stress, 19, 122, 186
stroke, 70, 190
structural changes, 145, 159
structure, 11, 13, 18, 19, 28, 57, 58, 60, 61, 62, 67, 74, 76, 86, 87, 94, 97
subgroups, 139, 141, 148
sub-Saharan Africa, 72
sulfate, 138
suppression, 39, 73
surface area, 2, 186
survival, 61, 70, 73, 115, 117, 119, 181, 188
survival rate, 115
susceptibility, 40, 64, 72, 189, 200
suspensions, 37
swelling, 92, 155
sympathetic nervous system, 130
symptoms, 5, 6, 11, 46, 66, 131
syndromic NS, 71
Synechiae, 172
synthesis, 4, 12, 13, 16, 17, 26, 28, 60, 107, 130, 188
syphilis, 130, 136, 157
systemic lupus erythematosus, 54, 105, 130
systolic blood pressure, 153

T

T cell(s), 5, 16
T lymphocytes, 12, 17, 24
T regulatory cells, 5
Taiwan, 36, 40
target, 4, 21, 23, 29, 31, 35, 37, 39, 50
taxonomy, 99
TBM, 152
techniques, 34, 113, 127, 161, 162, 167
TEM, 132, 139, 141, 142, 143, 148, 149, 152, 163, 164, 165, 166
tensile strength, 151
testing, 9
testis, 151
texture, 138
TGF, 22, 171, 184, 192
Thailand, 113
therapeutic agents, 41
therapeutic effects, 53
therapeutic interventions, 41
therapeutic targets, 118
therapy, 22, 36, 49, 57, 58, 63, 65, 74, 100, 119, 178, 180, 181, 182, 183, 194, 195, 197, 199
thinning, 152
threonine, 69
thrombocytopenia, 51
thrombocytopenic purpura, 155
thrombomodulin, 51
thrombosis, 6, 7, 10, 63, 111, 152
thrombotic microangiopathy, 155
thrombus, 51
thymus, 183, 197
thyroglobulin, 110
tip variant, 134
tissue, 15, 17, 18, 23, 25, 35, 41, 42, 50, 51, 54, 58, 73, 111, 134, 163, 165, 166
tissue plasminogen activator, 15
TNF, 171, 184
TNF-α, 184
topology, 63
total cholesterol, 2
toxic effect, 19, 184
toxic waste, 166
toxicity, 11, 12, 153, 179, 180, 182
trafficking, 11, 13, 26, 62, 63
transcription, 5, 42, 60, 62, 66, 67, 68, 78, 186
transcription factors, 42, 60
transferrin, 14, 52
transformation, 34, 115, 132, 135, 141, 142, 143, 180, 183
transmission, 164, 188
transplant, 32, 162, 163, 164, 167, 180, 182, 198
transplantation, 5, 16, 24, 39, 51, 59, 64, 69, 71, 73, 92, 109, 133, 141, 160, 182, 183, 186, 188, 190, 196, 197
transport, 14, 17, 18, 21, 22, 26
transport processes, 18
trauma, 182
treatment, 1, 2, 7, 8, 9, 12, 13, 14, 15, 17, 21, 34, 41, 49, 50, 51, 58, 59, 64, 65, 71, 73, 74, 76, 83, 98, 102, 103, 104, 106, 107, 117, 118, 123, 127, 147, 164, 169, 181, 183, 194, 195, 196, 198
treatment agents, 41
trial, 82, 124
triglycerides, 184
trypanosomiasis, 72
trypsin, 22
tuberculosis, 149
tumor(s), 14, 16, 23, 62, 66, 68, 69, 73, 78, 84, 95, 161, 164, 171, 190, 200, 201
tumor growth, 171
tumor necrosis factor, 14, 23, 171
tumorigenesis, 73
tumours, 22
Turkey, 113
twins, 201
type 1 collagen, 52
tyrosine, 15, 71

U

UK, 74, 118, 163, 165
UN, 121
unilateral renal agenesis, 108, 133, 174
United States (USA), 8, 34, 64, 143
uPAR, vii, 12, 13, 15, 16, 17, 19, 24, 25, 59
urinary tract, 67, 186
urine, 1, 2, 4, 6, 12, 13, 18, 19, 21, 24, 46, 50, 55, 73, 101, 102, 149
urokinase, 9, 11, 12, 13, 14, 15, 16, 23, 24, 25, 26, 59, 75, 130

V

vascular diseases, 82
vascular endothelial growth factor (VEGF), 171
vasculature, 27, 149
vasculitis, 42, 50, 55, 118, 152, 155
vasculopathy, 105
vaso-occlusion, 156
vasopressin, 18
vein, 6, 7, 10, 111
venules, 156
vessels, 50

viral infection, 32, 52, 91, 169, 170
virus infection, 94, 190
viruses, 133, 170
viscosity, 19, 20
vitamin D, 7
vomiting, 186

W

WAGR syndrome, 69
waste disposal, 48
water, 11, 12, 13, 14, 16, 17, 18, 20, 59, 130, 166
western blot, 35
World Health Organization (WHO), 47, 154
WT1, 60, 61, 62, 66, 68, 69, 73, 75, 78, 120, 133, 187, 190, 201

X

X-linked inheritance, 151
X-ray diffraction, 163

Y

yolk, 39
young adults, 113, 139

Z

zinc, 68, 78